Big Data Analytics and Artificial Intelligence in the Healthcare Industry

José Machado
Centro ALGORITMI, Universidade do Minho, Portugal

Hugo Peixoto
Centro ALGORITMI, Universidade do Minho, Portugal

Regina Sousa
Centro ALGORITMI, Universidade do Minho, Portugal

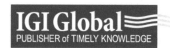

A volume in the Advances in
Medical Technologies and Clinical
Practice (AMTCP) Book Series

Published in the United States of America by
    IGI Global
    Medical Information Science Reference (an imprint of IGI Global)
    701 E. Chocolate Avenue
    Hershey PA, USA 17033
    Tel: 717-533-8845
    Fax: 717-533-8661
    E-mail: cust@igi-global.com
    Web site: http://www.igi-global.com

Library of Congress Cataloging-in-Publication Data

Names: Machado, José Manuel editor. | Peixoto, Hugo, 1985- editor. |
   Sousa, Regina, editor.
Title: Big data analytics and artificial intelligence in the healthcare
   industry / Jose Manuel Machado, Hugo Peixoto, Regina Sousa, editors.
Description: Hershey, PA : Medical Information Science Reference, [2022] |
   Includes bibliographical references and index. | Summary: "The main goal
   of this book is to contribute to the development of new approaches and
   reliable enabling technologies in the healthcare industry that will
   enhance not only human quality of life, but also will lead to healthier,
   innovative, and secure societies as an all"-- Provided by publisher.
Identifiers: LCCN 2022001654 (print) | LCCN 2022001655 (ebook) | ISBN
   9781799891727 (hardcover) | ISBN 9781799891734 (ebook)
Subjects: MESH: Artificial Intelligence | Big Data | Data Analysis |
   Medical Informatics--methods
Classification: LCC R855.3 (print) | LCC R855.3 (ebook) | NLM W 26.55.A7
   | DDC 610.285--dc23/eng/20220127
LC record available at https://lccn.loc.gov/2022001654
LC ebook record available at https://lccn.loc.gov/2022001655

This book is published in the IGI Global book series Advances in Medical Technologies and Clinical Practice (AMTCP) (ISSN: 2327-9354; eISSN: 2327-9370)

British Cataloguing in Publication Data
A Cataloguing in Publication record for this book is available from the British Library.

All work contributed to this book is new, previously-unpublished material.
The views expressed in this book are those of the authors, but not necessarily of the publisher.

For electronic access to this publication, please contact: eresources@igi-global.com.

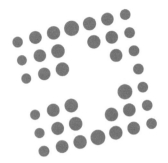

Advances in Medical Technologies and Clinical Practice (AMTCP) Book Series

ISSN:2327-9354
EISSN:2327-9370

Editor-in-Chief: Srikanta Patnaik, SOA University, India, Priti Das, S.C.B. Medical College, India

MISSION

Medical technological innovation continues to provide avenues of research for faster and safer diagnosis and treatments for patients. Practitioners must stay up to date with these latest advancements to provide the best care for nursing and clinical practices.

The **Advances in Medical Technologies and Clinical Practice (AMTCP) Book Series** brings together the most recent research on the latest technology used in areas of nursing informatics, clinical technology, biomedicine, diagnostic technologies, and more. Researchers, students, and practitioners in this field will benefit from this fundamental coverage on the use of technology in clinical practices.

COVERAGE

- Nursing Informatics
- Nutrition
- Biometrics
- Biomedical Applications
- Clinical Nutrition
- Telemedicine
- Biomechanics
- Medical Imaging
- Patient-Centered Care
- Medical Informatics

IGI Global is currently accepting manuscripts for publication within this series. To submit a proposal for a volume in this series, please contact our Acquisition Editors at Acquisitions@igi-global.com or visit: http://www.igi-global.com/publish/.

Titles in this Series

For a list of additional titles in this series, please visit:
http://www.igi-global.com/book-series/advances-medical-technologies-clinical-practice/73682

For an entire list of titles in this series, please visit:
http://www.igi-global.com/book-series/advances-medical-technologies-clinical-practice/73682

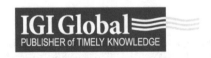

701 East Chocolate Avenue, Hershey, PA 17033, USA
Tel: 717-533-8845 x100 ● Fax: 717-533-8661
E-Mail: cust@igi-global.com ● www.igi-global.com

Table of Contents

Chapter 13

Detailed Table of Contents

    Rui Santos, Centro ALGORITMI, Universidade do Minho, Portugal
    Ana Regina Sousa, Centro ALGORITMI, Universidade do Minho,
        Portugal
    Manuel Filipe Santos, Centro ALGORITMI, Universidade do Minho,
        Portugal
    António Abelha, Centro ALGORITMI, Universidade do Minho, Portugal
    Hugo Peixoto, Centro ALGORITMI, Universidade do Minho, Portugal

The importance of collecting and presenting data/events in real time from monitors in the intensive care units (ICU) demands constant research. Moreover, improvements in the systems are critical, thus adjusting their behavior to the new requests. The high amount of IoTs present results in the term big data in healthcare, where the most traditional technologies become invalid or operate with high difficulties. This chapter aims to propose an alternative system, quicker and above all, scalable, to allow for an improvement in the retrieval and presentation of data from different monitors. To this end, emergent technologies will be used, such as Apache Kafka. This technology has increasingly been put to use in healthcare due to its scalability, safety, and speed. Real datasets that simulate several types of data, like heartbeat, blood pressure, among others, will be used to obtain results. Furthermore, they also display fault and warning logs.

Cardiovascular disease (CVD) is a broad term encompassing a group of heart and blood vessel abnormalities that is the leading cause of death worldwide. The most popular and low-cost diagnostic tool for assessing the heart electrical impulses is an electrocardiogram (ECG). Automation is required to reduce errors and human burden while interpreting ECG signals. In recent years, deep learning shows better performance in ECG classification and has also shown that automated classification of ECG signals can improve accuracy and efficiency. In this chapter, the authors review the research work on ECG signals using deep learning methods like deep belief network (DBNK), convolutional neural network (CNNK), long short-term memory (LSTMY), recurrent neural network (RNNK), and gated recurrent unit (GRUT). In the research articles published between 2017 and 2021, CNNK was found to be the most appropriate technique for feature extraction.

Big data analytics is frequently termed as the complicated operation of analysing the big data to unfold the information like market trends, correlations, customer preferences, and hidden patterns which might be helpful for the organisations to make decisions. On the other hand, data analytic techniques and technologies provide organisations methods to analyse data sets and to collect new data. With right garage and analytical tools in hand, the data and insights derived from big data could make the critical social infrastructure additives and offerings. In healthcare the usage of artificial intelligence has the capability to help healthcare companies in lots of factors of administrative processes and patient care. Artificial intelligence has converted companies across the world and has the capability to appreciably regulate the sphere of healthcare. Most of the AI and healthcare technology have strong relevance to the healthcare field; however, the procedures they help can range significantly.

Chapter 4

Erman Çakıt, Department of Industrial Engineering, Gazi University,
Ankara, Turkey

A variety of fuzzy logic approaches have been employed in order to handle uncertainty by examining the capability of fuzzy logic techniques and improve effectiveness in various aspects of the COVID-19 pandemic. After an inclusion-exclusion procedure, a total of 52 articles were chosen from a set of 399 articles. The objectives of this study were 1) to introduce briefly the fuzzy logic concepts, 2) to review the literature, 3) to classify the literature based on the applications of fuzzy logic to COVID-19 pandemic, 4) to emphasize future developments and trends. The application of fuzzy logic includes screening, diagnostics, and forecasting the COVID-19 outbreak. ANFIS approach and its modified models were revealed to be the most commonly employed for estimation of COVID-19 pandemic. Furthermore, the study found that fuzzy decision-making approaches have mostly been used for detection and diagnosis. In this regard, it is anticipated that the findings of this study will provide decison makers with new tools and ideas for combating the COVID-19 epidemic using fuzzy logic.

Chapter 5

Tiago Guimarães, Centro ALGORITMI, Universidade do Minho,
Portugal
Inês Afonso Quesado, Centro ALGORITMI, Universidade do Minho,
Portugal
Inês Tavares, Centro ALGORITMI, Universidade do Minho, Portugal
Maria Passos, Centro ALGORITMI, Universidade do Minho, Portugal
Júlio Duarte, Centro ALGORITMI, Universidade do Minho, Portugal
Manuel Filipe Santos, Centro ALGORITMI, Universidade do Minho,
Portugal
Álvaro Silva, Centro Hospitalar, Universitário do Porto, Portugal

Due to ICU critical environment, where seriously ill patients must be constantly monitored, it is imperative to make quick but assertive decisions. Several studies have shown that continuous monitorization of ICU patients result in large amounts of data, from which knowledge can be extracted and better decisions made. This chapter aims to analyse and visualize the data obtained by an ICU, so that conclusions can be deduced regarding patients' outcome, clinical errors, as well as healthcare service quality. To achieve the objective, initially, the data was acquired and collected from several data sources such as bedside monitors and electronic nursing records. Secondly, the raw data was transformed so that it could be used in visualization.

Finally, interactive charts were built so that data could be forecasted and patterns discovered. The results allow one to draw conclusions such as the source of data gaps, the correlation between medication and vital signs, as well as the importance of SAPS regarding patient outcomes.

Chapter 6

   Marcelo Marreiros, Centro ALGORITMI, Universidade do Minho,
       Portugal
   Diana Ferreira, Centro ALGORITMI, Universidade do Minho, Portugal
   Cristiana Neto, Universidade do Minho, Portugal
   Deden Witarsyah, Telkom University, Indonesia
   José Machado, Centro ALGORITMI, Universidade do Minho, Portugal

Polycystic ovarian syndrome (PCOS) is the most common endocrine pathology in reproductive-age women worldwide. Research has shown that the application of machine learning (ML) and data mining (DM) can have a positive impact in this condition's diagnosis. This study aims to develop a model to identify patients with PCOS using different scenarios based on correlation weights. Five DM techniques were applied, namely random forest (RF), decision tree (DT), naive bayes (NB), logistic regression (LR), and artificial neural network (ANN), to determine the best model, which was the RF classifier. Additionally, the results show that the model was able to predict PCOS with 93.06% of accuracy, 92.66% of precision, 93.52% of sensitivity, and 92.59% of specificity. Compared with a previous work conducted by the authors, the feature selection-based solo on the correlation weight decreased the accuracy values by 1.9%, precision by 3.7%, sensitivity by 0.3%, and specificity by 3.6%.

Today's metrics for women housework work (WHW) operate at a quantitative level, specifically measuring time expended on a task and the totality of tasks women perform, not considering that it is a process that is eminently qualitative in nature. To fill this gap, an innovative framework for representing and thinking about big data or knowledge is presented, borrowing from the field of artificial intelligence the methods and methodologies for problem solving, from logic programming the artifacts to improve practice through theory, and from the laws of thermodynamics the construct of entropy, interpreted as the degree of disorder or unpredictability in a system, a principle that may be used to understand system evolution. Last but not least, it also considers the relationship among the disciplines of psychometrics and psychology or sociology (i.e., how certain psychological and sociological concepts such as cognition, knowledge and personality affect WHW satisfaction).

The growth of electronic health records (EHR) produced by health facilities has been exponential, leading to massive and heterogeneous data storage. This raises the need for secure, continuous, and interoperable data structuring between different legacy systems. The OpenEHR standard provides open data specifications that aim to overcome recognized gaps in the collection, storage, and management of clinical records. In this sense, this chapter describes a case study applied in an emergency context, where 14-year clinical records were restructured to an interoperable and standardized environment, according to the OpenEHR specifications.

Drugs are a marvel of modern medicine. With the huge drug market present in the world today, there is also a huge bane to the existence of drugs which is the presence of counterfeit drugs in the market that may cause irreversible damage to us. This chapter proposes a solution to counter this menace and save lives. After exploring the existing solutions in the global market and reviewing academic literature, it was found that such a comprehensive solution has not yet been implemented in India or the world. A comprehensive, affordable, easily accessible mobile application and website is proposed as the outcome of this research work. The application can provide the consumer with necessary details like the constituent salts, side effects, age barrier, safe consumption limit, and the purpose of the drug. To achieve this, a database of all known drugs and their images will be created and will be continuously updated with the help of machine learning and artificial intelligence. The chapter also discusses the business model to make it commercially viable.

Artificial intelligence is growing, but techniques like deep learning require more data than is usually available, especially in the medical context. Usually, the available data sets are not representative of reality, meaning that more samples have to be acquired, which is very costly. The demand for tools that can generate as much data as needed has increased. Traditional data augmentation tools are used to expand the available data, but they are not able to generate new data. The use of generative adversarial networks to generate synthetic data has proven revolutionary for big data as it increases the amount of available data without much cost. To this end, an adaptation of alpha-GAN for 3D MRI scans was developed to create a pipeline for generating as many synthetic scans of rat brains as needed. The applicability of the synthetic data was tested in a segmentation test and the realism by visual assessment.

Chapter 11

B. Hemavathi, Sri Padmavati Mahila Visvavidyalayam, India
Depuru Bharathi, Sri Padmavati Mahila Visvavidyalayam, India
A. Suvarna Latha, Sri Padmavati Mahila Visvavidyalayam, India

E-health plays a significant role in giving valuable information to the people about human life. E-health is commercial and protected use of data about the health, information and communication technology (ICT), and its associates with the health-related directions and human health activities. ICT or e-health includes different interventions like telehealth, telemedicine, m-health (mobile health) e-health registers (EHR), big data, wearables, and uniform artificial intelligence. In life there is no time for paper and pen work in the countries, and they are change completely to the digitalization and sharing health information and patient health data through the online mode, which is more simple and successful healthcare improvements. Such healthcare apps are useful to us to lead better, well, and more fruitful lives. E-health can be one of the important hopeful aspects for providing community health benefits which incorporates a predictable medical system.

Chapter 12

Ana Cecilia Coimbra, Centro ALGORITMI, Universidade do Minho,
*   Portugal*
Filipe Miranda, Centro ALGORITMI, Universidade do Minho, Portugal
Nicolas F. Lori, Universidade do Minho, Portugal
Júlio Duarte, Centro ALGORITMI, Universidade do Minho, Portugal
Luis Mendes Gomes, University of the Azores, Portugal

At the University of Porto Hospital (Centro Hospitalar Universitário do Porto [CHUP]), a tool for computerized clinical coding was developed to assist in the codification of hospital discharge. However, for this tool to be useful, it is necessary to have a process to manage the entire coding process. Thus, a platform was developed to help manage the coding of hospital dis-charge episodes. The biggest advantage of the existence of this platform is to better organize the entire coding process in order to improve the quantity and quality of work performed by CHUP's health professionals.

Chapter 13

Filipe Manuel Mota Miranda, Centro ALGORITMI, Universidade do
    Minho, Portugal
Cecilia Coimbra, Centro ALGORITMI, Universidade do Minho,
    Portugal

The main goal of the present case study is to infer the possibility of introducing the Apache Kafka paradigm to the exchange of healthcare information. Initially, a simple HL7 message generated in accordance with documentation was used as message origin message. Then that message should reach destination using the FHIR standard. As communication middle and handler, the Apache Kafka was implemented featuring a Confluent docker image. To map between HL7 versions, the Python language converts the original message into a JSON object. Then the Kafka API handles the socket interface between structures. Considering the charge test, the results were very positive considering a 6000-message integration under one minute and with an offset of 500 messages. Also, the systems are capable of maintaining the order of messages and recover in case of errors. So, it is possible to use Kafka to share JSON objects under FHIR standard but having in mind a prior definition of the topic, consumer, and producer configuration.

Preface

HEALTH INFORMATION SYSTEMS

Medicine's first real contact with technology was in 1989, with the discovery of the X-ray. Since then, medicine has been inseparably linked to technology. Even more so today, medicine depends on informatics and technologies (Kalender, W. A., 2006).

The innovations have emerged since then have provided significant improvements in the quality of life of the community as well as cost reductions in the services provided to it. If, apparently, everything is advantageous and associated with evolution, the increase in the average life expectancy has created the need for more significant investments in the health area. All this, coupled with tragic and striking events, such as the pandemic that began in 2019 (Sars-CoV-2), has caused the philosophy of institutions and healthcare practice to change dramatically. Today, instead of the traditional interpretation of symptoms to solve as quickly as possible, the focus is on preventive and even predictive medicine (Auffray, C., Charron, D., & Hood, L., 2010).

As such, and with this new approach in mind, there is enormous potential for using the data collected daily to transform healthcare. As a result, institutions have begun to focus on data to apply it to analysis, machine learning algorithms, and artificial intelligence with the goal of identifying patterns and correlations and, therefore, implementing preventive medicine and, later, prediction (Neves, J., Vicente, H., Esteves, M., Ferraz, F., Abelha, A., Machado, J., ... & Sampaio, L).

Every day, in every healthcare institution, a vast amount of data is generated in different sectors: hospital and electronic health record data, healthcare providers' data, medical insurance, medical equipments, life sciences and medical research, among many others. Thus, the concept of "Big Data" emerges (Wang, Y., Kung, L., & Byrd, T. A., 2018).

THE DATA OVERLOAD

Every day, individuals, and organizations all over the world generate massive amounts of data.

Data science is concerned with a variety of issues, including data management and analysis, in order to gain deeper insights and improve the functionality or services of a system (e.g. healthcare and transportation system) (Sousa, R., Miranda, R., Moreira, A., Alves, C., Lori, N., & Machado, J., 2021).

Furthermore, with the availability of some of the most creative and meaningful ways to visualize Big Data post-analysis, understanding the workings of any complex system has become easier.

As a greater proportion of society becomes aware of and involved in the generation of Big Data, it is necessary to define what Big Data is (Wilson, T. D., 2001).

DEFINING BIG DATA

Big Data is more than just large amounts of information. The "big" part of Big Data denotes its sheer volume. However, this definition encompasses the terms speed and diversity in addition to volume. The storage, processing and analytical power of this new universe beats that of previous universes.

Although there are various definitions for Big Data, Douglas Laney's is the most prominent and widely recognized. Laney saw that (large) data was expanding in three dimensions: volume, velocity, and variety (also known as the 3 Vs) (Laney, D., 2001).

According to Laney's definition, velocity in the 3Vs model refers to both the rate of data generation and the speed of analysis required. Variety is one of the more complex characteristics because it corresponds to the various types of data, both organized and unorganized (for example, video, audio, text, registration forms, etc.).

These three v's form the foundation of the Big Data model. However, other authors crossed these lines, adding several other V's to this definition, such as value, veracity, visualization, and viscosity, among others (De Mauro, A., Greco, M., & Grimaldi, M., 2016). Without a doubt, the most consensual "V" is Veracity.

The first major question in this data universe is whether we can manage what we can't measure.

CHALLENGES ASSOCIATED WITH BIG DATA IN HEALTHCARE

Several gaps have been identified as priority research needs as a result of the emergence of several companies interested in the research and use of Big Data in healthcare institutions.

The branches with the most identified needs are:

- Research support in a general context;
- Data transformation into information and even Knowledge;
- Self-care support.

Despite all the efforts, investigating these issues is not always an easy process. This is largely due to the resistance to change that exists in the nature of healthcare professionals accustomed to making decisions without the aid of other technologies. Moreover, even if information technology is health-related, investment initiatives in this area are rarer than we would like, as it requires significant investments with uncertain returns (Bates, D. W., Saria, S., Ohno-Machado, L., Shah, A., & Escobar, G., 2014).

Lately, the issues of protection, information security, and information proprietorship have been added to these two difficulties, requiring extraordinary consideration with regards to getting to and taking care of outsider information (Kruse, C. S., Goswamy, R., Raval, Y. J., & Marawi, S., 2016).

All things considered, throughout the long term, a few objectives have been set as to the improvement of data frameworks. Objectives, for example, expanding the effectiveness of medical care suppliers, diminishing expenses and blunders, patient-focused and avoidance situated medication, and customized medication stand out and speculation (Raghupathi, W., & Raghupathi, V.,2014).

Advanced frameworks developed for Big Data enjoy an unmistakable upper hand over more established advances and approaches, permitting information to be examined, overseen, and handled paying little mind to design. Along these lines, a similar device or handling innovation can be utilized for organized, unstructured, or semi-organized information, prompting significant information working for medical services foundations and experts.

TARGET AUDIENCE

The book delves into topics of great interest in the healthcare domain, such as Big Data and artificial intelligence.

As a result, its primary target audience includes stakeholders in health information and technology, stakeholder groups, and those who contribute to the healthcare research ecosystem.

It is associated with themes like Information Systems, Computer Science, Healthcare, and Medicine.

The target audience is composed by Health Organizations, Hospitals, Health Professionals, Biomedical Engineers, Informatics Engineers and researchers from related disciplines with a focus on IoT, Machine Learning, Artificial Intelligence, Health standards, and Decision support Systems.

ORGANIZATION OF THE BOOK

The book is composed of 13 chapters, each of which contains a unique study on a different topic related to the main scope. The following sections provide an overview of each one of them, where the main goals, a brief description of the methodology and methods used, and the achieved results are presented.

Real-Time UCI Monitoring Using Apache Kafka

This first manuscript focuses on the relevance of gathering and displaying data or even events from monitors in Intensive Care Units (ICU) in real-time. It covers new system enhancements that are essential for adapting the systems' behavior to new requirements. Due to the large number of IoT devices now in use, the term "Big Data" has been coined in the healthcare industry, where the most conventional technologies have become obsolete or function with great difficulty. With this work, authors try to suggest an alternative approach that is faster and, most importantly, scalable, in order to enhance data retrieval and presentation from several displays. Emergent technologies, such as Apache Kafka, were employed to achieve this goal. Because of its scalability, safety, and speed, this technology is rapidly being used in healthcare. To acquire findings, real datasets that imitate various sorts of data, such as heartbeat and blood pressure, were employed.

A Review on Artificial Intelligence for Electrocardiogram Signal Analysis

The second work in this book brings attention to cardiovascular disease, which is the world's leading cause of death, and refers to a range of heart and blood vessel disorders. An electrocardiogram (ECG) is the most common and low-cost diagnostic technique for monitoring cardiac electrical impulses and when it comes to analyzing ECG data, automation is necessary to eliminate mistakes and human stress. New Deep Learning (DL) techniques are studied, and their aim is to improve performance in ECG classification, as well as increase the ability of automated ECG signal categorization to enhance accuracy and efficiency. In this article, authors look at how deep learning approaches including the Deep Belief Network (DBNK), Convolutional Neural Network (CNNK), Long Short-Term Memory (LSTMY), Recurrent Neural Network (RNNK), and Gated Recurrent Unit (GRUT) can be used to study ECG data. Authors identified CNNK to be the best acceptable approach for feature extraction, based on comprehensive bibliographic research that gathered publications between 2017 and 2021.

A Review on Big data and Artificial Intelligence for Healthcare Domain

Chapter number three comprises a study that makes a comprehensive review on Big Data and Artificial Intelligence. Indeed, it states that Big Data analytics is often referred to as a difficult process of analyzing large amounts of data to uncover information such as market trends, correlations, client preferences, and hidden patterns that may assist businesses in making choices. Data analytic techniques and technologies, on the other hand, provide a method for organizations to analyze data sets and collect new data. The data and insights gained from Big Data might be used to create important social infrastructure enhancements and offers if the necessary garage and analytical tools are in place. Artificial intelligence has the potential to assist healthcare organizations in a variety of administrative procedures as well as patient care. Artificial intelligence has transformed businesses all over the globe and has the potential to significantly control the healthcare industry. The majority of AI and healthcare technology has a strong connection to the healthcare profession, however authors state that beyond this there are several applications to these fields.

A Systematic Review of Fuzzy Logic Applications for COVID-19 Pandemic

The fourth manuscript explores the capabilities of fuzzy logic methods to improve efficacy in many elements of the COVID-19 epidemic. To address uncertainty, a variety of fuzzy logic approaches have been used. A total of 52 papers were picked from a total of 399 articles through an inclusion-exclusion technique. The goals of this research were to: i) explain fuzzy logic ideas briefly, ii) evaluate the literature, iii) categorize the literature based on fuzzy logic applications to the COVID-19 pandemic, and iv) highlight future advancements and trends. The use of fuzzy logic in the COVID-19 epidemic covers screening, diagnosis, and forecasting. The

ANFIS technique and its modified models were found to be the most widely used for COVID-19 pandemic estimates.

Knowledge Extraction From ICU Data Using Data Visualization

Authors from the fifth chapter, focus their study on the crucial nature of the intensive care unit (ICU), where critically sick patients must be continually watched, and where it is vital to make swift but firm choices. Indeed, several studies have demonstrated that continuous monitoring of ICU patients generates significant volumes of data, which may be used to extract information and make better choices. This chapter tries to analyze and show data collected by an ICU so that judgments about patient outcomes, clinical mistakes, and healthcare service quality may be drawn. To accomplish the goal, data was first gathered from a variety of sources, including bedside monitors and computerized nursing records. Second, the raw data was translated into a format that could be seen. Finally, interactive charts were created in order to predict data and uncover trends. The findings enable researchers to make inferences about the cause of data gaps, the relationship between medicine and vital signs, and the significance of SAPS in terms of patient outcome.

Classification of Polycystic Ovary Syndrome Based on Correlation Weight Using Machine Learning

Work number six talks about Polycystic Ovarian Syndrome (PCOS), and identify it has the most prevalent endocrine disease in women of reproductive age all over the globe. They introduce Machine Learning (ML) and Data Mining (DM) have favorable tools that influence on the diagnosis of this illness. The goal of this research is to create a model that can be used to detect patients with polycystic ovarian syndrome utilizing various scenarios based on correlation weights. To find the best model, the RF classifier, five DM approaches were used: Random Forest (RF), Decision Tree (DT), Naive Bayes (NB), Logistic Regression (LR), and Artificial Neural Network (ANN). Furthermore, the model was able to predict PCOS with 93.06 percent accuracy, 92.66 percent precision, 93.52 percent sensitivity, and 92.59 percent specificity, according to the findings. The feature selection based simply on the correlation weight dropped the accuracy values by 1.9 percent, precision by 3.7 percent, sensitivity by 0.3 percent, and specificity by 3.6 percent when compared to the authors' earlier work.

A Psychometrics Approach to Entropy

In manuscript number seven authors focus on a Psychometrics Approach to Entropy. Today's metrics for Women Housework Work (WHW) are quantitative in nature, notably assessing the amount of time spent on a job and the total number of chores performed by women, without taking into account the fact that it is an essentially qualitative process. To address this gap, an innovative framework for representing and thinking about large amounts of data or knowledge is presented, borrowing methods and methodologies for problem solving from the field of Artificial Intelligence, artifacts for improving practice through theory from Logic Programming, and the concept of Entropy from the Laws of Thermodynamics, interpreted as the degree of disorder or unpredictability in a system, a principle that can be used to understand system evolution. In the end authors examine the link between Psychometrics and Psychology or Sociology, specifically how particular psychological and social concepts such as cognition, knowledge, and personality influence WHW satisfaction.

Electronic Health Records Structuring
Based on the OpenEHR Standard

Chapter number eight reflects on the growth of Electronic Health Records (EHR) produced by health facilities and how it has resulted in vast and diverse data storage. The manuscript highlights the need for safe, continuous, and interoperable data structure across legacy systems. The OpenEHR is brought to action, and as standard defines open data requirements that attempt to overcome known gaps in healthcare record gathering, storage, and administration. In this regard, this chapter outlines a case study conducted in an emergency setting, in which 14-year clinical records were reconstructed into an interoperable and standardized environment using OpenEHR criteria.

A New Approach to E-Health Application Using Blockchain

Authors from chapter number nine cover the drug market and its contribution to medicine. With the massive drug industry that exists in the modern world, there is also a massive impediment to the existence of medications: the availability of counterfeit drugs on the market, which may bring permanent harm to humans.

Generation of Synthetic Data: A Generative Adversarial Networks Approach

As discussed in Chapter 10, artificial intelligence is progressing. However, Deep Learning approaches demand more data than is often accessible, particularly in the medical setting. Typically, current data sets are not indicative of reality, necessitating the acquisition of more samples, which is quite expensive. The desire for instruments capable of generating an unlimited amount of data has skyrocketed. Traditional data augmentation techniques are used to supplement existing data, but they do not produce new data. The use of generative adversarial networks to produce synthetic data has been groundbreaking for Big Data since it significantly expands the accessible data without incurring significant costs. To this goal, a version of alpha-GAN for 3D MRI images was created to enable the generation of an unlimited number of synthetic rat brain scans. A segmentation test was also performed to determine the application of the synthetic data, and visual inspection was used to determine the realism.

Importance of E-Health in Human Life

Chapter eleven discusses E-health, and how it is critical in providing vital information to the public about human life. E-health is the commercial and protected use of health information, and communication technology, and is associated with health-related directions and human health activities. ICT and E-health encompasses a variety of approaches, including telehealth, telemedicine, M-health (mobile health), Electronic Health Records (EHR), Big Data, wearables, and standardized artificial intelligence. In today's world, there is no time for paper and pen work. As countries continue to embrace digitalization, they are sharing health information and patient health data via an online mode that is more convenient and effective for digital health care improvements. These health care apps help us live better, healthier, and more fruitful lives. Lastly, authors state that E-health has the potential to be a critical component in providing community health benefits while incorporating a predictable medical system.

Improving the Management of Hospital Discharges

Centro Hospitalar Universitário do Porto (CHUP) serves as a pilot for an automated clinical coding method to help with hospital discharge coding. This project is described in Chapter 12 by critically presenting the results obtained. To make this tool usable, however, authors propose a procedure for managing the whole coding process. As a result, a platform was built to assist in the management of hospital discharge events. The primary benefit of having this platform is that it improves the organization of the whole coding process, hence increasing the amount and quality of work completed by CHUP's health experts.

Message System to Healthcare Interoperability

In the last chapter of this book, authors define as their primary objective to deduce the feasibility of adopting the Apache Kafka paradigm to healthcare information sharing. Initially, the message origin message was a basic HL7 message created in line with the specification. The message should then be routed to its destination using the FHIR protocol. Apache Kafka was used as the communication middleware and handler, along with a Confluent docker image. To map between HL7 versions, the python programming language was utilized, which turns the original message to a JSON object. Then, the Kafka API handles the structure-to-structure socket interface. Regarding the charge test, the findings were quite good, given that a 6000-message integration took less than a minute and required just a 500-message offset. Additionally, the systems can preserve the sequence of messages and recover from faults. Thus, it is feasible to utilize Kafka to distribute JSON objects in accordance with the FHIR standard while maintaining a predefined topic, consumer, and producer setup. This is a practical approach to Big Data architecture and its application in healthcare sector.

CONCLUSION

All of the chapters above presented, show how Big Data and artificial intelligence can contribute to distinct areas within the healthcare domain. It is, without doubt, one of the most important topics in this research field, and the main conclusions achieved by each individual chapter contribute to a more widespread knowledge of these thematic. Indeed, this book ranges its coverage, from more practical approaches with proposed architectures and tools, such as presented, for example, in chapters one, five, and thirteen to systematic and comprehensive literature reviews and research has shown, for example, in chapters three, four, nine and eleven.

REFERENCES

Adler-milstein, J., & Pfeifer, E. (2017). Information blocking: Is it occurring and what policy strategies can address it? *The Milbank Quarterly*, *95*(1), 117–135. doi:10.1111/1468-0009.12247 PMID:28266065

Auffray, C., Charron, D., & Hood, L. (2010). Predictive, preventive, personalized and participatory medicine: Back to the future. *Genome Medicine*, 2(8), 1–3. doi:10.1186/gm178 PMID:20804580

Bates, D. W., Saria, S., Ohno-Machado, L., Shah, A., & Escobar, G. (2014). Big data in health care: Using analytics to identify and manage high-risk and high-cost patients. *Health Affairs*, 33(7), 1123–1131. doi:10.1377/hlthaff.2014.0041 PMID:25006137

Belle, A., Thiagarajan, R., Soroushmehr, S. M., Navidi, F., Beard, D. A., & Najarian, K. (2015). Big data analytics in healthcare. *BioMed Research International*. PMID:26229957

De Mauro, A., Greco, M., & Grimaldi, M. (2016). A formal definition of Big Data based on its essential features. *Library Review*, 65(3), 122–135. doi:10.1108/LR-06-2015-0061

Fromme, E. K., Eilers, K. M., Mori, M., Hsieh, Y. C., & Beer, T. M. (2004). How accurate is clinician reporting of chemotherapy adverse effects? A comparison with patient-reported symptoms from the Quality-of-Life Questionnaire C30. *Journal of Clinical Oncology*, 22(17), 3485–3490. doi:10.1200/JCO.2004.03.025 PMID:15337796

Gubbi, J., Buyya, R., Marusic, S., & Palaniswami, M. (2013). Internet of Things (IoT): A vision, architectural elements, and future directions. *Future Generation Computer Systems*, 29(7), 1645–1660. doi:10.1016/j.future.2013.01.010

Kalender, W. A. (2006). X-ray computed tomography. *Physics in Medicine and Biology*, 51(13), R29–R43. doi:10.1088/0031-9155/51/13/R03 PMID:16790909

Kruse, C. S., Goswamy, R., Raval, Y. J., & Marawi, S. (2016). Challenges and opportunities of Big Data in health care: A systematic review. *JMIR Medical Informatics*, 4(4), e5359. doi:10.2196/medinform.5359 PMID:27872036

Laney, D. (2001). 3D data management: Controlling data volume, velocity and variety. *META Group Research Note, 6*(70), 1.

Martins, B., Ferreira, D., Neto, C., Abelha, A., & Machado, J. (2021). Data mining for cardiovascular disease prediction. *Journal of Medical Systems*, 45(1), 1–8. doi:10.100710916-020-01682-8 PMID:33404894

Neves, J., Vicente, H., Esteves, M., Ferraz, F., Abelha, A., Machado, J., Machado, J., Neves, J., Ribeiro, J., & Sampaio, L. (2018). A deep-big data approach to health care in the AI age. *Mobile Networks and Applications*, 23(4), 1123–1128. doi:10.100711036-018-1071-6

Raghupathi, W., & Raghupathi, V. (2014). Big data analytics in healthcare: Promise and potential. *Health Information Science and Systems*, *2*(1), 1–10. doi:10.1186/2047-2501-2-3 PMID:25825667

Sousa, R., Miranda, R., Moreira, A., Alves, C., Lori, N., & Machado, J. (2021). Software Tools for Conducting Real-Time Information Processing and Visualization in Industry: An Up-to-Date Review. *Applied Sciences (Basel, Switzerland)*, *11*(11), 4800. doi:10.3390/app11114800

Wang, Y., Kung, L., & Byrd, T. A. (2018). Big data analytics: Understanding its capabilities and potential benefits for healthcare organizations. *Technological Forecasting and Social Change*, *126*, 3–13. doi:10.1016/j.techfore.2015.12.019

Wilson, T. D. (2001). Information overload: Implications for healthcare services. *Health Informatics Journal*, *7*(2), 112–117. doi:10.1177/146045820100700210

Chapter 1
Real-Time UCI Monitoring Using Apache Kafka

Rui Santos
Centro ALGORITMI, Universidade do Minho, Portugal

António Abelha
Centro ALGORITMI, Universidade do Minho, Portugal

Ana Regina Sousa
https://orcid.org/0000-0002-2988-196X
Centro ALGORITMI, Universidade do Minho, Portugal

Hugo Peixoto
https://orcid.org/0000-0003-3957-2121
Centro ALGORITMI, Universidade do Minho, Portugal

Manuel Filipe Santos
https://orcid.org/0000-0002-5441-3316
Centro ALGORITMI, Universidade do Minho, Portugal

ABSTRACT

The importance of collecting and presenting data/events in real time from monitors in the intensive care units (ICU) demands constant research. Moreover, improvements in the systems are critical, thus adjusting their behavior to the new requests. The high amount of IoTs present results in the term big data in healthcare, where the most traditional technologies become invalid or operate with high difficulties. This chapter aims to propose an alternative system, quicker and above all, scalable, to allow for an improvement in the retrieval and presentation of data from different monitors. To this end, emergent technologies will be used, such as Apache Kafka. This technology has increasingly been put to use in healthcare due to its scalability, safety, and speed. Real datasets that simulate several types of data, like heartbeat, blood pressure, among others, will be used to obtain results. Furthermore, they also display fault and warning logs.

DOI: 10.4018/978-1-7998-9172-7.ch001

INTRODUCTION

Information from the most diverse types of sources has been one of the key points for a better organization and development of society. The more information with quality, the better the results that will be achieved. For this reason, companies and organizations from different areas are increasingly recognizing its importance and need. (Hassan et al., 2020)

One of the areas where there is still space for evolution is healthcare, an area that we all depend on as a society. Every day, traditional health information systems produce a huge amount of data, making it complex and costly to manage. Additionally, new technologies are developing, and Internet of Things (IoT) has been taking over this area as well, generating even more data, thus making the whole process of collecting, storing, and making data available more difficult and complex. The growth of IoT has made it so that more traditional methods face more difficulties, which contributes to the emergence of the term Big Data. (Dash et al., 2019)

Data obtained by the various monitors must be presented in real-time, so that health professionals (doctors, nurses, etc.) can act accordingly, especially in an emergency.

However, to achieve better results, in addition to obtaining patient data, it is necessary to carry out several innovative strategies throughout the development cycle, namely in **data ingestion**, that is, in the way the data reaches the processing; in **verifying the data**, to certify that there is no invalid or fraudulent data; in the **processing of data** and, finally, in its **presentation**.

Furthermore, when developing healthcare software, which may be responsible for processing large amounts of information, it is important that an architecture is prepared to deal with the concept of Big Data but also with scalability issues, such as the introduction of new features and/or increased load/response capacity.

A solution provided and adopted in other industries, has been to change systems based on monolithic architectures to systems based on microservices architectures. The latter has been gaining prominence in scientific articles, blogs and conferences. A microservices architecture is based on a distributed development, where an application is divided into small services that communicate with each other through Application Programming Interface (API). Each service can be developed, implemented, and scaled completely independently without directly affecting other services in the application. (Richardson & Smith, 2016) Figure 1 represents the difference between monolithic architectures and microservices architectures.

Figure 1. Monolithic Architectures versus Microservices Architectures Source: (Sanjaya, 2020)

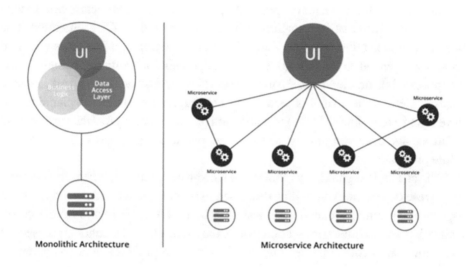

Allied to microservices architectures, there are several problems that can become complex, namely the communication between the services of an application. There are different forms of communication, however, a bad approach can make an application based on microservices become a monolithic distributed solution, thus not enjoying its advantages. Among the various types of communication, the Messaging that employs a Message Broker stands out. (Newman, 2020)

One of the most used Message Brokers, employed by 35% of Fortune 500 companies, is Apache Kafka, an open-source platform for event streaming, initially developed by LinkedIn. It allows communications with latencies below 2ms, is tolerant to the most diverse failures that may occur during communication and can be scaled horizontally. Apache Kafka has evolved and today has a complete ecosystem, which can be used to help in various areas, such as Apache Kafka Streams and Apache Kafka Connect. (Narkhede et al., 2017)

Therefore, the main objective of this article is the proposal of an architecture that is based on the resolution of the above presented adversities. However, there are some challenges inherent in carrying out this project. Data collection must be done quickly, securely, and able to easily scale with increasing devices. Storage, due to the huge amount of data produced, is demanding. In turn, the treatment/ processing, as well as the visualization of the data, must be presented in real time, to detect possible alterations to the millisecond.

This chapter has as its main objective the investigation of the following possibility: Is the use of architectures based on microservices and technologies such as Apache Kafka a viable alternative for the processing of messages in healthcare, with special focus in the transfer of information in intensive care units (ICU) where the flow of information is rather critical? Through the construction of a prototype with real data, it is intended to be able to demonstrate potential advantages, namely in the reception of information from the most diverse health providers, which may later be used. Therefore, the formal objectives of this chapter are designing, planning and developing a real-time ICU data visualization prototype, using real data available in a dataset, and evaluating the prototype developed in order to assess the suitability of the proposal.

This article is organized as follows: a background section, where the contexts of the research carried out will be described in order to better understand the main aspects of the study; a related work section, where a literature review is performed; a materials and technologies section, where the resources and technologies used are mentioned; an architecture section, which shows the problems and controversies as well as the architecture used and the way it was constructed in which everything was thought; a development section, where it is described the development process applied in the architecture previously presented; an evaluation section, in which the tests are described, exposed and the results are commented; a discussion section, with an analysis of the results obtains in the evaluation section, through a SWOT analysis; and, a conclusion section dedicated to the conclusions, as well as the future work to be developed.

BACKGROUND

Big Data

The term big data has grown immensely in recent years and has become recurrent in several sectors, mainly those related to information and communication technology. This concept refers to the effort required to handle the processing and storage of large amounts of data. It is often data with a high size and complexity, which more traditional technologies have difficulty responding to. This high amount of data produced by organizations is directly related to the various sources existing today, such as IoT devices (sensors, mobile devices), banking transactions, industrial equipment, amongst others. (*"Big Data: What it is and why it matters"*, n.d.)

One of the most challenging difficulties in managing big data is how data can surge. There are three types of classification for data, namely: (Ohri, 2021)

- Structured data;
- Unstructured data; and
- Semi-structured data.

Healthcare as a broad concept can be defined has a set of healthcare services aimed at treating diseases and preserving the health of human beings. This sector, which is in constant evolution, generates a large amount of data from the large number of sources present in hospital units. These data sources are varied and may include: Electronic health record (EHR); medical imaging; wearables; and medical devices, such as the intensive care unit monitors present in the intensive care units. The ability to process Big Data, not just in healthcare, brings several benefits. With the information from the data analysis, healthcare professionals can have the help of an external intelligence to assist in decision making. (Catalyst, 2018)

Intensive Medicine

Intensive Medicine is an area that depends on quick, effective and under great pressure decisions by health professionals, based mainly on the information obtained through the large number of devices existing in these units. Thus, these data contribute to the perception of the current status of patients, as well as helps in decision making, especially in these cases, where the health status of patients is complex, requiring up-to-the-minute follow-up. This continuous tracking of highly unstable users results in an exponential increase in devices in these services. (Peixoto et al., 2020)

Microservices Architecture

A microservices based architecture is the decomposition of an entire app by basic functions, where each function is named microservice and can be created and run in a totally independent manner. (Dragoni et al., 2017)

Making each microservice autonomous, allows for it to be developed, implemented, run, and scaled without affecting the functioning of the other services of the app. Moreover, there isn't an excess of coupling, since the other services do not share any type of codes amongst themselves. The communications through APIs are well defined. (Dragoni et al., 2017)

Another important fact is that microservices are specialized, meaning each service is projected for a specific functionality dedicated to the solution of a problem. In case there is a need to add new functionalities to a specific service increasing its complexity, the same can be later divided into smaller services allowing for a horizontal scaling. (Dragoni et al., 2017) Horizontal scaling is directly linked to adding new machines while vertical scaling is related to adding more power, RAM, memory and more to a single existing machine. By managing to have a horizontal scaling, it is possible for a company or organization to save resources, namely in terms of capital and also in terms of organization, since it is possible to divide the software by different machines, facilitating its maintenance. (*Scaling Horizontally vs. Scaling Vertically*, 2020)

Martin Fowler identified a set of characteristics that are directly linked with microservices architecture. However, despite the similarities, not all apps that employ this architecture share all the characteristics detailed below. The set of features is: Componentization via Services, that is, the possibility of building a complete application composed of small totally independent services; Organized around Business Capabilities, that is, the development teams are organized around the business and not around development parts as usual; Products not Projects, because a team is responsible for a product during its development and production process, being in permanent contact with the product in order to improve it for the end customers; Smart Endpoints and Dumb Pipes, for the reason that the communication between the various microservices must be simple, fast and uncomplicated through the use of simple asynchronous or synchronous protocols such as Request/Response and Publish/Subscribe; Decentralized Governance, since it is possible to use the most suitable technology for each functionality, without the restriction of technologies that occur in other types of architectures; Infrastructure Automation, since the process must be agile and fast, it is common to use several techniques for the DevOps part, such as Continuous Integration and Continuous Delivery; and Design for Failure, because an application is composed of several services, it must be prepared for eventual communication failures, having to exist secondary plans that come into action when one or more services fail. (Lewis & Fowler, 2014)

Choreography versus Orchestration

Associated with microservices architectures, there is much discussion regarding the type of coordination logic in the communication between the various services of an architecture. There are two types of approaches: Orchestration and Choreography. (Dragoni et al., 2017)

Orchestration promotes the coordination of logic through a centralized approach using a central service. This central service is primarily responsible for communicating with each of the services, then monitoring the results and returning the response to the front-end. This coordination technique is quite common in SOA architectures through the use of the ESB. Although with Orchestration you get rigider control of all the steps, this more centralized approach makes the services dependent on each other and has a single point of failure. Figure 2 represents the Orchestration approach in microservices architectures. (Heusser, 2020)

Figure 2. Orchestration approach Source: (Sucaria, 2021)

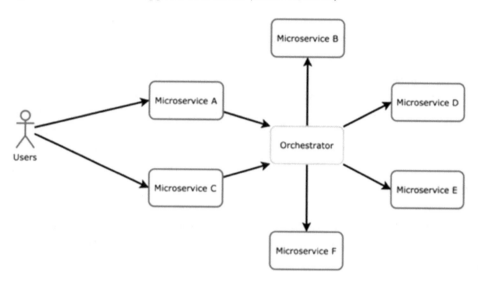

In the Choreography approach there is no longer a central service responsible for coordinating communication between the various microservices. In this approach, the application services work independently and are not blocked waiting for information from other services. It is common to use an Event Broker that distributes the work among the various components. In this sense, there is no longer a single point of failure but, the development complexity increases. Figure 3 represents the Choreography approach in microservices architectures. (Heusser, 2020)

Figure 3. Choreography approach Source: (Sucaria, 2021)

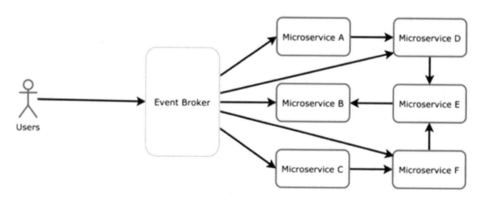

Inter-Process Communication

Since microservices architecture is a distributed system, one of the focal points is precisely the communication between the various services. In monolithic services, the communication is made through call functions between modules. The same is not possible for microservices. (Richardson & Smith, 2016)

Microservices need to communicate amongst each other through a mechanism of communication between processes. There are several approaches that can be used for the interaction between microservices. (Richardson & Smith, 2016)

Event Based

A service publishes a message that will be consumed by one or more services. An example of this type of communication is RabbitMQ and Apache Kafka. (Richardson & Smith, 2016)

As seen in figure 4 when microservice A wants to send information to two other microservices, namely B and C, it publishes a message in a Broker. Later it will then be consumed by microservice B and C. In this way, it is possible to guarantee that, even if microservice B and C are offline, the message will not be lost, being consumed when the microservices are back online.

Figure 4. Event based communication Source: (de la Torre et al., 2019)

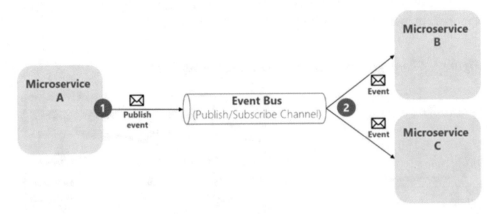

RELATED WORK

In this chapter, two companies are analyzed, Humana Inc. and Babylon Health, which stand out for multiple factors. The most important factors are the fact that they operate in the healthcare area and process a large volume of data. This choice was also due to the fact that these companies are at very different stages of development. Babylon Health is a startup while Humana Inc. already has a consolidated presence in the area.

Humana Inc.

Humana Inc. is a healthcare-related company, founded by David A. Jones and Wendell Cherry in 1961. It is currently headquartered in Louisville (United States of America) and integrates insurance, health, and wellness services as main areas of its job market. This company works with several segments, including: Retail, Employer Group and Health and Well Being Services. (*Humana (HUM)*, 2021)

The Health and Well-Being Services segment involves services offered to health plan subscribers, as well as third parties, which include pharmacy solutions, provider services, clinical care, predictive modeling and informatics services to other Humana businesses, as well as external health plan members, external health plans, and other employers. (*Humana (HUM)*, 2021)

Due to the multiple areas involved in Humana Inc.'s job market, it is difficult to link all clinical data of patients, so that they are updated. This data may be present in several providers, such as: the pharmacy record, the home healthcare visit, the specialists' recommendations, the electronic medical record at the local hospital, and others. If the data is out of date, it may trigger an incomplete perception of health professionals with regard to the clinical data of patients, implying their decision-making. Ultimately it could have serious repercussions, inclusively fatal. (Combs, 2020)

Levi Bailey, current Associate Vice President and Cloud Architecture at Humana Inc., said: *"When we think of a better healthcare ecosystem, we need to think about the opportunity to exchange data in a seamless way, where all participants can freely integrate that data to help drive the outcomes and the experience within their organizations."* In order to overcome this adversity, the solution found by Levi Bailey and Humana Inc., went through the use of Event-driven mechanisms in the cloud, namely Apache Kafka. (Confluent, 2020) This type of mechanism changed the concept of certain actions, such as sales or a customer service interaction for events. Data from these events can be used to provide real-time recommendations and decisions. (Combs, 2020)

The use of this type of mechanisms allows Humana Inc. the ability to scale to a hyperconnected data ecosystem, thus managing to gather all data, optimize it and subsequently make it available for the intended services. In addition, it provides another benefit, allowing the existence of a history of events, which makes it easier to understand the implications of changes. (Combs, 2020)

All the changes made allowed Humana Inc. and its patients to obtain a more complete view of their information, including lab data and diagnostic codes, ensuring, above all, an accurate and current assessment by healthcare professionals. (Combs, 2020)

Babylon Health

Babylon Health is a healthcare company, founded in 2013 in the UK by Ali Parsa. The main objective of the company is to make healthcare accessible to all citizens worldwide. In order to achieve this, it applies innovative technologies and Artificial Intelligence, in order to relieve the doctors work, allowing them to focus on the patients who need it most. (Babylon Health, 2013)

In addition to developing its products, Babylon Health is present at several conferences such as Big Data LDN [1] and KafkaSummit (led by Confluent)[2]. During these events, Babylon Health explains how it applies microservices architectures and Event Streaming to develop its products. At the Freeing up Kafka conference engineering resources to scale with DataOps for Big Data LDN, Jeremy Frenay, the Data Operation Engineer of Babylon Health, showcased Babylon Health's evolution from a low-service startup to a healthcare unicorn as well as the resulting challenges. (Stevenson & Frenay, 2019)

Since Babylon Health intends to revolutionize the healthcare area with Artificial Intelligence techniques, the need arose to aggregate a set of data present in various services, as represented in Figure 5. (Stevenson & Frenay, 2019)

Figure 5. Babylon Architecture before the introduction of Apache Kafka Ad: (Stevenson & Frenay, 2019)

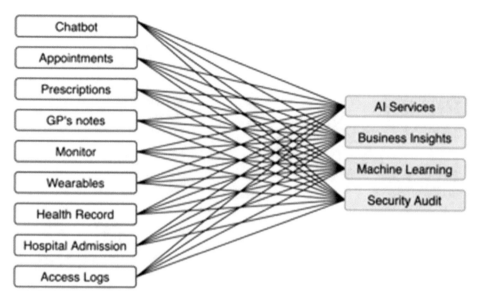

To be able to aggregate, filter and anonymize data from the various services, in order to obtain better insights, models and security, it was necessary to outline a new style of development based on the development of microservices. Furthermore, it chose to use Apache Kafka to aggregate all the data quickly and efficiently. Figure 6 represents the role of microservices and Apache Kafka at Babylon Health. (Stevenson & Frenay, 2019)

Figure 6. Babylon Architecture after the introduction of Apache Kafka Source: (Noble & Nobilia, 2019)

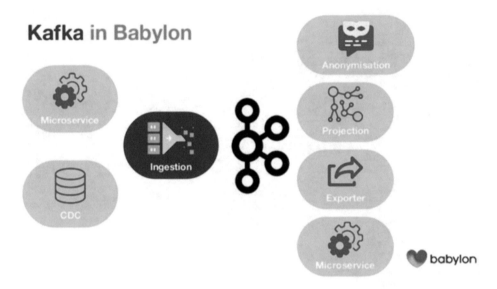

Related Articles

The authors of (Peixoto et al., 2020) proposed a modular architecture that aims to improve scalability for future implementations. This is composed of several components, including a Gateway, a set of Middewares and a database. The processed data is stored and subsequently made available to Electronic Health Records and Knowledge Discovery. Containerization is suggested by the authors in order to provide isolation and management of resources on the server as well as balancing traffic and data load across the various containers, making the architecture adjustable and scalable. This is due to the fact that, when running a software inside a container, this makes the processing somewhat isolated from other software. In addition, it allows for easy migration and restoration of data, since the storage is allocated in the hard disk from the host. In the event that there is any change in a container, it is only necessary to restart that specific container, not there being a need to restart the rest of the architecture. Nextgen Connect was also used. It is an open-source tool specialized in the integration of health data and which provides channels for data input and output through TCP's, database and files. In addition, the HL7, an international communication standard that enables the sharing of electronic health information, in version 2, was used as a message standard.

The authors of (Cruz et al., 2021) suggested an architecture similar to the described above (Peixoto et al., 2020). The authors of (Peixoto et al., 2020) and

(Cruz et al., 2021), chose to follow the same strategy, namely in the data reception and processing component, since the Gateway, Nextgen Connect and Middleware components are present in both. However, the latter opted for another approach with regard to data visualization, namely through the use of Kibana and Grafana. Once the data has been stored in ElasticSearch, it is possible to visualize the data in real time, as well as present it in the form of a graph. In addition, it also has alert features via email and SMS.

The two articles (Peixoto et al., 2020) and (Cruz et al., 2021) served as a starting point for the architecture that will be presented in the next sections. These articles were able to expose the difficulties existing in hospital units, such as the high amount of processed data as well as the speed with which they appear. Furthermore, articles (Peixoto et al., 2020) and (Cruz et al., 2021) managed to expose some advantages that are used in the present architecture, namely in the use of containers as well as in the use of a NoSQL database.

Both companies analysed in the related work use the microservices architecture together with some sort of event-driven (in this specific case the Apache Kafka). However, and despite the successful results achieved by these companies, none of them have their business focus related to Intensive Medicine. In this sense, the architecture presented in the section called Architecture has as its main goal to explore open points of these architectures and redirect and adapt them to Intensive Medicine, where speed and security are fundamental.

About the articles under review, the use of Mirth or Nextgen Connect is one of the common points in both architectures (Peixoto et al., 2020) and (Cruz et al., 2021). However, these softwares, in addition to having a non intuitive interface, can becameslow when the number of messages sent increases.

MATERIALS AND TECHNOLOGIES

MIMIC Database

To assist the study presented in this chapter, a public dataset that is available on PhysioNet was used. This platform is managed by members of the MIT Laboratory for Computational Physiology, whose purpose is to offer large datasets of clinical data for research and studies. (Goldberger et al., 2000) The selected dataset was the MIMIC Database version 1.0.0, which contains data from 72 patients present in the ICU. (Moody and Mark, 1992) Each patient in the dataset has a corresponding folder that is identified by a unique ID (ex. 301, 209) and where all their files available in different formats, such as: txt; dat; and hea. Each file represents ten minutes of measurements, resulting in twenty or more hours of periodic signals and measurements that may vary between patients. Thus, there are a total of 200 days of vital signs recorded in the dataset.

In the current chapter, txt files were used, which have the following format:

Figure 7. Example of a txt file format Source: (Goldberger et al., 2000)

```
[11:27:45 14/08/1994]      03700001.txt
RESP       46
ABP        64          82          53
HR         122
SpO2       0
PULSE      0
```

The first line of each file corresponds to the identification of the date and time of the first measurement. Subsequently, the periodic measurements of the patient are found, where, in this specific case, each 5 lines represent 1 second of the 10 minutes presented in each file. Each line displays a measurement of the sensors present on the monitor, initially identified by the signal type name, followed by one or more values. Values can be simple (1 single value) or composite (+ than one value). The types of sensors shown may vary by patient.

There are several types of data present in the files, such as:

- NBP – Noninvasive blood pressure;
- Arterial Blood Pressure (ABP);
- HR – Heart rate;
- SpO2 – Peripheral Oxygen Saturation.

In addition to the above-mentioned data types, notes corresponding to changes in the monitor's operation as well as changes in the patient's condition are also presented. Changes can be of various types (Inactivity, incorrect sensor reading and Alarm).

Apache Kafka

Apache Kafka is an open-source platform of distributed transmission of events, developed in the programming languages Java and Scala. Initially developed by

LinkedIn, with the goal of processing 1.4 trillion messages a day, it was launched in January 2011. Currently, it is kept and explored by the company Confluent, under the stewardship of the Apache Foundation. (Narkhede et al., 2017)

Of the many characteristics of the Apache Kafka, four can be highlighted: High Performance, since the delivery of messages has a latency of around 2 milliseconds; Horizontal Scalability - it is possible to expand up to hundreds of brokers and process millions of messages by the second; Failure tolerant, thanks to its distributed system, in which messages are duplicated and stored in different locations; and High availability, since it is possible to have clusters in several parts of the world. (Narkhede et al., 2017)

Apache Kafka supports different types of use cases categories, such as: the publish-subscribe message system; Website Activity tracking; Gather Metrics from many different locations; Log Aggregation; Stream Processing; Event Sourcing; and Commit Log. (Narkhede et al., 2017)

The main concepts of Apache Kafka are related to:

- Kafka Cluster and Kafka Brokers, where a Kafka Cluster consists of one or more Kafka servers (also called kafka brokers);
- Messages, where the content to be published is stored.
  - A Message is composed by a Key, that identifies in which partition the message will be stored, a Value, where the content is stored (it can be a simple number or a string to an object in JavaScript Object Notation), and a timestamp, that identifies the hour in which a message was sent to a specific topic. (Narkhede et al., 2017)
- Topic - The term topic in Apache Kafka signifies a category or a name of a flow in which messages are published. It is identified through a single name that usually references the flow of data for which it was created. It is composed by a specific number of partitions that should be introduced by the user when it creates the topic. The messages are stored in the partitions in an ordained and immutable way, where each is attributed, a single incremental identifier called Offset. (*Apache Kafka Documentation*, n.d.)
- Producers are the applications responsible for producing and publishing messages in one or more topics.
- Consumers are the applications responsible for consuming messages from one or more topics.

Initially Apache Kafka was essentially, what was previously described, there being, the existence of Producers, Consumers, Topics and Messages. However, throughout its existence it has evolved to a complete ecosystem build and sustained to help companies that use this system. Some of the products that have helped build the ecosystem are the Apache Kafka Connect and the Apache Kafka Streams. (Sax, 2018)

The Apache Kafka Connect was created in November 2015 during an update of the Apache Kafka. Its goal is to simplify what, often, is very repetitive. It allows to fetch data from a source (e.g., MongoDB, MySQL), and to publish it in one or more Kafka topics, without there being a need to type a single line of code. Furthermore, another product was created, Apache Kafka Connect Sinks, that does the exact opposite. It fetches data from a topic and places it in a Sink, that can be anything from an ElasticSearch or a text file. (Sax, 2018)

Besides Apache Kafka Connect there is also the Apache Kafka Streams, a library produced in Java and launched in 2016. It aims to help in the processing and transformation of data in real time. In other words, Apache Kafka Streams is a library capable of consuming data from a topic, processing it, and, per a condition, sending it a specific topic. (Sax, 2018)

Besides the two variables presented previously, Apache Kafka contains a wide range of options that can help companies in the most varied of occasions.

Apache Kafka is present in the most diverse business areas such as banks, telecommunications and hospitals. Currently, it is employed by more than 200 companies, including 80% of all Fortune 100 companies. (*Apache Kafka*, n.d.)

Mongo DB

MongoDB is an open-source document database that provides high performance, high availability, and easy scaling. It is one of the NoSQL databases available on the market, which is currently part of the group of the most used. Applies to many use cases, such as: Big Data; Content Management and Delivery; Mobile and Social Infrastructure; User Data Management; and Data Hub. Furthermore, this database is known for its simplicity of use when it comes to data representation, since its key concepts are related to: Document, where the data is stored; and Collection, a set of several Documents. (Maksimovic, 2017)

A Document in MongoDB is a data structure made up of field and value pairs. The representation format of a Document is very similar to the JSON format, however, MongoDB stores the information internally in BSON format. BSON in turn, represents a JSON in binary format and its use in MongoDB allows it to be analysed faster. (*"JSON and BSON,"* n.d.)

A Collection in MongoDB is the location where Documents are stored. Each Document in the Collection, unless specified, has an "_id" automatically assigned by MondoDB. Inside a Collection, contrary to what happens in a traditional SQL database, there is no specific format, that is, a Collection can have different Document formats, which simplifies the storage of unstructured or semi-structured data. By default, all Documents in a Collection have similar or directly related purposes. (*"MongoDB - Overview,"* n.d.) The example Document of figure 8 is composed of an _id, two fields (firstname and lastname), a sub-document address with four fields, and a field of type array with two values.

Figure 8. Example of a MongoDB document Source: (What is a Document Database?, n.d.)

```
{
  "_id": "5cf0029caff5056591b0ce7d",
  "firstname": "Jane",
  "lastname": "Wu",
  "address": {
    "street": "1 Circle Rd",
    "city": "Los Angeles",
    "state": "CA",
    "zip": "90404"
  }
  "hobbies": ["surfing", "coding"]
}
```

Architecture

The architecture of a healthcare-related system should address the purpose of its creation, methods that facilitate the inclusion of future functionalities, as well as communication with external elements from multiple service providers. In this sense, it is important to develop a prototype that presents an organized, well-designed, and efficient structure, so that it can respond to problems and facilitate future changes. In this way, it is possible to promote a better flow of data in the system and an efficient use by the end user.

Consequently, a prototype was created, which represents a real-time data visualization system of patients in an intensive care unit.

The prototype to be developed must be able to respond to a set of challenges that are often present in healthcare-related architectures, namely:

- The presence of **external suppliers**, that is, companies that provide services and that provide data through public APIs, making the communication process with the system difficult;
- The existence of **large amounts of data in short periods of time (Big Data)**, due to the excess of IoT devices (Medical Devices, bedside monitors) and users (Doctors, Nurses);
- The **reception, analysis and processing of data in real-time**, in order to prevent any anomalies/faults;
- **Large-scale data storage**, as they deal with clinical data, so it is extremely important to have a data history;
- The **representation of data through real-time graphics**, in order to support the medical decision and present alerts of possible changes (Alarms, Errors, etc.);
- The **horizontal scalability must be previously weighed** (instead of the vertical one) due to the high probability of a significant increase of devices and users.

The architecture of an ICU real-time clinical data visualization system comprises the communication between the IoT devices and the application responsible for the visualization, as well as the communication with other services for data analysis and storage. Thus, it is necessary to organize a structure capable of managing the data communication flow between the various components of the system.

The main features are described in the following steps:

1. The System must be able to carry out communication between the IoT devices (originated or not from external services) and the application itself. The data resulting from these devices can appear in different formats (structured, semi-structured or unstructured).
2. The application must be able to receive data quickly and securely and then present tools capable of processing and analysing it. Later, they can be provided for other resources (Front-end application, Data Knowledge) in a specific and known format: JSON.
3. Storage must be carried out in a database capable of quick and simple queries. At the same time, it must also adapt to the different types of data provided by the numerous sensors present.

4.   After processing and storing the data, they must be made available to the end user through a WEB application that presents them in an intuitive and dynamic way.

The diagram in Figure 9 illustrates the architecture proposed to solve the problem and demonstrates the sequence of interactions between the different components of the system, as well as the data flow that occurs in the process. This architecture was developed based on the proposal in article (Peixoto et al., 2020) where the main change is the replacement of Mirth Connect Engine Software for Apache Kafka. In addition, several microservices are used in order to support data analysis and visualization in real time.

Figure 9. Architecture diagram

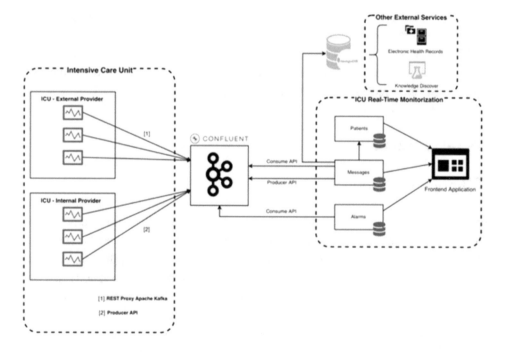

This architecture is based on event streaming technology, Apache Kafka, and microservices architectures. On the left side of figure 9 the monitors used in the Intensive Care Units are represented, which may come from external suppliers, and which are constantly producing new data. Then, this data is sent to a topic previously generated in the Apache Kafka cluster called "icu_messages". For this there are two possibilities: the REST Proxy provided by Apache Kafka or the Publisher-Subscriber

API. Apache Kafka brokers are located on the Confluent platform in order to get an overview of what is happening in the cluster.

Regarding the ICU Real-Time Monitorization (Backend and Frontend), which is the main focus of these thesis, there are a total of three microservices, as shown in Figure 9. The "Messages" microservice aims to consume the data published by bedside monitors and then validate the existence of any type of anomaly. In the event of an anomaly, the "Messages" microservice publishes a new message in an Apache Kafka topic called "icu_alarms". Later, this message will be consumed by the "Alarms" microservice and persisted in a database for this purpose. Regardless of the existence of an anomaly, the microservice "Messages" stores all data in a NoSQL database. In addition, this same data is also sent, through WebSockets, to a Frontend application, which allows it to be visualized in real time in the form of a graph or table.

The application responsible for displaying patient information, real-time value graphs and alarms that have already occurred, will consume the data through REST API and through WebSockets.

Through the storage of data, it is possible that it allows to assist in other aspects, given that, in addition to presenting data in real time, it allows for future availability for Data Science and Machine Learning techniques.

DEVELOPMENT

ICU Simulator Application

In order to continue the study of the surrounding architectural methods and technologies, the need arose to create applications that could reproduce the simulation of bedside monitors that are present in intensive care units. The application created to reproduce the simulators has the objective of reading the files of a specific patient from the MIMIC dataset, separating the data from each file, creating the message and, subsequently, sending it to the Apache Kafka cluster.

For the development of the simulation application, an object-oriented language, namely Java using JDK 11 together with Maven, was used. The choice of language was based on the fact that the support/documentation language used in Apache Kafka is Java.

In order to run the same application several times and for different patients, a mechanism was created that internally differentiates patients. To do so, when starting the application, it is necessary to indicate the path relative to the patient's folder in MIMIC Database v1.0. It is possible to indicate the path through arguments or, if there are no arguments, indicate the path at the beginning of the execution.

After validating the path of a specific patient, it is run through to start the process of reading each file. The files are in the format indicated above, where the first line has the indication of the time of the first measurement, the patient indicator and the name of the file being read. Since initially only the timestamp of the first measurement in the file was present, it was necessary to find a formula to calculate the timestamp of the remaining measurements. Each file has a total of ten minutes of measurements and the number of data may vary. The formula found was: (1), where x corresponds to the number of registers (lines) of the file and y the value in milliseconds that must be added to the timestamp of message to message. In addition, the values can be of different types, so it was necessary to carry out several validations, namely, about warnings, the composition of sensor values and alarms. At the end, the message is constructed in the following format:

$$y = \left(1 + \frac{600 - x}{x}\right) \times 1000 \tag{1}$$

Afterwards, with the message already created, it is necessary to send it to the Apache Kafka cluster. Apache Kafka offers two ways of sending messages: one through a REST API (Apache Kafka Rest Proxy); and another through the Producer/Consumer APIs.

Apache Kafka REST Proxy works as a REST API, which consists of sending an HTTP request with the POST method to a specific endpoint. This endpoint varies depending on the topic the message is sent to *(https://ip_address/topic/topic_name)*. In addition, it is necessary to add headers to the request, namely Accept and Content-Type. The request body must follow a specific format.

The other option, the most common one, works using the Apache Kafka library. For this, it is necessary to add this library to the project and perform the initial configuration indicating several properties, such as the IP Address of one of the Brokers in the Cluster, as well as the part related to authentication. After successful configurations, it is possible to use the various methods available in the library, such as the methods of class *KafkaProducer*, namely the *java.util.concurrent. Future<RecordMetadata> send(ProducerRecord<K,V> record, Callback callback)*. This method allows to send a message to the Apache Kafka cluster asynchronously. Since the messages can be distributed in different partitions of the Apache Kafka topic, it is necessary to add the Key, in order to guarantee the reading order. The Key used refers to the ID of each patient.

Analysis and Processing Application

To perform the reception, analysis, processing and availability of application data, the Java programming language was used together with the Spring Boot framework. The choice of this framework derives from the ease of integration of different modules (Apache Kafka, Databases, among others) and also to the use of concepts such as Inversion of Control and Dependency Injection that simplify and protect the way we program.

The data is published in the Apache Kafka cluster topics through the producers, which in the scope of this project are the bedside monitor simulators. Then, the consumers responsible for validating and processing the data - Message Service, start consuming them.

Through the use of the Spring Boot Framework, it is possible to connect to the Apache Kafka cluster in a simple and fast way, by installing the Spring for Apache Kafka module. Subsequently, and with the connection made to the cluster, it was necessary to create *KafkaListerner's* for the topics in which the information is intended to be consumed.

After receiving the data, there was the need to process the message in order to be able to verify the existence of anomalous values or alarms. For this purpose, tools such as ModelMapper were used, which allows mapping objects in a simple and practical way. After that, the treated message is stored in the MongoDB database and sent in JSON format through WebSockets to the Web interface. In the event of anomalies, it was important that they be stored permanently. For this, they were published in a topic of the Apache Kafka cluster with an extensive durability. Later, they will be consumed and persisted by the "Alarms" microservice. The message is sent to the web interface in the following format:

Figure 10. JSON structure with a patient's data

```
{
    "patientId":"037",
    "timestamp":"1994-08-14T09:27:45",
    "file":"03700001.txt",
    "values":[
        {
            "typeOfValue":"RESP",
            "values":[
                46
            ]
        },
        {
            "typeOfValue":"ABP",
            "values":[
                64,
                82,
                53
            ]
        },
        {
            "typeOfValue":"HR",
            "values":[
                122
            ]
        },
        {
            "typeOfValue":"SpO2",
            "values":[
                0
            ]
        },
        {
            "typeOfValue":"PULSE",
            "values":[
                0
            ]
        }
    ],
    "isAlarm":false
}
```

Finally, for all messages in which the existence of an anomaly is not verified, an expiration TTL is applied, which can be changed by the user through the Single Page Application (SPA).

Frontend Application

Regarding the WEB client, a SPA was used, where users can observe in real-time the graphics related to the sensors of the bedside monitors. This was developed using the JavaScript programming language together with the VueJS Framework. The choice of VueJS was based on five main factors: Learning curve; Speed of development; Speed of the app; and Code structure and Documentation. Additionally, and due to the speed of styling compared to other tools or CSS in its pure state, the Vuetify library was applied. Furthermore, and in order to develop intuitive, responsive and customizable charts, the Apex Charts library was chosen.

The application responsible for frontend communicated with the backend services through two methods: REST APIs and WebSockets. Since not all browsers support the WebSockets technology, it was necessary to overcome this problem using an emulator, in this case SockJS. In this sense, it was essential to make changes on the server side, using the STOMP protocol, which implied the use of a new library on the application side responsible for demonstrating the graphics. Webstomp-client was the library chosen.

For the construction of the charts and, as mentioned above, the Apex Charts library was used. It offers different types of charts, such as: Line Charts, Bar Charts, Area Charts, among others. In this specific case, we resorted to the use of Line Charts, adding DataLabels and Annotations. DataLabels are necessary to specify the values in more detail in a certain period, while Annotations serve to indicate the limit of values in the acceptable level.

In the following sections, the result of the application responsible for displaying the sensor graphics for each patient registered in the system will be demonstrated.

Demonstration

Using the microservices and the technologies discussed above, it was possible to develop the application as shown in the following figures.

Figure 11 illustrates a patient's data in real-time in the form of an interactive graph and in the form of cards.

Figure 11. Page responsible for the information of a patient with data

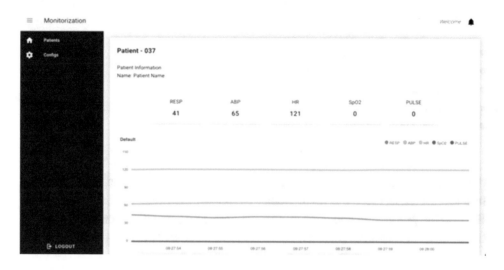

Evaluation

To evaluate the idealized architecture two types of tests were implemented: performance tests and message format tests. The performance tests aim to verify the processing capacity of reception and availability of messages, as well as, the number of stored messages. For these tests, different numbers of simulators were used in order to have a better perception of the performance, reaching a maximum of 40 simulators simultaneously.

As a comparison, in the National assessment of the situation of intensive care units (Penedo et al., 2013) report for the year 2013, the Braga Hospital of ARS Norte had 12 beds in intensive care units.

Regarding the message format tests, different formats were used, namely JSON and HL7v2. The choice of these formats was related, respectively, to popular use and, to representing the international standards for the representation and transfer of clinical and administrative data between health information systems.

Performance Tests

This subsection contains the performance tests performed on the developed prototype, along with the MIMIC Database dataset. For the development of these tests, a specific script was created to run several ICU simulators simultaneously. Tests were performed with 1, 3, 5, 20 and 40 simulators. To elaborate the discussion, during the tests different types of metrics were collected through the Apache Kafka dashboard and MongoDB. The metrics collected were:

- Production (bytes/sec avg over 1 min)
- Consumption (bytes/sec avg over 1 min)
- Storage
- Messages save
- Messages saved/sec.

Table 1 represents the data obtained with 1 ICU simulator. It is possible to see that the production values and the consumption values follow each other at the bytes/min level. That is, there was no difficulty in receiving the data from the consumers. Besides the production and consumption of data, and since it was only a simulator, the number of messages received and the average per second was as expected.

Table 1. Performance tests with 1 ICU simulator

Production	Consumption	Storage	Messages	Messages/sec
116	116			
327	383			
327	338			
332	327			
327	332			
332	327	202.43 kb	614	0.9
327	332			
332	327			
327	327			
330	375			
327	327			
51	51			

Table 2 illustrates the data obtained from the performance behavior of the prototype developed with 3 ICU simulators. Once again, the production and consumption values were similar, which means that there was no difficulty in making the data available for processing. The number of messages stored was higher in relation to the previous one, and the number of messages stored per second corresponds to the number of sends, i.e., 3 simulators correspond to 3 messages stored per second.

Table 2. Performance tests with 3 ICU simulator

Production	Consumption	Storage	Messages	Messages/sec
835	846			
959	948			
954	965			
959	948			
949	965			
966	949			
949	949	653.21 kb	2045	3.1
965	965			
947	947			
948	965			
965	959			
507	507			

According to the data obtained in the 5 simulators test (Table 3) it was possible to see, once again, that the prototype received data efficiently, with no significant differences between production and consumption. The number of messages stored was higher, reaching 3141 with an average of 4.8 messages per second.

Table 3. Performance tests with 5 ICU simulator

Production	Consumption	Storage	Messages	Messages/sec
427	441			
1.33k	1.32k			
1.31k	1.33k			
1.33k	1.32k			
1.32k	1.32k			
1.33k	1.33k			
1.32k	1.32k	853.62 kb	3141	4.8
1.32k	1.33k			
1.33k	1.32k			
1.32k	1.31k			
1.32k	1.33k			
595	586			

Observing Table 4, which represents data from 20 simultaneous ICU simulators, it is also possible to conclude that the developed prototype can easily respond to production and consumption values. The number of messages stored in the database is about 13381, which averages to 20.3 messages stored per second. This is a very considerable value for an ICU in Portugal.

Table 4. Performance tests with 20 ICU simulator

Production	Consumption	Storage	Messages	Messages/sec
5.97k	5.99k			
6.22k	6.22k			
6.23k	6.29k			
6.28k	6.22k			
6.23k	6.28k			
6.29k	6.24k	4.19 mb	13381	20.3
6.22k	6.23k			
6.24k	6.27k			
6.28k	6.24k			
6.22k	6.27k			
6.27k	6.25k			
3.12k	3.08k			

The last performance test was the most demanding and involved 40 ICU simulators (Table 5) running simultaneously. Despite the high number of messages stored, 25563, which gives an average of 38.7 messages stored per second, the prototype had no difficulty regarding the difference of bytes in production and in consumption. Table 5 represents the values collected during this experiment.

Table 5. Performance tests with 40 ICU simulator

Production	Consumption	Storage	Messages	Messages/sec
4.01k	4.1k			
12.5k	12.44k			
12.49k	12.51k			
12.5k	12.51k			
12.5k	12.48k			
12.48k	12.5k	8.01 mb	25563	38.7
12.52k	12.5k			
12.51k	12.52k			
12.5k	12.46k			
12.5k	12.49k			
12.47k	12.49k			
7.76k	7.72k			

Briefly, and with the data collected and analyzed during the various experiments performed, it is possible to conclude that the prototype can easily meet the requirement of 40 ICU simulators. The producer and consumer values during the various test scenarios are always similar, i.e., there is no difficulty regarding the data being produced and consumed. This makes it possible to always have the most up-to-date data in real-time. The storage values shown are related to Apache Kafka's internal storage, which gives the prototype extra storage security.

In the event that more than 40 ICU simulators were needed simultaneously and the consumer could not handle the data demand, it would only be necessary to add one more consumer and create a consumer group in order to split the reading of the received data. The strategy of coordinating the consumers would be done simply and automatically by Apache Kafka using Zookeeper.

Message Format Tests

As in other areas, healthcare can receive data in different formats, so it was necessary to check whether Apache Kafka can support them. To do this, messages were sent in several formats, such as: Txt, JSON XML, and HL7 v2.0. HL7 is an international community of health information experts that collaborate to develop standards for the exchange of health information and health systems interoperability.

The following table (6) shows the result of the tests when sending messages with different formats.

Table 6. Message Format tests

Message Format	Evaluation
TXT	Acceptable
XML	Acceptable
JSON	Acceptable
HL7	Acceptable

Although Apache Kafka accepts the different types of text format, it is necessary to configure the consumers to be able to interpret the data later.

DISCUSSION

In order to discuss the results obtained with the propose architecture, a SWOT analysis was performed. A SWOT analysis is a tool that aims to identify the strengths, opportunities, weaknesses, and threats of the object of study, through a rigorous analysis.
As **strengths** one can identify:

- Scalable

One of the key factors that decide the success of an architecture is the ability with which it handles the increased load/users. This increase in load/users must be handled in a simple, sustainable, and continuous way. With the use of microservices and Container technology, scaling the application/architecture to meet the increased load is possible by duplicating microservices and using a Load Balancer.

Another important factor is the eventuality that new features need to be added to the application. Solving this problem in the developed architecture is simple. It can be applied to an existing microservice or, if justified, opt to create a new microservice.

Regarding the growth of new IoT devices (Bedside Monitors, etc) or the addition of new external services, the developed architecture can respond to this growth by using Apache Kafka. If the existing Apache Kafka cluster is having trouble receiving and delivering data, it is only necessary to add a new Kafka Broker to the Cluster. Eventually, to be able to consume the data faster it may be useful to create consumer clusters.

- Reliable

Considering healthcare a critical market when it comes to data loss, this architecture becomes reliable due to the fact that it uses Apache Kafka as a data intermediary. Apache Kafka technology provides several ways to ensure that data can be received and made available. When it comes to receiving data, coming from IoT devices, it is possible to use Acks to prevent possible failures. Acks allow the Kafka Cluster to resend a message if it fails to receive it, until it succeeds. For the provision of messages, Apache Kafka provides three ways to perform the read commits. It is also possible to choose when the commit is performed, whether at the beginning or at the end of the provision of the message.

In addition to the security methods of writing and reading messages, Apache Kafka allows messages to be stored in a topic for a period defined by the administrator. This way, if an error happens, it is possible to re-consume the messages.

Another important aspect regarding reliability, is that Apache Kafka stores the same message in different partitions of the topic. These partitions are separated among the Kafka Brokers of the Kafka Cluster. That is, if one Kafka Broker is offline, the message is still available in another Kafka Broker for reading.

- High Availability

One of the main characteristics of microservice architectures is that microservices are totally independent from each other, with no dependencies between them. If one microservice is unavailable the others continue to work, thus not putting the application completely offline.

Another factor is that both Apache Kafka and microservices architectures must be based on Cloud Servers. This way it is possible to have clusters in different geographical locations.

Finally, Apache Kafka duplicates the messages received by different Kafka Brokers. If any Kafka Broker goes offline, there is guaranteed to be no problem due to the message still being present in the Cluster. This requires more than one Kafka Broker in a Kafka Cluster.

- High Throughput

In addition to the reliability aspect, healthcare has another important aspect, which is the speed in which data is made available to the end user. It is important that the data received by IoT devices is available quickly, both for checking anomalies/faults and for visualization. Apache Kafka allows the receival of data from various devices at high speeds as demonstrated in the previous section of this chapter.

- Diversity of Data

There are several types of formats in which data can be received. By using Apache Kafka to receive data from IoT devices, it is possible that data comes in several formats, such as TXT, JSON, HL7 v2, among others. It is only necessary to, subsequently, make changes at source code level in the part related to the Consumers, either through external libraries or own converters.

However, the architecture naturally has some weaknesses associated with it. **Weaknesses** include:

- Complexity

Regardless of the numerous advantages associated with microservices architectures and Apache Kafka, it is possible to realize that it is a complex concept and technology. The cost of learning and development is higher than for example in a Monolithic architecture because it involves the use of more concepts such as: the communication processes between microservices; CI and CD processes for DevOps automation; and the use of Cloud to put the application in production. In addition, and especially in Apache Kafka, because it is a complex technology with a large ecosystem, sometimes finding useful solutions to problems that may occur becomes complicated.

- High Costs

Since it is a distributed architecture and must be developed based on Cloud, it is natural that the costs related to the DevOps component are higher. Additionally, it is useful to use a tool to support the Apache Kafka cluster, as is the case of Confluent's tool, which allows us to simplify some of the existing complexity but has additional costs, which depending on the number of Brokers, could be high.

From an external perspective, the **Opportunities** identified are:

- Reuse of microservices

The use of microservices architecture allows microservices to be developed and used independently. That said, there is the opportunity in the future, and if necessary, to reuse the same microservice for another product that may be developed. This way it avoids the development of code that was already developed.

- Add new functionalities through the Apache Kafka ecosystem

Since Apache Kafka, in addition to what is presented in this chapter, has a vast ecosystem, it is possible to use some of its additional products to assist in troubleshooting. The use of Apache Kafka Connect and Apache Kafka Streams are two examples of Apache Kafka products and together they can serve to assist in the creation of ETL and ML processes.

Among the possible **Threats**, we can consider:

- Lack of technical resources

Since microservices architectures are a distributed architecture where microservices are developed and designed independently, it is important to assure that there are several teams developing different microservices of an application. Otherwise, if there is a lack of resources, microservices architectures may not pay off in the end, since it will take more time and more work from a small team.

- Lack of investment

As described earlier, one of the weaknesses of using microservices architectures and Apache Kafka is the high cost of development and production. This weakness can later mean lack of investment by government policies and put the development and design of the solution in question.

CONCLUSION

The proposed architecture represents a solid foundation to support critical care, making data available in real time, securely, quickly and above all, reliably. Using different technologies and paradigms such as the use of architectures based on microservices and event-sourcing, it was possible to build a modular system, capable of responding to the most diverse challenges. This architecture has high availability as its main feature, as well as the fact that it is scalable, secure, and reliable. These characteristics are demonstrated when employing Apache Kafka and microservices architectures.

Future Work

In order to continue the work done so far, there is a need to reflect on what could be developed and improved.

The next steps should go through the implementation of the architecture presented in the chapter in test and quality environments, in order to assess its potential. This type of testing should involve: testing against different message formats; speed tests, namely of reception and delivery of messages; downtime tests in the event of any failure with the technologies used; tests of alerts/notifications in the existence of any anomaly in the data obtained by the sensors; between others.

On the other hand, there is also the possibility of adapting to new challenges, such as the exploration of the Apache Kafka ecosystem, from Apache Kafka Connect to Apache Kafka Streams, and how both can be used in healthcare. Another important aspect is the use of analysis techniques and real-time Machine Learning, interacting with applications such as Apache Kafka and Apache Spark.

ACKNOWLEDGMENT

This work has been supported by "FCT–Fundação para a Ciência e Tecnologia" within the R&D Units Project Scope: UIDB/00319/2020.

REFERENCES

Apache Kafka Documentation. (n.d.). *Apache Kafka*. http://kafka.apache.org/090/documentation.html#intro_topics

Apache Kafka. (n.d.). https://kafka.apache.org/

Babylon Health. (2013). *About*. Babylon Health. https://www.babylonhealth.com/about/

Catalyst, N. (2018, January 1). *Healthcare Big Data and the Promise of Value-Based Care*. NEJM Catalyst. https://catalyst.nejm.org/doi/full/10.1056/CAT.18.0290

Combs, V. (2020, November 5). *Humana uses Azure and Kafka to make healthcare less frustrating for doctors and patients*. TechRepublic. https://www.techrepublic.com/article/humana-uses-azure-and-kafka-to-make-healthcare-less-frustrating-for-doctors-and-patients/

Confluent. (2020). *Humana Adopts Event Streaming and Interoperability Using Confluent. Confluent*. https://www.confluent.io/customers/humana/

Cruz, R., Guimarães, T., Peixoto, H., & Santos, M. F. (2021). Architecture for Intensive Care Data Processing and Visualization in Real-time. *Procedia Computer Science, 184*, 923–928. doi:10.1016/j.procs.2021.03.115

Dash, S., Shakyawar, S. K., Sharma, M., & Kaushik, S. (2019). Big data in healthcare: Management, analysis and future prospects. *Journal of Big Data, 6*(1), 54. Advance online publication. doi:10.118640537-019-0217-0 de la Torre, C., Wagner, B., & Rousos, M. (2019). *NET Microservices: Architecture for Containerized. NET Applications.* Microsoft Corporation. https://docs.microsoft.com/en-us/dotnet/architecture/microservices/

Dragoni, N., Giallorenzo, S., Lafuente, A. L., Mazzara, M., Montesi, F., Mustafin, R., & Safina, L. (2017). Microservices: Yesterday, Today, and Tomorrow. *Present and Ulterior Software Engineering*, 195–216. doi:10.1007/978-3-319-67425-4_12

Goldberger, A., Amaral, L., Glass, L., Hausdorff, J., Ivanov, P. C., Mark, R., Mietus, J. E., Moody, G. B., Peng, C.-K., & Stanley, H. E. (2000). PhysioBank, PhysioToolkit, and PhysioNet: Components of a new research resource for complex physiologic signals. *Circulation*, *101*(23), e215–e220. doi:10.1161/01.CIR.101.23.e215 PMID:10851218

Goldberger, A. L., Amaral, L. A. N., Glass, L., Hausdorff, J. M., Ivanov, P. Ch., Mark, R. G., Mietus, J. E., Moody, G. B., Peng, C.-K., & Stanley, H. E. (2000). PhysioBank, PhysioToolkit, and PhysioNet: Components of a new research resource for complex physiologic signals. *Circulation*, *101*(23), e215–e220. doi:10.1161/01.CIR.101.23.e215 PMID:10851218

Hassan, F. E. M., & Sahal, R. (2020). Real-Time Healthcare Monitoring System using Online Machine Learning and Spark Streaming. *International Journal of Advanced Computer Science and Applications*, *11*(9). Advance online publication. doi:10.14569/IJACSA.2020.0110977

Heusser, M. (2020, August 19). *Orchestration vs. choreography in microservices architecture.* SearchAppArchitecture. https://searchapparchitecture.techtarget.com/tip/Orchestration-vs-choreography-in-microservices-architecture

Humana (HUM). (2021). *Forbes.* https://www.forbes.com/companies/humana/?sh=5fce4cf04390

JSON and BSON. (n.d.). *MongoDB.* https://www.mongodb.com/json-and-bson

Lewis, J., & Fowler, M. (2014, March 25). *Microservices.* https://martinfowler.com/articles/microservices.html

Maksimovic, Z. (2017). *MongoDB 3 Succinctly.* Syncfusion Inc. https://s3.amazonaws.com/ebooks.syncfusion.com/downloads/MongoDB_3_Succinctly/MongoDB_3_Succinctly.pdf

MongoDB - Overview. (n.d.). *Tutorials Point.* https://www.tutorialspoint.com/mongodb/mongodb_overview.htm

Moody, G. B., & Mark, R. G. (1996). A Database to Support Development and Evaluation of Intelligent Intensive Care Monitoring. *Computers in Cardiology*, *23*, 657–660.

Narkhede, N., Shapira, G., & Palino, T. (2017). *Kafka: The definitive guide: Real-time data and stream processing at scale.* O'Reilly Media.

Newman, A. (2020, September 30). *Is your microservice a distributed monolith?* Gremelin. https://www.gremlin.com/blog/is-your-microservice-a-distributed-monolith/

Noble, R., & Nobilia, F. (2019, May 14). *One Key to Rule them All.* Confluent Kafka Summit London 2019. https://www.confluent.io/kafka-summit-lon19/one-key-to-rule-them-all/

Ohri, A. (2021, March 19). *Types Of Big Data: Simplified.* Jigsaw Academy. https://www.jigsawacademy.com/blogs/big-data-analytics/types-of-big-data#Semi-Structured-Data

Peixoto, H., Guimarães, T., & Santos, M. F. (2020). A New Architecture for Intelligent Clinical Decision Support for Intensive Medicine. *Procedia Computer Science*, *170*, 1035–1040. https://doi.org/10.1016/j.procs.2020.03.077

Penedo, J., Ribeiro, A., Lopes, H., Pimentel, J., Pedrosa, J., Vasconcelos e Sá, R., & Moreno, R. (2013). Avaliação da Situação Nacional das Unidades de Cuidados Intensivos. In *SNS - Serviço Nacional de Saúde*. Governo de Portugal, Ministério da Saúde. https://www.sns.gov.pt/wp-content/uploads/2016/05/Avalia%C3%A7%C3%A3o-nacional-da-situa%C3%A7%C3%A3o-das-unidades-de-cuidados-intensivos.pdf

Richardson, C., & Smith, F. (2016). *Microservices From Design to Deployment.* NGINX, Inc. https://www.nginx.com/resources/library/designing-deploying-microservices/

Sanjaya, H. (2020, March 11). *Monolith vs Microservices.* Hengky Sanjaya Blog. https://medium.com/hengky-sanjaya-blog/monolith-vs-microservices-b3953650dfd

Sax, M. J. (2018). Apache Kafka. *Encyclopedia of Big Data Technologies*, 1–8. doi:10.1007/978-3-319-63962-8_196-1

Scaling Horizontally vs. Scaling Vertically. (2020, July 24). *Section.* https://www.section.io/blog/scaling-horizontally-vs-vertically/

Stevenson, A., & Frenay, J. (2019, December 16). *Big Data LDN 2019: Freeing up engineering and infrastructure resources to scale with DataOps.* YouTube. https://www.youtube.com/watch?v=J7bEunZXkxc

Sucaria, D. (2021, April 23). *Microservices Architecture - orchestrator, choreography, hybrid... Which approach to use?* Diego Sucaria. https://diegosucaria.info/microservices-architecture-orchestrator-choreography-hybrid-which-approach-to-use/

What is a Document Database? (n.d.). *MongoDB.* https://www.mongodb.com/document-databases

ENDNOTES

[1]   Big Data LDN

[2]   Kafka Summit

Chapter 2
A Review on Artificial Intelligence for Electrocardiogram Signal Analysis

M Krishna Chaitanya
VIT AP University, India

Lakhan Dev Sharma
ⓘ https://orcid.org/0000-0002-5389-3928
VIT AP University, India

Amarjit Roy
Ghani Khan Choudhury Institute of Engineering and Technology, India

Jagdeep Rahul
ⓘ https://orcid.org/0000-0003-4890-1898
Rajiv Gandhi University, India

ABSTRACT

Cardiovascular disease (CVD) is a broad term encompassing a group of heart and blood vessel abnormalities that is the leading cause of death worldwide. The most popular and low-cost diagnostic tool for assessing the heart electrical impulses is an electrocardiogram (ECG). Automation is required to reduce errors and human burden while interpreting ECG signals. In recent years, deep learning shows better performance in ECG classification and has also shown that automated classification of ECG signals can improve accuracy and efficiency. In this chapter, the authors review the research work on ECG signals using deep learning methods like deep belief network (DBNK), convolutional neural network (CNNK), long short-term memory (LSTMY), recurrent neural network (RNNK), and gated recurrent unit (GRUT). In the research articles published between 2017 and 2021, CNNK was found to be the most appropriate technique for feature extraction.

DOI: 10.4018/978-1-7998-9172-7.ch002

INTRODUCTION

Cardio-Vascular Disease (CVD) is a broad term that refers to illnesses that affect the heart and blood arteries of a person's body. Damage to the arteries in organs such as the heart, brain, eyes, and kidneys is also a possibility. CVDs can cause blood vessel blockage and blood clot development, which can result in either cerebral or cardiac ischemia, necrosis resulting in myocardial infarction (MI). Every part present in the body may turn out to be congested and starved of oxygen as a result of the heart's long-term inefficient blood pumping, resulting in varying degrees of damage (Yu et al. 2015). Even among young people, CVD is one of the leading causes of death in many established and developing countries around the world. However, adopting a healthy lifestyle can greatly reduce the risk of developing it.

Electrocardiogram (ECG) is the best popular and low-cost investigative device for assessing the heart's electrical impulses and diagnosing cardiovascular health. The heart beats in a regular rhythm, with regular myocardial excitation, circulating blood to the entire body. During the practice, When the myocardium contracts, a little current is generated by the heart and carried to the surface of the body, generating potential modifications in every portion of the human body. The ECG is created by calculating the potential drift with the help of electrodes placed on the limbs and chest of the subject and recorded with electrocardiograph or a vector electrocardiograph (Liu et al. 2021). The aberrant activity of the heartbeat and rhythm can be demonstrated in this way. CVD, Coronary heart disease, and congestive heart failure can all be predicted using an ECG. Because several of these disorders are linked to an elevated liability of stroke or sometimes it can lead to death, early detection is critical. ECG has been shown to be helpful in determining both short- and long-term results in investigations. For individuals with MI, for instance, the sooner the irregular cardiac rhythm is diagnosed, the better the possibility of avoiding life-threatening complications and recovery (Lown et al. 1969). Hence the agile and precise diagnosis of ECG is essential clinically. Since signal analysis is a time-consuming and difficult operation, there is a risk of personal ambiguity and human mistakes during the analysis procedures, also for professionals who have been taught for years. As a result, it is critical to experiment with computer-assisted methods. Computer-assisted exploration can evaluate ECG signals more accurately and quickly without causing any differences (Liu et al. 2021).

The first computer-assisted ECG analysis, structure was created in the 1960s (Pipberger et al. 1961). Data preprocessing, feature extraction (FE), and categorization are the three essential processes in the completely automatic structure of the classic intelligent procedure for the analysis of ECG. In the preprocessing stage, data is denoised, added, or chopped into signal slices of the same length. For ECG signal categorization, the FE phase is critical. The geometry of the ECG signal not only in the time domain but also in the frequency domain, as well as the cardiac rhythm, can be utilized to excerpt features. Finally, based on the collected attributes, the signals are categorized as distinct types of heartbeat or sickness. The vision is to build algorithms that are exceptional in accuracy, efficiency, and stability while also reducing the strain on doctors.

Deep learning (DL), is a computer-assisted process with a significant capability of extracting features, was able to classify ECG signals with high accuracy (Murat et al. 2020). DL is accomplished through the formation of hierarchical artificial neural networks (Goodfellow et al. 2016). Deep learning, according to (Bengio et al. 2007), discovers subtle structure in big datasets by utilizing the backpropagation technique to determine how a model's internal weight values, which are utilized to generate the illustration in every layer, should evolve. As a result, DLs are allowed to possess fine culpability tolerance and avoid overfitting-induced errors. DL can automate FE and categorization by emulating the overall purpose of studying the human brain, whereas, in the past, these tasks required engineers to plan. In this approach, it can be learned that implicit knowledge was previously mastered by professionals, implying a significant human burden. The advancements in the central processing unit (CPU) reduce the execution and training time effectively. As a result, DL can now train enormous volumes of data and use more complicated algorithms, providing it with much more development potential.

In the DL area Stack auto-encoders (SAE) as well as deep belief network (DBN) are initial typical methods. Multiple Restricted Boltzmann Machine (RBM) layers are used to create DBNs. DBN is a prevailing learning prototype for modeling random variables that change over a period of time. Subsequently, with its success in visual perception, the convolutional neural network (CNN) has become the most popular method, and it has been applied to a variety of applications. The recurrent neural network (RNN) is an iterative network that excels at processing time-series data, making it excellent for categorizing ECG signals. Long short-term memory (LSTM) outperforms standard RNN in terms of long-term reliance, and it is becoming increasingly popular. Gated Recurrent Unit (GRU) is an enhanced and simple version of LSTM with faster training time and less computational complexity (Chung et al. 2014).

With no or little human aid, most DL approaches have attained high accuracy when compared with manual classification, effectively decreasing the stress on health care professionals. DL, in contrast to conventional methods, can evaluate raw ECG data without the need for primitive feature elicitation, resulting in improved efficacy and fewer stages of use. Though, in reality, the ECG signal acquired is always escorted by the noise, denoising in the preprocessing stage demands lot of computing resources. Hence, more prosperous prototypes with fewer constraints should be developed. In view of hypothetical advancement, the practical implementation of approaches should be given additional emphasis. Some reviews focused on the DL and ECG signal. In (Sharma et al. 2018), Segmentation of an ECG signal yields in early detection, and as a result treatment can be done in advance. In (Murat et al. 2020) heartbeat classification is being concentrated. RR interval based approach for cardiac arrhythmia categorization is proposed in (Rahul et al. 2021). It is mentioned in (Hong et al. 2020) that more than disease detection, DL has applications in all fields of ECG signal. The review of Faust covers studies on a variety of biological signals, with ECG being introduced in a small space (Faust et al. 2018).

To demonstrate the significance of DL in the area of ECG investigation this article is formulated in the following sections: methodology employed, fundamentals about the ECG signal and prevalent cardiovascular disorders, most commonly utilized databases, theoretical underpinning of DL, research and discussions, and conclusion subsections.

METHODOLOGY

The fundamental goal of this research is to critically evaluate existing arrhythmia classification algorithms on the published forums.

To download related research articles, main search terms that are used in the Google Scholar are: "arrhythmia classification" or "ECG" or "arrhythmia detection" or "electrocardiogram" or "cardiac arrhythmia" and "deep learning". Judging as well as selecting the appropriate publications that is relevant to our research is based on determining the most recent developments in arrhythmia classification approaches using deep neural networks.

ECG SIGNAL AND MEDICAL IDIOMS

ECG Signal

The heart is a four-chambered pump that consists of two atria for the purpose of blood collection and two ventricles for driving blood out. The resting or filling phase of a cardiac chamber is known as diastole; the contracting or pumping stage is termed systole. ECG is the electrical representation of the heart's contractile movement, and it is easily captured using exterior electrodes placed either on the chest or on the limbs. Perhaps the utmost famous, familiar, and utilized biological signal is the ECG. Counting the easily distinguishable waves can be used to determine the heart's rhythm in beats per minute (bpm) (Rangayyan 2015).

An ECG signal consists of three waves representing the three electrical events of the heart in the single cardiac cycle: P wave denotes atrial depolarization, QRS complex wave represents the ventral depolarization, and T wave shows repolarization (Acharya et al. 2017). The identification of a QRS complex on an ECG is a vital step in detecting a heart condition (Rahul et al. 2021). The components present in a single heartbeat are shown in Figure 1.

Figure 1. Components of a single heart beat

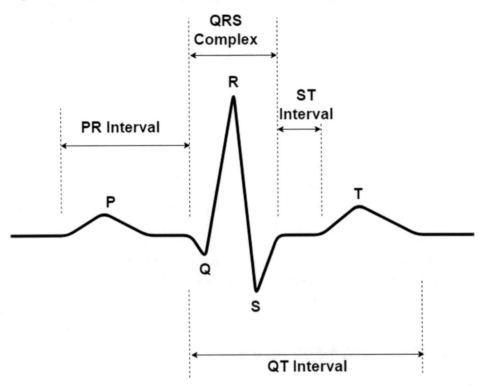

Based on the geometry of the ECG signal, many heart diseases can be determined. Some of the complications of the heart are coronary artery disease (COAD), myocardial infarction (MI), and various kinds of arrhythmia. The arrhythmias may be classified into 16 categories, including atrial fibrillation (AFN), ventricular arrhythmia (VA), supra-ventricular arrhythmia (SVA), bradycardia (BC), tachycardia (TC), etc.,

Medical Idioms

This section presents an outline of the common heart disorders that can be identified using an ECG signal. Any disturbance in the activity of the heart alters the ECG signals and is commonly referred to as arrhythmia. Common arrhythmias are discussed in the preceding sub-sections:

Myocardial Infarction (MI)

A myocardial infarction (MI), often referred to as a heart attack, arises when the supply of blood to the coronary artery of the heart is reduced or stopped, resulting in injury to the heart muscle. Chest pain or discomfort is the most prevalent symptom, which might spread to other parts of the body. It usually starts in the middle or left part of the chest and exists for a few minutes. The phenomenon of MI is depicted in Figure 2. the detection of MI disorder is proposed in (Sharma et al. 2020, Sharma et al. 2018).

Figure 2. Graph showing MI

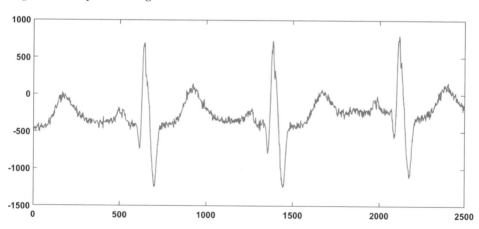

Atrial Fibrillation (AF)

The most common abnormal heart rhythm that begins in the atria is atrial fibrillation (AF). The atria cannot efficiently contract and/or squeeze blood into the ventricle, since the action potentials are so rapid and disorganized. As a result, P waves may be invisible as not only the atrial rate is high, but also the amplitude is too low. The phenomenon of AFN is depicted in the Figure 3.

Figure 3. Graph showing AFN

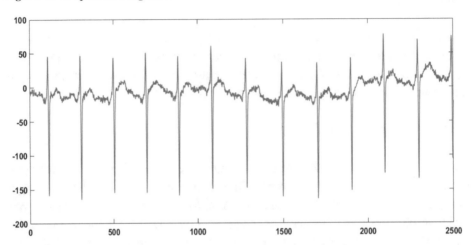

Ventricular Arrhythmia (VA)

VA is an irregular heartbeat that originates in the lower chamber of the heart (ventricles). Such arrhythmias may lead the heart to beat excessively quickly, preventing oxygen-rich blood from reaching the brain and body and perhaps leading to cardiac arrest. . The phenomenon of VA is depicted in Figure 4.

Figure 4. Graph showing VA

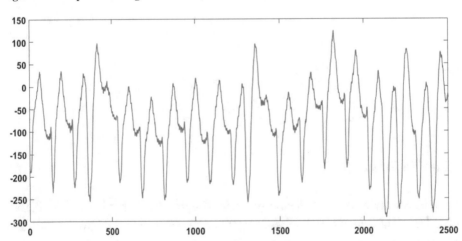

Supra-Ventricular Arrhythmia (SVA)

An SVA is characterized by an abnormal cardiac rate that starts above the ventricles of the heart. SVAs start in the heart's upper chambers (atria), although not all of them. As a result, the heart tends to beat erratically i.e., either too rapidly or too slowly. The phenomenon of SVA is depicted in Figure 5.

Figure 5. Graph showing SVA

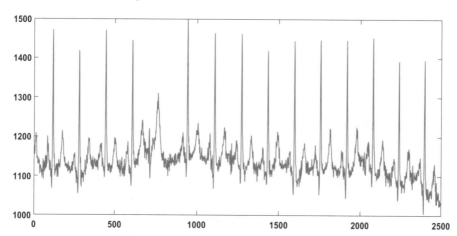

Normal Sinus Rhythm (NSR)

Heart rate and sinus rhythm are not all the same. The amount of times the heart beats in a minute is referred to as your heart rate, whereas the pattern of the heartbeat is referred to as sinus rhythm. NSR is the electrical impulse from the sinus node that is being properly transmitted. The phenomenon of SVA is depicted in Figure 6.

Figure 6. Graph showing NSR

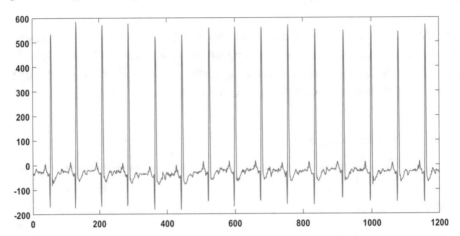

Bundle Branch Block (BBB)

BBB is an aberrant QRS morphology caused by a disruption in the usual conduction system. The right bundle usually depolarizes the right ventricle (RV). The right bundle is inactive in Right BBB. Instead, the impulse from the left bundle is diffused via the Left Ventricle (LV) and subsequently to the RV, depolarizing the RV. The left bundle usually depolarizes the LV. The left bundle is inactive in a Left BBB. Instead, the LV is depolarized by impulse spread from the right bundle is diffused through RV and then on to the LV. The phenomenon of Left BBB and Right BBB are depicted in Figures 7 and 8 respectively.

Figure 7. Graph showing Left BBB

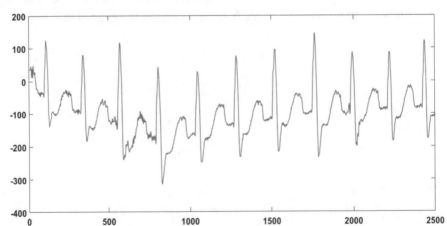

Figure 8. Graph showing Right BBB

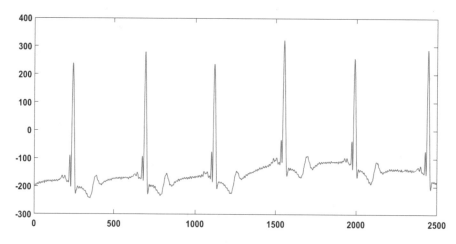

Database

The following databases were used in the majority of the studies we looked at. The features of some of the most regularly employed databases are outlined in Table 1. The most extensively used database is the MIT-BIH Database. It has nine sub-databases for various disorders; the most prominent is the MIT-BIH Arrhythmia Database (MITBIHDB) (Goldberger et al. 2000). The MITBIHDB includes an assembly of 48 completely labeled half-hour recordings of two-lead ECGs. The MITBIHDB is divided into two main categories. The first set shows representative waveforms and artifacts of arrhythmias that may be observed during diagnosis. Supraventricular arrhythmia, complex ventricular arrhythmia, and junctional arrhythmia, as well as conduction anomalies, fall into the second category.

The 12-lead Arrhythmia Dataset at the St. Petersburg Institute of cardiological technics (Goldberger et al. 2000) is made up of people who have been diagnosed or accused of having COAD. This dataset is inevitably labeled and physically rectified using an algorithm. The PhysioNet Computing Cardiology Challenge 2017 (PCCC17) (Goldberger et al. 2000) database comprises 8528 inadequately relatively brief ECG recordings aimed at rhythm level. In recent times the PCCC17 is the next most prominent database.

Table 1. Synopsis of ECG datasets

Database	Number of Records	Length	Sampling frequency (Hz)	Disorder
PCCC17 (Goldberger et al. 2000)	8528 training, 3658 testing	30 sec	300	AFN
MITBIHDB (Goldberger et al. 2000)	48	30 min	360	Complex Ventricular arrhythmia, SVA Conduction abnormalities
Physikalisch-Technische Bundesanstalt (PTB) (Goldberger et al. 2000)	549	38 min	1000	MI
MIT-BIH Supraventricular Arrhythmia Database (Goldberger et al. 2000)	78	30 min	128	VEBS, SVEBS
PhysioNet, The ECG-ID Database (Goldberger et al. 2000)	310	20 min	500	Normal Sinus Rhythm (NSR), AFN
The MIT-BIH Atrial Fibrillation Database (MIT-BIHAF) (Goldberger et al. 2000)	25	63 min	250	NSR, AFN
Creighton University VT Database (CUDB) (Goldberger et al. 2000)	35	08 min	250	Sustained Ventricular Tachycardia (VT), Ventricular fibrillation (VFB)
MIT-BIH Malignant Ventricular Arrhythmia Database (VFDB) (Goldberger et al. 2000)	22	30 min	250	Sustained Ventricular Tachycardia (VT), Ventricular fibrillation (VFB)
The UCI cardiac arrhythmia (Dua, 2017)	279	Attributes:279	-	NSR, Old Inferior MI, Sinus Bradycardia, Right buldle branch block (RBBBK)
Long Term ST Database (LTSTDB) (Goldberger et al. 2000)	86	63 min	250	NSR, SVEBS, VEBS
CinC Challenge 2000 Datasets. (Goldberger et al. 2000)	70	7 hrs – 10hrs	100	Sleep Apnea, NSR
The PAF Prediction Challenge Database (Goldberger et al. 2000)	50	30 min	128	Paroxysmal Atrial Fibrillation (PAFN)
St.-Petersburg Institute of Cardiological Technics 12-lead Arrhythmia Database (NCART) (Goldberger et al. 2000)	75	120 min	257	Acute MI, Prior MI, COAD with Hypertension, Sinus Node Dysfunction, Supraventricular ectopy, Pre-Excitation (WPW), AFN, Bundle Branch Block (BBB)
Fantasia Database- PhysioBank (Goldberger et al. 2000)	40	63 min	250	NSR while watching a Fantasia movie
The MIT-BIH Normal Sinus Rhythm (NSR) Database (Goldberger et al. 2000)	18	126 min	-	NSR
BIDMC PPG and Respiration Dataset (Goldberger et al. 2000)	53	8 min	125	-

History of Deep Learning (DL)

Warren McCulloch and Walter Pitts introduced the term "artificial neural network (ANNK)" and "artificial neuron mathematical model," ushering in a new phase of ANNK research (Liu et al. 2021). In the recent decade, the use of artificial intelligence (AI) in the automatic arrangement of several cardiac arrhythmias has expanded dramatically (Rahul et al. 2022). Existing AI technology can be divided into two types: machine learning (ML) and deep learning (DL). The algorithms used in the ML method are used to categorize the arrhythmias existing in the cardiovascular system, whereas algorithms used in DL have the ability to automatically detect and classify arrhythmias in the cardiovascular system.

DL is a concept that relates to research in knowledge extraction, prediction, and intelligent decision making, or, in other words, identifying complicated patterns by using a set of data known as training data. Deep Neural Network (DNN) is more scalable than traditional learning techniques because improved accuracy is typically attained by expanding the capacity of the network or training database. DL has produced excellent outcomes in various application sectors, despite its limitations, demonstrating its enormous promise. This rejuvenation kicked off with unsupervised feature learning containing deep belief network (DBN) and stacked auto-encoders (SAE). Thereafter, AlexNet (Krizhevsky et al. 2012) reintroduced the convolutional neural network (CNN), and CNN was followed by the recurrent neural network (RNN). DL has been used to solve a variety of problems, such as semantic segmentation (Guo et al. 2018, Garcia-Garcia et al. 2018), object identification (Zhao et al. 2019), and background diminution (Minematsu et al. 2018, Bouwmans et al. 2019).

Stacked Auto-Encoders (SAE)

SAE is a type of DNN, which consists of not only various layers of autoencoder (AE)s but also classifiers and is shown in Figure 9. Denoising AE and sparse AE are two other AE versions that are used in ECG classification. In (Vincent et al. 2010), they developed a denoising AE to extract strong features from a contaminated input and perform denoising, and they used it to recognize handwritten digits and images. In (Makhzani et al. 2013), they developed a k-sparse AE that can excerpt deep features in a graded manner while preventing the system from overfitting, and they verified it in the identification of the handwritten digit and object detection. AE consists of one input, one output, and one hidden layer. The layer-wised training method is used by SAE. Each AE is initialized before the neural network is trained. The first AE uses input to forecast itself, resulting in the discovery of the first parameter. Following that, each auto-hidden encoder's layer likewise aids as the input layer for the next AE. The remaining AEs are trained in this manner. Following pretraining, labeled training sets are employed to tune the performance finely. The cost function is reduced and the constraints are well-tuned using backpropagation. In the autoencoder, let e be the input, g is extracted feature while f being the reconstructed signal and are represented by the equations 1 and 2

$$g = \epsilon(Ze * E + ue_{)} \tag{1}$$

$$f = \epsilon(Zd * g + ub_{)} \tag{2}$$

Figure 9. Architecture of SAE

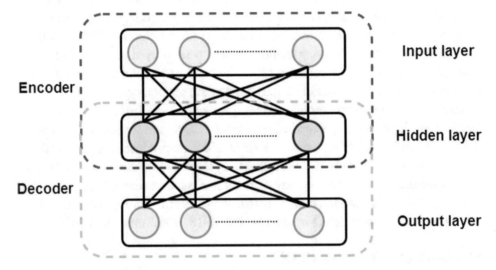

Deep Belief Network (DBN)

Deep belief networks (DBNs) are generative neural networks that are made up of unsupervised basic learning modules (Hinton et al. 2006). As seen in Figure 10, DBNs are built by utilizing stacked restricted Boltzmann machines and a classifier. Associative memory is formed by undirected connections between the top two levels. Directional connections exist between the lower layers. On the basis of the original RBM framework, a number of enhancements have been implemented. Conditional Restricted Boltzmann Machines (CRBMs) was proposed in (Mnih et al. 2012) to cope with multi-label organization and picture denoising. RBM (Restricted Boltzmann machine) is a bi-directionally coupled stochastic neural network that can forecast the likelihood function across its input (Fischer et al. 2012). A bipartite graph with one visible and one hidden layer is known as an RBM. The visible and concealed layers are intended to accept and excerpt characteristics, respectively (Larochelle et al. 2012). RBM training's purpose is to retain as much of the input probability distribution as possible. $E(p,q)$ is an energy function defined as follows:

$$E(p,q) = p'Zq - x'_p - x'_q q \tag{3}$$

Where p and q denotes activation matrix of visible and concealed layers correspondingly, Z represents weight that the visible layer is connected to hidden layer, p' denotes transpose of p.

Figure 10. Architecture of DBN

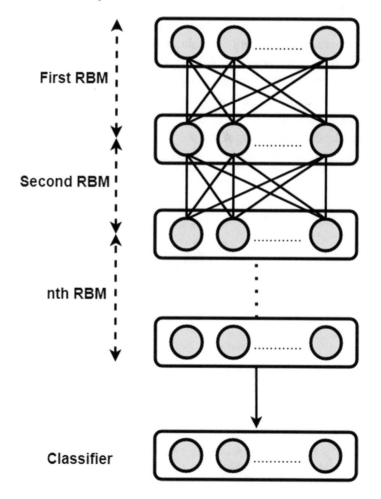

Convolutional Neural Network (CNN)

The CNN is hierarchical feedforward neural network (Chua 1998). CNN presents learning filters, which apply operations to each of the input sub-regions, rather than completely linked layers like normal neural networks. A CNN normally includes convolutional layers, pooling layers, and fully linked layers in terms of network topology (LeCun et al. 1995). CNN is a component of several common deep learning networks. Alexnet (Krizhevsky et al. 2012) presents a new deep structure and washout approach, which deepens the network and improves the performance of LeNet-5. Thereafter, with a smaller convolution kernel and deeper layers, VGG-net (Simonyan et al. 2014) is presented, and its execution in picture identification is comparable with humans. Next, DenseNet (Iandola et al. 2014) and ResNet (He et al. 2016) include dense networks and cluster convolution, respectively, and demonstrate decent object detection presentation. The convolutional layer utilizes a filter kernel to convolve with every input sub-region, extracting features from the preceding layer's input. The pooling layer is always positioned behind the convolutional layer and conducts a block downsampling process. By highlighting or suppressing features, it is used to minimize the size of the topographies and choose the most illustrative area. A single output is generated for each little chunk of data. After the convolutional and pooling layers, the resulting topographies of each sub-region are compressed into a 1-dimensional vector as the input to the fully connected layer. The supplied data are mapped into multiple classes in this section. The architecture of CNN is shown in the Figure 11.

Figure 11. Structure of CNN

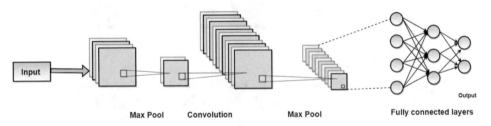

Recurrent Neural Network (RNN)

RNN is a variant of Artificial Neural Network (ANNK) which has communal weights across time. It is the best learning framework for training sequential input data and time-series data categorization, in which the feedback and current value are fed back into the system, and the output consists of addition of elements in the memory (Liu et al. 2018). The RNN gets an input at every time unit, modifies its concealed state, and generates an estimate. The weights of an RNN are trained using a gradient descent approach over time. The RNN's underlying architecture is portrayed in Figure 12.

Figure 12. Structure of RNN

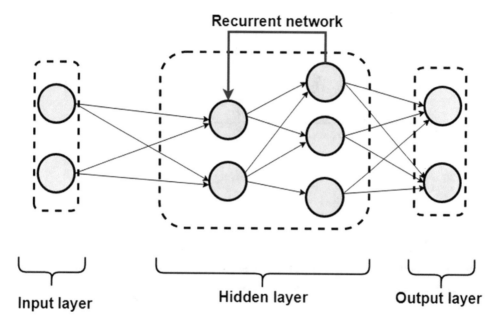

Recurrent network

Input layer   Hidden layer   Output layer

Long Short-Term Memory (LSTM)

In (Hochreiter et al. 1997), Hochreiter and Schmidhuber presented a method to mitigate the effect of the RNN becoming weak when confronted with long-term dependence. The LSTM's main concept is to continuously update the memory in memory cells, allowing relevant information to be kept and superfluous information to be abandoned. To achieve this every input has to pass via three gates viz. input, output, and forget gates respectively, and is depicted with the help of Figure 13.

Figure 13. Architecture of LSTM

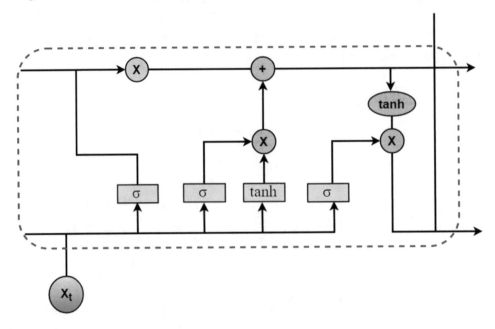

Bidirectional LSTM (Bi-LSTM), the combination of forward LSTM and backward LSTM is intended to find any point in a sequence with the help of data from the past and future, which has been proven to work in phonemes (Schuster et al. 1997).

Gated Recurrent Unit (GRU)

GRU is a more advanced form of LSTM that allows for a faster training phase (Chung et al. 2014). GRU is made up of gates that are jointly engaged in matching the information movement inside the components. The input and the forget gates are added to generate a new gate known as the update gate. The update gate is primarily concerned with adjusting the states of the previous and candidate activations. The structure of GRU is depicted in Figure 14.

Figure 14. Structure of GRU

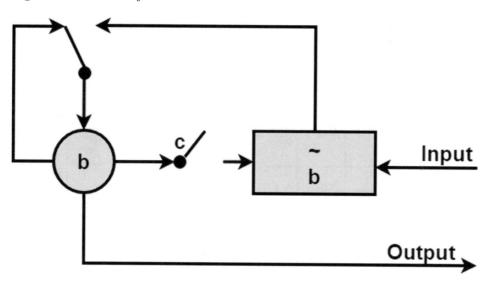

RESEARCHES AND DISCUSSION

Researches

Active learning (AL) is introduced in some research (Al Rahhal et al. 2016, Luo et al. 2017). AL is widely used to finely tune the categorization procedure in the ECG. For each iteration, AL criteria are typically used to pick up the most dubious and significant samples for experts to identify, with the labeled data being returned to enrich the training set in the subsequent iteration. For long-term ECG diagnosis, in contrast to AL, the training strategy is partitioned global and patient-specific training is applied (Al Rahhal et al. 2016).

DL methods for categorizing ECGs are introduced in this part based on their algorithm. A summary of the works performed with ECG signals with the help of DL algorithms is depicted in Table 2.

Table 2. Summary of research performed by DL algorithms with ECG signals

Author	Database	Input	Preprocessing	DL algorithm	Application	Result
Luo et al. 2017	MITBIHDB	ECG Signal and its Image	Two median filters (MF)	Stacked denoising auto-encoders	Heartbeat classification and monitoring	Accuracy (ACC) 97.5%
Rahhal et al. 2016	MITBIHDB	ECG Signal	Two MF and one low pass filter (LPF)	Stacked denoising auto-encoders with sparsity constraint	Heartbeat classification (interpatient)	ACC 99.7%
Yang et al. 2018	MITBIHDB	ECG Signal	-	Stacked sparse auto-encoders	Arrhythmia classification	ACC 99.5% Sensitivity (SEN) 99.2%
Farhadi et al. 2018	MITBIHDB	ECG Signal	-	Stacked sparse auto-encoders	AFN classification	ACC 99.5%
Hou et al. 2019	MITBIHDB	ECG Signal	-	LSTM-based auto-encoder	Arrhythmia Classification	ACC 99.74% SEN 99.35%
Nurmaini et al. 2020	MITBIHDB; MIT-BIH noise stress test database	ECG Signal	Denoising autoencoders (DAEs)	Stacked auto-encoders, Deep neural network	Contaminated arrhythmia classification	ACC 99.34% SEN 93.83%
Altan et al. 2016	MITBIHDB	ECG Signal	Two MF	DBN-based multistage Algorithm	Arrhythmia Classification	ACC 96.10%
Song et al. 2019	MITBIHDB	ECG Signal	-	DBN	Heartbeat Classification	ACC 98.49%
Taji et al. 2017	MIT-BIHAF	ECG Signal	Band pass filter (BPF)	DBN	AFN	ACC 81%
Kiranyaz et al. 2015	MITBIHDB	ECG Signal	BPF	1-D CNN	Arrhythmia classification and monitoring	ACC 97.05%
Acharya et al. 2018	MITBIHDB; MIT-BIH VFDB; CUDB	ECG Signal	Discrete wavelet transforms (DWT) (Daubechies wavelet 6 (db6))	1-D CNN	Shockable and non-shockable ventricular arrhythmias	ACC 93.1% SEN 95.32%
Acharya et al. 2017	PTB	ECG Signal	DWT (Daubechies wavelet 6 (db6))	1-D CNN	MI Detection	ACC 93.53%
Liu et al. 2018	PTB	ECG Signal	DWT (Daubechies wavelet 6 (db6))	Multiple Feature Branch CNN (MFB-CNN)	MI detection and localization	ACC 99.95%
Zhai and Tin 2018	MITBIHDB	ECG Signal	BPF	2-D CNN	MI detection and localization	ACC 97.3% SEN 89.3%
Yildirim 2018	MITBIHDB	ECG Signal	BPF	LSTM	Arrhythmia Classification	ACC 99.39%

Continued on following page

Table 2. Continued

Author	Database	Input	Preprocessing	DL algorithm	Application	Result
Tan et al. 2018	Fantasia; NCART	ECG Signal	DWT (Daubechies wavelet 6 (db6))	LSTM,CNN	Coronary artery Classification	ACC 99.85%
Guo et al. 2019	MITBIHDB	ECG Signal	MF followed by moving average filter	GRU,CNN	Interpatient arrhythmia classification	F1 score 61.25 for SVEBS
Faust et al. 2018	MITBIHDB	ECG Signal	100 beat window 99 beats overlap	LSTM,CNN	Arrhythmia Classification	ACC 98.10% SEN 97.50%
Andersen et al. 2019	MITBIHDB, MIT-BIHAF, MIT-BIH noise stress test database	ECG Signal	Raw ECG recordings are converted to RR interval (RRI) sequences	LSTM,CNN	AFN detection and monitoring	ACC 97.80% SEN 98.98%
Saadatnejad et al. 2019	MITBIHDB	ECG Signal	DWT (Daubechies wavelet 6 (db6))	RNN	Arrhythmia Classification	ACC 99.3%
Sun et al. 2020	Long-term AF Database; AF terminal challenge Database	ECG Signal	-	LSTM	AFN Prediction	ACC 92%
Lih et al. 2020	NCART; PTB; Fantasia	ECG Signal	-	LSTM,CNN	Myocardial infarction, congestive heart failure	ACC 98.51% SEN 97.85%
Labati et al. 2019	PTB	ECG Signal	Notch IIR filter followed by high pass butterworth filter	CNN	Biometric Recognition	ACC 100%
Takalo-Mattila et al. 2018	MITBIHDB	ECG Signal	High pass filter, band stop filter, low pass filter and normalization	AFIB	NSR, VEBS, SVEBS	SEN 92% (NSR); SEN 62% (SVEBS); SEN 89% (VEBS)
Xia et al 2018	MITDB: MIT-BIH Atrial Fibrillation database	ECG Signal	Elliptical bandpass filter	CNN	AFN	ACC 98.24% SEN 98.34%
Kamaleswaran et al. 2018	PhysioNet/ Computing in Cardiology Challenge	ECG Signal	Low pass filter	CNN, Multilayer perception	NSR, AFN, other abnormal rhythms	ACC 76.79%
Zhong et al. 2018	PhysioNet Challenge 2013	ECG Signal	Notch filter and band pass Butterworth filter	CNN+Fully convolutional network (FCNN)	Fetal QRS complex detection	Precision: 75.33%

Continued on following page

57

Table 2. Continued

Author	Database	Input	Preprocessing	DL algorithm	Application	Result
Isin and Ozdalili 2017	MITBIHDB	ECG Signal	10 point moving average filter	CNN+FCNN	NSR, Left bundle branch block, Paced Beats	ACC 92.4%
Savalia and Emamian 2018	PhysioBank	ECG Signal	-	FCNN	NSR, Ventricular Tachycardia, AFN, Ventricular Bigeminy	ACC 88%
Sodmann et al. 2018	PhysioNet, MIT-BIH PhysioNet/ CinC Challenge 2017	ECG Signal	DWT (Daubechies wavelet 4 (db4))	FCNN	NSR, AFN	F1 score(Avg.) 89%
Sujadevi et al. 2017	MITBIHDB	ECG Signal	No preprocessing	RNN	NSR, AFN	ACC 95%
Liu and Kim 2018	CinC Challenge (Apnea)	ECG Signal	Symbolic Aggregate approXimation (SAX)	LSTM	Sleep Apnea	ACC 98.4%
Tseng KK et al. 2021	PhysioNet, MIT-BIH PhysioNet/ CinC Challenge 2017	ECG Signal	Butterworth band stop filter, DWT (Daubechies wavelet 8 (db8)) and moving window MF	Sliding Large Kernel Network (LKNet)	AFN	F1 score 84.16%
Ramaraj 2021	PTB-XL	ECG Signal	-	GRU, Extreme Learning Machine (ELM)	Classification of CVDs	ACC 89%
Tong et al. 2021	MITBIHDB	ECG Signal	DWT	CNN	Abnormal heartbeat detection	ACC 99.22%
Radhakrishnan et al. 2021	MITBIHDB	ECG Signal	Butter-worth high-pass filter and notch filter	Bidirectional long short-term memory	AFN	ACC 90%
Rahul J 2022	MITBIHDB, MIT-BIH normal sinus rhythm database	ECG signal and its image	Two stage MF and least square smoothening filter	Bidirectional long short-term memory	Atrial fibrillation	ACC 98.85%

Discussion

DL is capable of producing faster and more consistent diagnoses in physiological signals, despite the fact that it is still in its early phases. That potency could prompt a move away from commonly used decision support approaches like a Support Vector Machine (SVM) and K-Nearest Neighbor (K-NN) in favor of deep learning (Faust et al. 2018). In (Faust et al. 2018), it is mentioned that the use of deep learning in ECG signals resulted in promising diagnostic capabilities. This is due to the created

DL model's ability to capture the unique characteristics of ECG data. As a result, albeit without significant data, the network may be trained using these learnt features, resulting in acceptable diagnostic performance. The automatic analysis of EMG and EEG signals, on the other hand, is more difficult due to their chaotic character. As a result, learning from the hidden and delicate information inherent in such signals is much more difficult for the network.

Feature selection in traditional machine learning algorithms takes a long time and exertion. In terms of generating the optimum diagnostic performance, these characteristics should retrieve useful information from large and diverse data sets. Furthermore, the optimum methodology is uncertain, necessitating a great deal of trial and error to find the best feature extraction algorithms and classification methods in order to construct robust and effective decision support systems for physiological signals. DL, on the other hand, does away with the necessity for feature extraction and feature selection. All evidence presented in (Min et al. 2017) can be considered by the decision-making algorithm.

The characteristics of DL architecture include the number, size, and type of the layers (Bouwmans et al. 2019). Good expressiveness can be achieved by selecting the right architecture. A fundamental difficulty in structure is inadequate interpretability. To begin with, there are few systematic approaches to aid in the adjustment of architecture in experiments, necessitating a series of tests in order to identify an efficient model. Furthermore, the consequences of an inaccurate conclusion might be severe in some areas, such as autonomous driving and medical aspects, making uncertainty practically intolerable. As a result, understanding how deep learning works is critical. Mathematical justification and visualization. The mathematic theory behind can help to justify the properties of deep learning (Vidal et al. 2017). There are two major techniques to visualize a network: viewing the strongest feature map activations and training images to increase the activation of certain neurons. Techniques for extracting more details from picture feature maps are introduced, shedding light on how networks use knowledge (Wang et al. 2018). DL can be applied to various physiological signals. The use of deep learning in ECG signals resulted in promising diagnostic capabilities, as shown in Table: 2. this is due to the created model's ability to capture the unique characteristics of ECG data. As a result, even without significant data, the network may be trained using these learned features, resulting in acceptable diagnostic performance. From Table: 2 we infer that CNN is used 18 times and hence makes it a very popular DL algorithm, while LKNet is the least used DL algorithm. Furthermore, CNN is combined with other techniques like multilayer perception or LSTM or GRU, or FCNN and obtained fairly good accuracy and sensitivity. A one- dimensional CNN is used in (Acharya et al. 2018, Acharya et al. 2017) and achieved an accuracy of approximately 93% whereas a two-dimensional CNN is used in (Zhai et al. 2018) and obtained an accuracy of nearly 97%. Moreover, MFs are used in the preprocessing stages in eight articles. DWT is the other most famous data preprocessing technique that is being employed in approximately eight articles. From Table: 2 we observe that in (Sujadevi et al. 2017) no preprocessing techniques were employed on the data from MITBIHDB and have achieved an appreciable F1 score.

The timefrequency image for heartbeat signal was originally produced using the modified frequency slice wavelet transform (MFSWT) in (Luo et al. 2017). The heartbeat classification was done using the DL approach that combines automatic feature abstraction with a DNN classifier. In (Al Rahhal et al. 2016), unsupervised learning is utilized to learn an appropriate feature representation from raw ECG data using stacked denoising autoencoders (SDAEs) with sparsity constraints. After this feature learning step, the DNN is created by layering a softmax regression layer on top of the resulting hidden representation layer. The expert is allowed to name the most significant and unclear ECG beats on the test record during the interaction phase, which is then utilized to update the DNN weights. (Yang et al. 2018) Proposes an ECG arrhythmia classification method based on stacked sparse auto-encoders (SSAEs) and a softmax regression (SF) model. The purpose of the SSAEs used in (Yang et al. 2018) is to extract high-level features from a large amount of ECG data in a hierarchical manner. (Farhadi et al. 2018) Uses a DL approach called stacked auto encoder in conjunction with a DL method called stacked autoencoder to classify AF. Spectral, temporal, and non-linear properties are derived from ECG signals from the MIT-BIH database. First, statistical tests and analysis of variance (ANOVA) were used to analyze extracted features, and then selected important features were employed in a stacked autoencoder as a parallel form to categorize AF and normal samples.

A novel DL based approach for ECG arrhythmias categorization that integrates LSTM based auto encoder (AE) network with SVM is described in (Hou et al. 2019).The LSTM-ased AE network (LSTM-AE) is used to extract features from ECG arrhythmia signals, and the SVM is used to categorize the signals based on the extracted features. DL is proposed in the pre-training and fine-tuning phases to produce an automated feature representation for multi-class classification of arrhythmia conditions (Nurmaini et al. 2020). In the pre-training phase, stacked denoising autoencoders (DAEs) and autoencoders (AEs) are used for feature learning; in the fine-tuning phase, DNNs are implemented as a classifier. The suggested model in (Altan et al. 2016) combines a DBN classifier with a greedy layer-wise training with RBM technique to create a multi-stage classification system that uses ECG waveforms and Second Order Difference Plot (SODP) data. The MITBIHDB heartbeats were divided into five primary groups using the multistage DBN model, which was based on ANSI/AAMI standards. In (Song et al. 2019), The morphological characteristics of ECG signals are automatically extracted from the designed generative restricted Boltzmann machine (GRBM), followed by the introduction of the discriminative restricted Boltzmann machine (DRBM) with feature learning and classification ability, and arrhythmia classification is performed using the extracted morphological features and RR interval features. A new method for reducing the number of false alarms (FA) caused by low-quality ECG data measurement during the identification of AF. To distinguish between acceptable and undesirable ECG segments, a deep belief network is used in (Taji et al. 2017).

A patient-specific ECG heartbeat classifier that uses an adaptive 1-D CNN implementation to combine the two key blocks of traditional ECG classification into a single learning body proposes feature extraction and classification in (Kiranyaz et al. 2015). A novel technique for automatic separation of shockable and non-shockable ventricular arrhythmias in two seconds ECG segments were proposed in (Acharya et al. 2018). An eleven-layer CNN model is used to process segmented ECGs. CNN structures (Net 1 and Net 2) with four convolutional layers, four pooling layers, and three fully-connected layers were constructed in (Acharya et al. 2017) to detect two classes (normal and coronary artery disease). A Generic Convolutional Neural Network (GCNN) is first trained using a large number of heartbeats without discriminating between patients is developed in (Li et al. 2018). A fine-tuning technique is used to convert the GCNN into a Tuned Dedicated CNN (TDCNN) for the relevant individual based on the GCNN. Notably, instead of shared training data, just the GCNN must be saved in wearable devices. In (Zhai et al. 2018), according to the changing heartbeat rate, a single channel ECG data were divided into heartbeats. As 2-D inputs to the CNN classifier, the beats were transformed into dual beat coupling matrices, which represented both beat shape and beat-to-beat correlation in the ECG. In order to improve classification performance, a systematic training beat selection approach was devised, which automatically includes the most representative beats in the training set. In (Yildirim 2018), for the identification of ECG data, a new model for deep bidirectional LSTM network-based a wavelet sequence titled DBLSTM-WS was proposed. A novel wavelet-based layer is used to produce ECG signal sequences for this objective. In this layer, the ECG signals were split into frequency sub-bands at various scales. A stacked CNN-LSTM technique is used in (Tan et al. 2018) to diagnose coronary artery disease using ECG signals. The system is fully automatic and requires minimum hand-engineering to train the algorithm.

In (Guo et al. 2019), densely connected convolutional neural network (DenseNet) and GRU for addressing the inter-patient ECG classification problem. The results clearly indicate that the model presented in (Guo et al. 2019) excelled in classifying the supraventricular (SVEB) and ventricular (VEB) arrhythmias. A DL system consisting of Deep RNN and LSTM to detect AF beats in Heart Rate (HR) signals are used in (Faust et al. 2018). The data were partitioned with a sliding window of 100 beats. The resulting signal blocks were directly fed into a DL method developed.

Automatic identification of atrial fibrillation (AF) from long-term ECG data using a DL technique that combines CNN and RNN to extract high-level characteristics from RR intervals (RRIs) and classify them as AF or normal sinus rhythm (NSR) is proposed in (Andersen et al. 2019). For the categorization of ECG utilized for continuous cardiac monitoring on wearable devices, the suggested method in (Saadatnejad et al. 2019) uses a unique DL architecture comprising of wavelet transform and several LSTM recurrent neural networks. For AF prediction, the technique developed in (Sun et al. 2020) uses a recurrent neural network (RNN) built of stacked LSTMs termed as SLAP. This model efficiently avoids the gradient explosion and the gradient explosion of standard RNNs, allowing it to learn features more effectively. (Lih et al. 2020) Developed the CNN, followed by hybrid CNN and LSTM models, as the most useful architectures for categorizing ECG signals into coronary artery disorders, MI, and congestive heart failure situations. In (Labati et al. 2019), Deep-ECG uses a deep CNN to extract key features from one or more leads and then compares biometric templates using simple and quick distance functions, resulting in higher accuracy for identifying, verifying, and periodic re-authentication. (Takalo-Mattila et al. 2018) proposes a completely automated interpatient ECG signal categorization approach based on deep CNN. In the inter-patient arrhythmia classification method, different patient data is used in the training and test phases. In (Xia et al. 2018), to acquire two-dimensional (2-D) matrix input suitable for deep convolutional neural networks, ECG segments was analyzed using the short-term Fourier transform (STFT) and stationary wavelet transform (SWT). Then, for the STFT and SWT outputs, two distinct deep convolutional neural network models were created.

A deep learning-based design capable of detecting aberrant heart rhythms from single-lead ECG records are proposed in (Kamaleswaran et al. 2018). In (Zhong et al. 2018), the features of non-invasive fetal electrocardiography (NI-FECG) signals are corrected before being input to a CNN classifier for detecting the fetal QRS complex. It is mentioned in (Isin et al. 2017) that by classifying patient ECGs into relevant cardiac states, a DL framework previously trained on a general picture data set is transferred to carry out automatic ECG arrhythmia diagnosis. As a feature extractor, a very deep convolutional neural network (AlexNet) is utilized, and the extracted features are fed into a simple backpropagation neural network to do the final classification. Several cardiac arrhythmias are classified by using deep neural network algorithms such as multi-layer perception and CNN (Savalia et al. 2018). In (Sodmann et al. 2018), Waveforms from the PhysioNet databases to train a CNN to annotate QRS complexes, P waves, T waves, noise, and interbeat ECG segments that distinguish the essences of normal and irregular heartbeats. In (Sujadevi et al. 2017), to detect AF faster in ECG traces, deep learning approaches such as RNN, LSTM, and GRU are used. A method for classification of heart diseases based on

ECG by using LSTM by analyzing ECG signals DL is used in (Liu et al. 2018). A novel diagnostic framework for mobile ECG signals is proposed in (Tseng et al. 2021), along with two improved approaches. The sliding segmentation strategy improves the model's generalization capacity, while the large-scale convolution kernel of a one-dimensional neural network is built for mobile ECG signals and is more resistant to the sparseness and noise concerns. (Ramaraj et al. 2021) uses a GRU-based feature extractor to create a suitable set of feature vectors. Finally, a classification model based on the Extreme Learning Machine model is used to select the proper class label for the test ECG data. An effective auxiliary diagnostic system is one that can extract useful information from an ECG. A unique multi-instance neural network (MINN) model capable of recognizing abnormal ECG segments and locating abnormal heartbeats in them was described in (Tong et al. 2021). A novel time-frequency domain DL-based technique for detecting AF and classifying terminating and non-terminating AF episodes using ECG data is proposed in (Radhakrishnan et al. 2021). The chirplet transform is used to evaluate the time-frequency representation (TFR) of ECG data in this method. Using time-frequency pictures of ECG data, the two-dimensional (2D) deep convolutional bidirectional LSTM neural network model is utilized to detect and categorize AF events. A novel method is proposed in (Rahul et al. 2022) for the identification of AF using both 1-D ECG signal and its time-frequency representation as an image (2D). In (Rasti-Meymandi et al. 2022), a 2D signal is created by stacking ECG cardiac cycles and feeding them to a CNN model. As a result, the connection between cardiac cycles can be leveraged; yielding in ECG denoising that is both efficient and resilient. To account for the correlation between the cycles, the proposed CNN model includes a novel local/non-local cycle observation (LNC) module. In (Panganiban et al. 2021), without undergoing ECG visual examination such as R-peak or P-peak identification developed a classification approach for ECG arrhythmia using the CNN with images based on spectrograms. DNN, one-dimensional (1D) CNN, two-dimensional (2D) CNN, RNN, LSTM, and GRU are six deep learning algorithms that were devised and deployed in (Erdenebayar et al. 2019) for autonomous detection of sleep apnea occurrences. In (Banerjee et al. 2021) a new approach of ECG steganography of hiding patients' confidential information is proposed. After decryption of hidden data, to predict original sample values of modified TP-segments, an LSTM-RNN was used which efficiently reduced the error between the original and predicted signal. A DNN model proposed in (Murat et al. 2021) was used on the data set during the extraction of the features of the ECG inputs.

The main advantage of the DL is that it does away with the necessity for feature extraction and selection. All evidence presented can be considered by the decision-making algorithm (Min et al. 2017). DL systems training algorithms have a significant computational burden. As a result, there is a high level of run-time intricacy, which corresponds to a protracted training period (Dean et al. 2012, Tokui et al. 2015, and Chatfield et al. 2014). The tuning parameters must be modified after the architecture has been chosen. The model will be influenced by both selection of structure and parameter adjustments. As a result, multiple test runs are required. Limiting the training period of the DL models is an effective research area (Erhan et al. 2010). The purpose of a parallel distributed processing structure (Chen et al. 2014) is to make the training process go faster. Graphics processing units (GPUs) can aid in network latency reduction (Bergstra et al. 2011). Training time may be an issue with this cutting-edge technology, as it can influence model selection tactics. To be more explicit, none of the publications examined used statistical methods like cross-validation (Schaffer 1993) to approach the model selection process. We can only infer that the DL architectures utilized in the scientific papers under review were chosen based on a single run trial. Similarly, we must assume that the hyper parameters were optimized after the network was trained once. This is a significant flaw as statistical validation procedures diminish sample selection bias (Zadrozny 2004, Huang et al. 2006).

CONCLUSION

We analyzed 42 papers on DL approaches for healthcare applications based on physiological cues in this study. The investigation was divided into two parts. The bibliometric search assessment based on the co-occurrence map was the initial phase. The relationship between the themes covered in the evaluated papers is shown in this step of the analysis. Four unique clusters were discovered, one for every physiological signal. This finding aided us in structuring the next analytical stage, which is concerned with the content of the article. As a result, the paper's content was determined by retrieving the information on the particular application field, the DL method, the performance of the system, and the sorts of datasets utilized to cultivate the system. To be more explicit, 36 studies do not reflect the whole range of physiological signal-based healthcare applications. More improved DL algorithms aimed at timely diagnosis of abnormalities employing physiological signals may be developed in the future.

Conflict of Interest

None.

REFERENCES

Acharya, U. R., Fujita, H., Lih, O. S., Adam, M., Tan, J. H., & Chua, C. K. (2017). Automated detection of coronary artery disease using different durations of ECG segments with convolutional neural network. *Knowledge-Based Systems*, *132*, 62–71.

Acharya, U. R., Fujita, H., Oh, S. L., Raghavendra, U., Tan, J. H., Adam, M., ... Hagiwara, Y. (2018). Automated identification of shockable and non-shockable life-threatening ventricular arrhythmias using convolutional neural network. *Future Generation Computer Systems*, *79*, 952–959.

Acharya, U. R., Oh, S. L., Hagiwara, Y., Tan, J. H., Adam, M., Gertych, A., & San Tan, R. (2017). A deep convolutional neural network model to classify heartbeats. *Computers in Biology and Medicine*, *89*, 389–396.

Al Rahhal, M. M., Bazi, Y., AlHichri, H., Alajlan, N., Melgani, F., & Yager, R. R. (2016). Deep learning approach for active classification of electrocardiogram signals. *Information Sciences*, *345*, 340–354.

Altan, G., Kutlu, Y., & Allahverdi, N. (2016). A multistage deep belief networks application on arrhythmia classification. *International Journal of Intelligent Systems and Applications in Engineering*, 222-228.

Andersen, R. S., Peimankar, A., & Puthusserypady, S. (2019). A deep learning approach for real-time detection of atrial fibrillation. *Expert Systems with Applications*, *115*, 465–473.

Banerjee, S., & Singh, G. K. (2021). A new approach of ECG steganography and prediction using deep learning. *Biomedical Signal Processing and Control*, *64*, 102151.

Bengio, Y., & LeCun, Y. (2007). Scaling learning algorithms towards AI. *Large-Scale Kernel Machines, 34*(5), 1-41.

Bergstra, J., Bastien, F., Breuleux, O., Lamblin, P., Pascanu, R., Delalleau, O., & Bengio, Y. (2011). Theano: Deep learning on gpus with python. In *NIPS 2011, BigLearning Workshop, Granada, Spain* (Vol. 3, pp. 1–48). Citeseer.

Bouwmans, T., Javed, S., Sultana, M., & Jung, S. K. (2019). Deep neural network concepts for background subtraction: A systematic review and comparative evaluation. *Neural Networks*, *117*, 8–66.

Chatfield, K., Simonyan, K., Vedaldi, A., & Zisserman, A. (2014). *Return of the devil in the details: Delving deep into convolutional nets.* arXiv preprint arXiv:1405.3531.

Chen, X. W., & Lin, X. (2014). Big data deep learning: Challenges and perspectives. *IEEE Access: Practical Innovations, Open Solutions*, *2*, 514–525.

Chua, L. O. (1998). *CNN: A paradigm for complexity* (Vol. 31). World Scientific.

Chung, J., Gulcehre, C., Cho, K., & Bengio, Y. (2014). *Empirical evaluation of gated recurrent neural networks on sequence modeling*. arXiv preprint arXiv:1412.3555.

Dean, J., Corrado, G., Monga, R., Chen, K., Devin, M., Mao, M., ... Ng, A. (2012). Large scale distributed deep networks. *Advances in Neural Information Processing Systems*, 25.

Dua, D., & Graff, C. (2017). *UCI machine learning repository*. Academic Press.

Erdenebayar, U., Kim, Y. J., Park, J. U., Joo, E. Y., & Lee, K. J. (2019). Deep learning approaches for automatic detection of sleep apnea events from an electrocardiogram. *Computer Methods and Programs in Biomedicine*, *180*, 105001.

Erhan, D., Courville, A., Bengio, Y., & Vincent, P. (2010, March). Why does unsupervised pre-training help deep learning? In *Proceedings of the thirteenth international conference on artificial intelligence and statistics* (pp. 201-208). JMLR Workshop and Conference Proceedings.

Farhadi, J., Attarodi, G., Dabanloo, N. J., Mohandespoor, M., & Eslamizadeh, M. (2018, September). Classification of atrial fibrillation using stacked auto encoders neural networks. In *2018 Computing in cardiology conference (CinC)* (Vol. 45, pp. 1-3). IEEE.

Faust, O. (2018). Documenting and predicting topic changes in Computers in Biology and Medicine: A bibliometric keyword analysis from 1990 to 2017. *Informatics in Medicine Unlocked*, *11*, 15–27.

Faust, O., Hagiwara, Y., Hong, T. J., Lih, O. S., & Acharya, U. R. (2018). Deep learning for healthcare applications based on physiological signals: A review. *Computer Methods and Programs in Biomedicine*, *161*, 1–13.

Faust, O., Shenfield, A., Kareem, M., San, T. R., Fujita, H., & Acharya, U. R. (2018). Automated detection of atrial fibrillation using long short-term memory network with RR interval signals. *Computers in Biology and Medicine*, *102*, 327–335.

Fischer, A., & Igel, C. (2012, September). An introduction to restricted Boltzmann machines. In *Iberoamerican congress on pattern recognition* (pp. 14–36). Springer.

Garcia-Garcia, A., Orts-Escolano, S., Oprea, S., Villena-Martinez, V., Martinez-Gonzalez, P., & Garcia-Rodriguez, J. (2018). A survey on deep learning techniques for image and video semantic segmentation. *Applied Soft Computing*, *70*, 41–65.

Goldberger, A. L., Amaral, L. A., Glass, L., Hausdorff, J. M., Ivanov, P. C., Mark, R. G., ... & Stanley, H. E. (2000). PhysioBank, PhysioToolkit, and PhysioNet: components of a new research resource for complex physiologic signals. *Circulation, 101*(23), e215-e220.

Goodfellow, I., Bengio, Y., & Courville, A. (2016). *Deep learning*. MIT press.

Guo, L., Sim, G., & Matuszewski, B. (2019). Inter-patient ECG classification with convolutional and recurrent neural networks. *Biocybernetics and Biomedical Engineering*, *39*(3), 868–879.

Guo, Y., Liu, Y., Georgiou, T., & Lew, M. S. (2018). A review of semantic segmentation using deep neural networks. *International Journal of Multimedia Information Retrieval*, *7*(2), 87–93.

He, K., Zhang, X., Ren, S., & Sun, J. (2016). Deep residual learning for image recognition. In *Proceedings of the IEEE conference on computer vision and pattern recognition* (pp. 770-778). IEEE.

Hinton, G. E., & Salakhutdinov, R. R. (2006). Reducing the dimensionality of data with neural networks. *Science, 313*(5786), 504-507.

Hochreiter, S., & Schmidhuber, J. (1997). Long short-term memory. *Neural Computation*, *9*(8), 1735–1780.

Hong, S., Zhou, Y., Shang, J., Xiao, C., & Sun, J. (2020). Opportunities and challenges of deep learning methods for electrocardiogram data: A systematic review. *Computers in Biology and Medicine*, *122*, 103801.

Hou, B., Yang, J., Wang, P., & Yan, R. (2019). LSTM-based auto-encoder model for ECG arrhythmias classification. *IEEE Transactions on Instrumentation and Measurement*, *69*(4), 1232–1240.

Huang, J., Gretton, A., Borgwardt, K., Schölkopf, B., & Smola, A. (2006). Correcting sample selection bias by unlabeled data. *Advances in Neural Information Processing Systems*, 19.

Iandola, F., Moskewicz, M., Karayev, S., Girshick, R., Darrell, T., & Keutzer, K. (2014). *Densenet: Implementing efficient convnet descriptor pyramids*. arXiv preprint arXiv:1404.1869.

Isin, A., & Ozdalili, S. (2017). Cardiac arrhythmia detection using deep learning. *Procedia Computer Science*, *120*, 268–275.

Kamaleswaran, R., Mahajan, R., & Akbilgic, O. (2018). A robust deep convolutional neural network for the classification of abnormal cardiac rhythm using single lead electrocardiograms of variable length. *Physiological Measurement*, *39*(3), 035006.

Kiranyaz, S., Ince, T., & Gabbouj, M. (2015). Real-time patient-specific ECG classification by 1-D convolutional neural networks. *IEEE Transactions on Biomedical Engineering*, *63*(3), 664–675.

Krizhevsky, A., Sutskever, I., & Hinton, G. E. (2012). Imagenet classification with deep convolutional neural networks. *Advances in Neural Information Processing Systems*, 25.

Labati, R. D., Muñoz, E., Piuri, V., Sassi, R., & Scotti, F. (2019). Deep-ECG: Convolutional neural networks for ECG biometric recognition. *Pattern Recognition Letters*, *126*, 78–85.

Larochelle, H., Mandel, M., Pascanu, R., & Bengio, Y. (2012). Learning algorithms for the classification restricted Boltzmann machine. *Journal of Machine Learning Research*, *13*(1), 643–669.

LeCun, Y., & Bengio, Y. (1995). Convolutional networks for images, speech, and time series. The handbook of brain theory and neural networks, 3361(10).

Li, Y., Pang, Y., Wang, J., & Li, X. (2018). Patient-specific ECG classification by deeper CNN from generic to dedicated. *Neurocomputing*, *314*, 336–346.

Lih, O. S., Jahmunah, V., San, T. R., Ciaccio, E. J., Yamakawa, T., Tanabe, M., ... Acharya, U. R. (2020). Comprehensive electrocardiographic diagnosis based on deep learning. *Artificial Intelligence in Medicine*, *103*, 101789.

Liu, M., & Kim, Y. (2018, July). Classification of heart diseases based on ECG signals using long short-term memory. In *2018 40th Annual International Conference of the IEEE Engineering in Medicine and Biology Society (EMBC)* (pp. 2707-2710). IEEE.

Liu, X., Wang, H., Li, Z., & Qin, L. (2021). Deep learning in ECG diagnosis: A review. *Knowledge-Based Systems*, *227*, 107187.

Lown, B., Klein, M. D., & Hershberg, P. I. (1969). Coronary and precoronary care. *The American Journal of Medicine*, *46*(5), 705–724.

Luo, K., Li, J., Wang, Z., & Cuschieri, A. (2017). Patient-specific deep architectural model for ECG classification. *Journal of Healthcare Engineering*.

Makhzani, A., & Frey, B. (2013). *K-sparse autoencoders*. arXiv preprint arXiv:1312.5663.

Min, S., Lee, B., & Yoon, S. (2017). Deep learning in bioinformatics. *Briefings in Bioinformatics, 18*(5), 851–869.

Minematsu, T., Shimada, A., Uchiyama, H., & Taniguchi, R. I. (2018). Analytics of deep neural network-based background subtraction. *Journal of Imaging, 4*(6), 78.

Mnih, V., Larochelle, H., & Hinton, G. E. (2012). *Conditional restricted boltzmann machines for structured output prediction*. arXiv preprint arXiv:1202.3748.

Murat, F., Yildirim, O., Talo, M., Baloglu, U. B., Demir, Y., & Acharya, U. R. (2020). Application of deep learning techniques for heartbeats detection using ECG signals-analysis and review. *Computers in Biology and Medicine, 120*, 103726.

Murat, F., Yildirim, O., Talo, M., Demir, Y., Tan, R. S., Ciaccio, E. J., & Acharya, U. R. (2021). Exploring deep features and ECG attributes to detect cardiac rhythm classes. *Knowledge-Based Systems, 232*, 107473.

Nurmaini, S., Darmawahyuni, A., Sakti Mukti, A. N., Rachmatullah, M. N., Firdaus, F., & Tutuko, B. (2020). Deep learning-based stacked denoising and autoencoder for ECG heartbeat classification. *Electronics (Basel), 9*(1), 135.

Panganiban, E. B., Paglinawan, A. C., Chung, W. Y., & Paa, G. L. S. (2021). ECG diagnostic support system (EDSS): A deep learning neural network based classification system for detecting ECG abnormal rhythms from a low-powered wearable biosensors. *Sensing and Bio-Sensing Research, 31*, 100398.

Pipberger, H. V., Arms, R. J., & Stallmann, F. W. (1961). Automatic Screening of Normal and Abnormal Electrocardiograms by Means of a Digital Electronic Computer. *Proceedings of the Society for Experimental Biology and Medicine, 106*(1), 130–132.

Radhakrishnan, T., Karhade, J., Ghosh, S. K., Muduli, P. R., Tripathy, R. K., & Acharya, U. R. (2021). AFCNNet: Automated detection of AF using chirplet transform and deep convolutional bidirectional long short term memory network with ECG signals. *Computers in Biology and Medicine, 137*, 104783.

Rahul, J., & Sharma, L. D. (2022). Artificial intelligence-based approach for atrial fibrillation detection using normalised and short-duration time-frequency ECG. *Biomedical Signal Processing and Control, 71*, 103270.

Rahul, J., Sora, M., & Sharma, L. D. (2021). Dynamic thresholding based efficient QRS complex detection with low computational overhead. *Biomedical Signal Processing and Control*, *67*, 102519.

Rahul, J., Sora, M., Sharma, L. D., & Bohat, V. K. (2021). An improved cardiac arrhythmia classification using an RR interval-based approach. *Biocybernetics and Biomedical Engineering*, *41*(2), 656–666.

Ramaraj, E. (2021). A novel deep learning based gated recurrent unit with extreme learning machine for electrocardiogram (ECG) signal recognition. *Biomedical Signal Processing and Control*, *68*, 102779.

Rangayyan, R. M. (2015). *Biomedical signal analysis*. John Wiley & Sons.

Rasti-Meymandi, A., & Ghaffari, A. (2022). A deep learning-based framework For ECG signal denoising based on stacked cardiac cycle tensor. *Biomedical Signal Processing and Control*, *71*, 103275.

Saadatnejad, S., Oveisi, M., & Hashemi, M. (2019). LSTM-based ECG classification for continuous monitoring on personal wearable devices. *IEEE Journal of Biomedical and Health Informatics*, *24*(2), 515–523.

Savalia, S., & Emamian, V. (2018). Cardiac arrhythmia classification by multi-layer perceptron and convolution neural networks. *Bioengineering (Basel, Switzerland)*, *5*(2), 35.

Schaffer, C. (1993). Selecting a classification method by cross-validation. *Machine Learning*, *13*(1), 135–143.

Schuster, M., & Paliwal, K. K. (1997). Bidirectional recurrent neural networks. *IEEE Transactions on Signal Processing*, *45*(11), 2673–2681.

Sharma, L. D., & Sunkaria, R. K. (2018a). Stationary wavelet transform based technique for automated external defibrillator using optimally selected classifiers. *Measurement*, *125*, 29–36.

Sharma, L. D., & Sunkaria, R. K. (2018b). Inferior myocardial infarction detection using stationary wavelet transform and machine learning approach. *Signal, Image and Video Processing*, *12*(2), 199–206.

Sharma, L. D., & Sunkaria, R. K. (2020). Myocardial infarction detection and localization using optimal features based lead specific approach. *IRBM*, *41*(1), 58–70.

Simonyan, K., & Zisserman, A. (2014). *Very deep convolutional networks for large-scale image recognition*. arXiv preprint arXiv:1409.1556.

Sodmann, P., Vollmer, M., Nath, N., & Kaderali, L. (2018). A convolutional neural network for ECG annotation as the basis for classification of cardiac rhythms. *Physiological Measurement, 39*(10), 104005.

Song, L., Sun, D., Wang, Q., & Wang, Y. (2019). Automatic classification method of arrhythmia based on discriminative deep belief networks. *Sheng wu yi xue gong cheng xue za zhi = Journal of biomedical engineering = Shengwu yixue gongchengxue zazhi, 36*(3), 444-452.

Sujadevi, V. G., Soman, K. P., & Vinayakumar, R. (2017, September). Real-time detection of atrial fibrillation from short time single lead ECG traces using recurrent neural networks. In *The International Symposium on Intelligent Systems Technologies and Applications* (pp. 212-221). Springer.

Sun, L., Wang, Y., He, J., Li, H., Peng, D., & Wang, Y. (2020). A stacked LSTM for atrial fibrillation prediction based on multivariate ECGs. *Health Information Science and Systems, 8*(1), 1–7.

Taji, B., Chan, A. D., & Shirmohammadi, S. (2017). False alarm reduction in atrial fibrillation detection using deep belief networks. *IEEE Transactions on Instrumentation and Measurement, 67*(5), 1124–1131.

Takalo-Mattila, J., Kiljander, J., & Soininen, J. P. (2018, August). Inter-patient ECG classification using deep convolutional neural networks. In *2018 21st Euromicro Conference on Digital System Design (DSD)* (pp. 421-425). IEEE.

Tan, J. H., Hagiwara, Y., Pang, W., Lim, I., Oh, S. L., Adam, M., ... Acharya, U. R. (2018). Application of stacked convolutional and long short-term memory network for accurate identification of CAD ECG signals. *Computers in Biology and Medicine, 94*, 19–26.

Tokui, S., Oono, K., Hido, S., & Clayton, J. (2015, December). Chainer: a next-generation open source framework for deep learning. In *Proceedings of workshop on machine learning systems (LearningSys) in the twenty-ninth annual conference on neural information processing systems (NIPS)* (*Vol. 5*, pp. 1-6). Academic Press.

Tong, Y., Sun, Y., Zhou, P., Shen, Y., Jiang, H., Sha, X., & Chang, S. (2021). Locating abnormal heartbeats in ECG segments based on deep weakly supervised learning. *Biomedical Signal Processing and Control, 68*, 102674.

Tseng, K. K., Wang, C., Xiao, T., Chen, C. M., Hassan, M. M., & de Albuquerque, V. H. C. (2021). Sliding large kernel of deep learning algorithm for mobile electrocardiogram diagnosis. *Computers & Electrical Engineering, 96*, 107521.

Vidal, R., Bruna, J., Giryes, R., & Soatto, S. (2017). *Mathematics of deep learning.* arXiv preprint arXiv:1712.04741.

Vincent, P., Larochelle, H., Lajoie, I., Bengio, Y., Manzagol, P. A., & Bottou, L. (2010). Stacked denoising autoencoders: Learning useful representations in a deep network with a local denoising criterion. *Journal of Machine Learning Research, 11*(12).

Wang, F., Liu, H., & Cheng, J. (2018). Visualizing deep neural network by alternately image blurring and deblurring. *Neural Networks, 97,* 162–172.

Xia, Y., Wulan, N., Wang, K., & Zhang, H. (2018). Detecting atrial fibrillation by deep convolutional neural networks. *Computers in Biology and Medicine, 93,* 84–92.

Yang, J., Bai, Y., Lin, F., Liu, M., Hou, Z., & Liu, X. (2018). A novel electrocardiogram arrhythmia classification method based on stacked sparse auto-encoders and softmax regression. *International Journal of Machine Learning and Cybernetics, 9*(10), 1733–1740.

Yildirim, Ö. (2018). A novel wavelet sequence based on deep bidirectional LSTM network model for ECG signal classification. *Computers in Biology and Medicine, 96,* 189–202.

Yu, Y. H., Chasman, D. I., Buring, J. E., Rose, L., & Ridker, P. M. (2015). Cardiovascular risks associated with incident and prevalent periodontal disease. *Journal of Clinical Periodontology, 42*(1), 21–28. doi:10.1111/jcpe.12335 PMID:25385537

Zadrozny, B. (2004, July). Learning and evaluating classifiers under sample selection bias. In *Proceedings of the twenty-first international conference on Machine learning* (p. 114). Academic Press.

Zhai, X., & Tin, C. (2018). Automated ECG classification using dual heartbeat coupling based on convolutional neural network. *IEEE Access: Practical Innovations, Open Solutions, 6,* 27465–27472.

Zhao, Z. Q., Zheng, P., Xu, S. T., & Wu, X. (2019). Object detection with deep learning: A review. *IEEE Transactions on Neural Networks and Learning Systems, 30*(11), 3212–3232.

Zhong, W., Liao, L., Guo, X., & Wang, G. (2018). A deep learning approach for fetal QRS complex detection. *Physiological Measurement, 39*(4), 045004.

Chapter 3

A Review on Big Data and Artificial Intelligence for the Healthcare Domain

A. V. Senthil Kumar
Hindusthan College of Arts and Sciences, India

Kavitha V.
Hindusthan College of Arts and Science, India

Malavika B.
Hindusthan College of Arts and Science, India

Parameshwari S.
Hindusthan College of Arts and Science, India

ABSTRACT

Big data analytics is frequently termed as the complicated operation of analysing the big data to unfold the information like market trends, correlations, customer preferences, and hidden patterns which might be helpful for the organisations to make decisions. On the other hand, data analytic techniques and technologies provide organisations methods to analyse data sets and to collect new data. With right garage and analytical tools in hand, the data and insights derived from big data could make the critical social infrastructure additives and offerings. In healthcare the usage of artificial intelligence has the capability to help healthcare companies in lots of factors of administrative processes and patient care. Artificial intelligence has converted companies across the world and has the capability to appreciably regulate the sphere of healthcare. Most of the AI and healthcare technology have strong relevance to the healthcare field; however, the procedures they help can range significantly.

DOI: 10.4018/978-1-7998-9172-7.ch003

INTRODUCTION

The volumes, symbols, or characters on those functions are finished i[th] the aid of using a computer system, that can be saved and transferred with inside the shape of electrical alerts and captured on mechanical, magnetic, or optical recording entity. Big Data is a set of information this is big in quantity, but developing extremely with time. It is an information with so massive length and complex data where none of conventional information control equipment can keep it or operate it efficiently. Big information is likewise an information however with big length. The time period Big Data termed to massive-scale statistics control and evaluation technology that out-do the functionality of conventional information operating technology (Chadwick, Ruth, 2017).

Big Data is distinct from conventional technology in 3 ways: the quantity of information (volume), the charge of information era and transferring speed (velocity), and the sorts of established and the unstructured information (variety) Big Data analytics is defined as the method of studying and mining Big Data – can provide functional and commercial enterprise information at an extraordinary specificity and scale. The major purpose to investigate and attachment fashion information accrued with the aid of using groups is one of the predominant entities for Big Data evaluation equipment. The technical developments in processing, storage, and evaluation of Big Data include:

- The unexpectedly reducing fee of garage and the CPU strength in latest decades.
- the ability and fee-efficiency of data enterprises and cloud computing for flexible calculation and garage.
- the improvement of recent platforms which includes Hadoop, this Hadoop permit customers to have benefit of those dispensed calculating structures keeping huge portions of records thru bendy collateral processing.

These advance features have invested numerous variations among Big Data analytics and conventional analytics.

The intention of Big Data analytics to ensure the safety is to attain efficiently acting as intellectual in actual time. Even though Big Data analytics always have a sizable assurance, there are some of demanding situations which should be conquered to recognize its real capability. The below mentioned are just a few of the queries that want to be shot out:

1.   Data provenance: The major property called integrity and authenticity of statistics utilized for analytics. When Big Data grows the resources of statistics it may

be used, the credibility of every statistics supply desire to be established and the incorporation of thoughts including opposed device gaining knowledge of should be experienced for one topic k out maliciously added statistics.

2. Privacy: People always want periodic motivations and technical machineries to reduce the quantity of results that Big Data customers could create. CSA has a collection devoted to isolation in Big Data and has cooperation with the NIST's Big Data running organization on safety and isolation. The researchers schedules to provide new suggestions and blank pages to explore the technical approach and the high-quality ideas for decreasing isolation occupations springing up from Big Data analytics.

3. Securing the Big Data storages: this file targeted on the use of Big Data to provide safety; however the different aspect of the key is the safety of Big Data. CSA has provided files on safety in Cloud Computing and additionally has running companies specializing in figuring out the high-quality plans to ensure the security in Big Data.

4. The Human-computer interaction: Big Data may provide the evaluation of various resources of statistics; however a human data analyst nevertheless has to explore almost all the results. As compared to other technical methods advanced for storage and appropriate calculations, the human-computer interaction along with the Big Data have obtained much less interest and that is a place that desires to develop. A suitable initial step on this course is using visualization equipment to assist the data analysts apprehend the statistics in their computer systems.

Big records is producing a sizable quantity of interest amongst enterprise, media or even the customers, together with the analytics, and cloud primarily based totally technology. These are all part of the present day eco-device developed through the era of major-trends. Big records has emerged as a chief subject matter or the topic of this decade's media, it has additionally created its manner into a number of accessories and in inner surveillance (White House,2019).

In 2014, a Survey called Global Forensic Data Analysis, the researchers found a rate of 72% from defendants who agree that rising massive records technology can enrol a major function in fraud detection and prevention. And least of few approximately 7% of defendants have been privy to any particular massive records technology, and simplest only a few approximately 2 percent of them have been clearly made use of them. Forensic records analysis technology is to assist the corporations to preserve the tempo along with growing records at a drastic speed in huge quantities (volumes), in addition to enterprise complexities.

Big Data is extensive and encloses numerous developments and fresh era implementations, the pinnacle ten rising technology which might be assisting customers deal with and manage Big Data in a price-effective way (NITRD et al, 2019).

1. Column oriented database conventional, row oriented databases are known to be exquisite for the web transmissions operating with the excessive replace velocities, however they indulge quickly within the question overall performance as extra records quantity increases and as records will become unstructured.

2. No SQL database or Schema-less database there are numerous databases which sorts according to the category, together with main price storage and record database, responsiveness on garage and delivery of massive quantities of records that's both unstructured, semi-structured, or it might be structured records too.

3. Map Reduce: This is a programming pattern that permits for large activity operations scalability in opposition to hundreds of attendants or group of servers. Slightly Map Reduce application includes tasks: The "Map" undertaking, wherein an enter dataset is transformed right into a distinctive set of key/cost pairs, or tuples. The "Reduce "undertaking, wherein numerous of the outcomes of the "Map" undertaking are blended to shape a discounted set of tuples .

4. Hadoop: Hadoop is the first-rate and the maximum famous application of map reduce, existence a wholly an exposed supply display place for managing of massive records. It is bendy sufficient which will paintings with more than one record's source. It has numerous distinctive programs, however one of the pinnacle use instances is for massive volumes of continuously converting records, together with location based records from climate or visitor's sensors.

5. Hive:Hive is defined as a SQL-LIKE connection which permits traditional BI software to run commands in opposition to a Hadoop cluster. It turned into advanced in the beginning through Facebook, however it has been developed foran exposed supply for a while, and it is a higher-degree abstraction of the Hadoop framework which permits all and sundry to create commands in opposition to records saved in a Hadoop cluster simply as though they have been changing a traditional records database.

6. Pig: PIG turned into advanced through Yahoo .PIG is bond which attempts to carry Hadoop toward the authenticities of builders and enterprise customers, much like Hive. Dissimilar to Hive, nevertheless, PIG includes a "Perl-like" programming language which permits for question implementation through records saved on the Hadoop cluster, in preference to a SQL-like language.

7. WibiData:Wibi records is a mixture of net data analytics by means of Hadoop its miles been constructed at the pinnacle of HBase on Hadoop is a database layer.

8.   Sky Tree: It is an excessive overall performance system gaining knowledge of and records analytics display place concentrated in particular at the managing of massive records. system gaining knowledge of is a completely critical a part of massive records, because the records quantity create guide examination.

Big Data and Big Data Analatics

The term big data is explained as a huge quantity or volume of data. These data can be structured or unstructured or it might be a mixture. These data are used in growth of decision making in various sectors like business, education, healthcare, e-governance, transport etc., Big data contains wide variety of data which will be increasing the volume with the time; thus it have greater volume, velocity and variety(Flores, 2013).

Figure 1. The types of big data

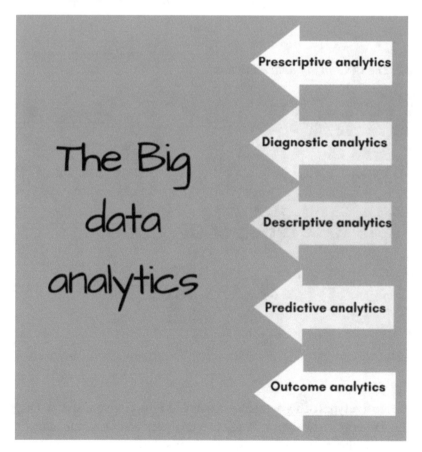

There are three types of big data namely structured, unstructured and semi-structured. The structured data is the form of well-defined data which was transformed and formatted. The weblog, statistics, quantity, barcodes, spreadsheets are some common examples of the structured data. On the other hand, various websites, social medias, document collections are in a section called unstructured big data. The unstructured data is termed as the absolute raw data, which is those data are neither formatted nor transformed, thus these data are creating a difficult task for processing. And here arrives the last category called semi-structured big data; this includes partially structured data. For example, the delimited file is a best example of semi structured data.

After preparation of the data it must be brought to the condition for processing. This process of extraction is called as big data analytics. The meaningful information must be extracted from the big data for an efficient learning. The big data analytics reduces the complexity of the problems in the processing. The big data analytics is an important feature, this is needed to take decisions using the big data analytics (United Healthcare uses Hadoop to Detect Health Care Fraud, Waste and Abuse, 2018).

Figure 2. The types in big data analytics

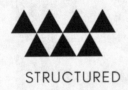
STRUCTURED

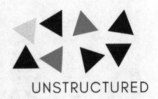
UNSTRUCTURED

Types of Big data

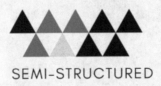
SEMI-STRUCTURED

There are five types of big data analytics such as Prescriptive analytics, Diagnostic analytics, Descriptive analytics, Predictive analytics and Outcome analytics. The prescriptive analytics are used to find the best solution and it also alleviates the future risk. For investigating foremost agitate pointers and process with the trends Diagnostic analytics are used. Similarly for every type of analytics there exist its own dedicated purposes.

There are many big data analytics tools such as Mango DB, Hadoop, Talend, Cassandra, Apache spark etc., The Apache Spark is considered as the most powerful big data analytics tool because it has 80 high level operators. These analytics are much easier when it is applied with machines, Thus AI also plays an important role in big data. AI analytics is another useful branch for big data analytics. While using machines the task will be easier, efficient and faster (Mian, M, 2014).

Big Data Life Cycle

Big records is a big object of diverse datasets. Nowadays massive records performs an critical function in people everyday life, on or after the fingertip programs to the massive companies it's miles "massive records". When so ever the records is amassed there originates some other canopy time period referred to as cyber-security. In the meantime each unstructured records is valuable and have to be stored exclusive from the attackers or hackers. In advance period the records turned into noted within side the papers and books which turned into a disappointment (Marks, Harry M. 2000).

As the time stimulated the inscribed facts modified to the virtual repeoples, and now in this period human clutches an idea of IoT wherein people can immediately talk with the digital machineries with none greater program design facts. The IoT goes to be the approaching rebellion wherein it is composed of latest vocabularies like Smart towns.

Artificial Intelligence

The term artificial intelligence was coined by Professor emeritus of computer science at Stanford named John McCarthy. The artificial intelligence is defined as "Machine imitating human behave people". The machine are implemented to ease the work pressure of the humans. AI contains keen technologies talented to carry out errands which classically need human intellect. These machines are capable to think humanly and rationally also to act according to it.

Till 1949, computer systems ought to implement queries, however people couldn't consider what people did as these people had been now no longer capable of saving those queries. In the year of 1950, A scientist named Alan Turing mentioned the way to construct clever machineries and took a look at this intellect in which scientist Alan tuning's paper "Computing Machinery and Intelligence". After five years, the primary artificial intelligence programs changed into supplied on the Dartmouth Summer Research Project on Artificial Intelligence (DSPRAI). This occasion changed into the booster for artificial intelligence studies for the following couple of years (Wilkinson, M. D, 2016).

Computers have become faster, less expensive and greater handy among the years of 1957 and 1974. Machine gaining knowledge of step by step procedures progressed and, in the year of 1970, one of the representatives of DSPRAI informed in the Life Magazine which there might be a device with the overall intellect of a median person in 3 to 8 years. On spite of their success, computer systems' lack of ability to efficaciously save or quick manner facts created as the barriers with inside the shadowing of artificial intellect for the subsequent decade of years.

Artificial intelligence technology is significant for the reason which it allows human competences like perception, planning, understanding, reasoning and communication to be recognized by software program progressively efficiently, proficiently and at less price. Artificial intelligence is touch on the upcoming days of practically every single manufacturing unit and every one human being. Artificial intelligence has act on behalf of the key motorist of developing concepts like robotics, IoT and big data (Pramanik, P. K. D & Choudhury, P, 2018).

Figure 3. Different phases of Artificial intelligence

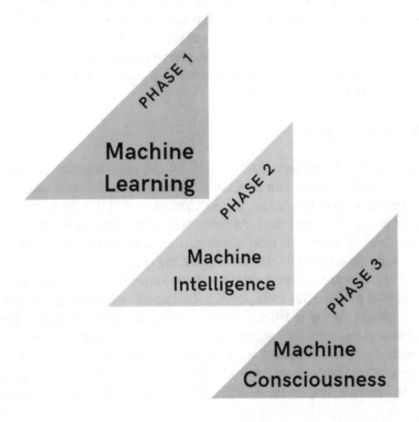

There are mainly three phases of AI such as machine learning, machine intelligence and machine consciousness. In machine learning, the main objective of the system will be to solve a single problem and will be concentrated on one area. Thus it is also termed as ANI(artificial narrow intelligence).Since the phase 2 is described as machine intelligence, which refer a computer system as smart as a human brain through the network it is also called as Artificial general intelligence, AGI in short. The final phase is called machine consciousness because it is an brain power which is smarter than powerful human brain so called in every sector.

Why is artificial intelligence an important concept?

Artificial intelligence systematizes monotonous knowledge and detection through facts. In its place of systematizing lab people-intensive responsibilities, artificial intelligence accomplishes recurrent, huge-volume, high-tech responsibilities. And it prepares so dependably and with a deprivation of exhaustion. Of peoples, humans are motionlessly indispensable to set up the arrangement and enquire the right queries. Artificial intelligence increments intellect to current goods. Numerous goods people even now makes use will be grown with artificial intelligence capacities, much similar to Siri was incremented as a fresh feature to a new peer group of Apple goods. Computerization, informal stages, bots and shrewd machineries can be accompanied with huge quantity of facts and data to make an improvement in number of machineries. Advancements at personal home and in the public workspace, ranging from safe keeping intellect and shrewd cameras to venture examination (Jorland, 2005).

Artificial intelligence become accustomed through broadminded knowledge step by step procedures to lease the facts do the user interface design. artificial intelligence discoveries assembly and symmetries in data so which step by step procedures can obtain services. Fair as a step by step procedure can communicate the problem to show the gaming like chess, it can communicate the issue which what invention to mention in upcoming through online. And the representations familiarize when assumed fresh fact. Artificial intelligence analyses supplementary and cavernous data by means of neural networks which have number of masked layers. Constructing a fraud detection system using five masked layers utilised to be not possible (Mian, M., 2014). All which has exchanged with unbelievable super computer supremacy and big data. One should gain huge quantity of data to equip deep learning representations for the reason which they study unswervingly from the collected facts.

Importance of Healthcare Industry

The term healthcare industry additionally known as the medical industry or health economy which is an assemblage and combination of companies in the financial machine which offers items and offerings to deal with sufferers with corrective, precautious, recoverable, and palliative super vision. It consists of the era and capitalization of products and offerings providing themselves for keeping and re-setting up fitness. The present day healthcare enterprise consists of 3 crucial portions which can be products, finance and services and can be separated into number sections and classes and relies upon at the multidisciplinary groups of educated specialists and such people to fulfil fitness wishes of populations and people.

Figure 4. Benefits of healthcare industry

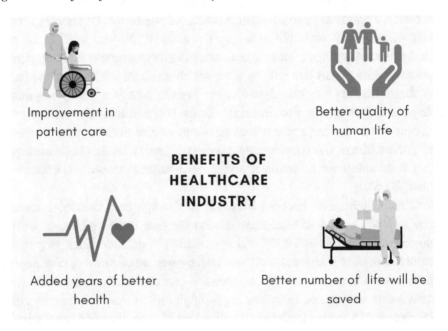

The above figure illustrates the major benefits of healthcare industry, the healthcare industry helps the healthcare providers to show an improvement in patient care, which intern leads to many other advantages like; saving many patients, improving quality of human life etc., In the United States the health care archaeologically engrossed on come across in the means by the care and pick up the check on disease as it ascends somewhat than averting it, is now experiencing an all encompassing alteration in the direction of a supplementary inhabitants health–oriented method.

This alteration is up-to-the-minute through a sequence of variations in compensation. Amongst these variations are numerous ages of be able to care and capitated inhabitants' administration examinations and growths in compensation for value-based care and anticipation, in cooperation of which effort to bring about the complete health of the enduring patient out there behave people of illness(Flores, 2013).

WHY TO IMPLEMENT ARTIFICIAL INTELLIGENCE AND BIG DATA ANALATICS IN HEALTH CARE INDUSTRY?

Recently, implementing the disciplines of Artificial Intelligence with big data are more general in healthcare industry. The pharmacy along with Artificial Intelligence is a current trend in the sector of health care in considered still in its infancy. Mostly the people thought which when they hear about AI in medical care may be connected to the Star Wars movies, where there are no mankind doctors. All kinds of medical activities are done through intelligent robots and systems. Big data together with the purpose of sophisticated analytical approaches similar to AI have the potential to enhance medical conclusions and population health. Clinical data are routinely produced from smart medical devices and electronic medical records have become gradually cheaper and simpler to gather, analyse as well as process.

In current years this has provoked a considerable increase in the research of biomedical efforts. Big data mainly focuses on real domain information similar to consideration of innovative enhancements in AI and digital health care, electronic medical records and genomic medicine and also consulting ethical issues and considerations connected to information sharing. On the whole, it remains constructive which the studies of big data connected with the innovative technologies will maintain to guide novel, exciting research which will eventually enhance healthcare and clinical care in realistic which concerns about equity, privacy, security and promote to all (United Healthcare uses Hadoop to Detect Health Care Fraud, Waste and Abuse, 2018).

Artificial Intelligence connected with big data are utilized in an extensive range of domains in hospitals like cognitive computer systems are utilized to facilitate repetitive tasks and to generate model analyses in the context of the diagnostics of radiological. Some of the enhanced tools are utilized to establish the most credible time of death seriously suffered patents and the optimal treatments as a result, embracing the enabled patients to be transferred to painless care in the correct time in order to provide them a dignified send-off. Robotic based systems and surgical robots are the most relevant field of applications. The medical industry believes which the clinical robots will be crucial for elevated precision surgical treatments in further. The supreme challenge to Artificial Intelligence in healthcare is not based on the technologies will be proficient enough to be useful, but rather guaranteeing adoption in day by day medical practice (Pramanik, P. K. D & Choudhury, P, 2018).

Role of Big Data Analatics in Healthcare Industry

The healthcare industry is the most essential industry people need. What will be the volume of data in healthcare industry? And What are the data stored in the database of healthcare industry? By finding the answers for these queries can help a person to get an idea of the data available in the healthcare industry. Big data may be devastating for health care companies because of its extent and its range i.e., medical, and economic. But then again large facts can assist health care structures to recognize the developments and the styles in the facts and in flip enhance the nice care of sufferers and decrease healthcare costs. Many pharmaceutical and biotechnological organizations also are realising the energy of large facts for economic chance administration, supervisory acquiescence administration.

Big data in healthcare is a time period utilised to explain huge capacities of data fashioned with the aid of using the implementation of virtual technology that gather sufferers' information and assist in coping with sanatorium presentation, in any other case too big and complicated for conventional technology.

The healthcare region faces challenges, such as, grading virtual maintenance shipping processes for ambulant sufferers for that it's loads vigorous to secure, collect, analyse, and movement the facts to make positive affected person care selections and identifies (Shah, S, 2016).

Big data goes to produce a huge function in a COVID world, wherein healthcare companies will change their awareness to develop healthcare on hand and operative, irrespective of characteristics, mobility, and location.

"Big data analytics consumes facilitated healthcare enhance with the aid of using presenting customized medicinal drug and unbending analytics, medical chance interference and prognostic analytics, left-over and care erraticismlessening, automatic outside and inner reportage of affected person data, consistent clinical phrases and affected person archives and disjointed factor solution."

Big data analytics transportations a whole lot of wonderful and additionally life-saving effects in healthcare. The extensive portions of data shaped with the aid of using the digitization of the whole thing, that receives joint and studied with the aid of using precise technology references to large-type facts. When carried out to healthcare, it's going to utilise precise fitness facts of a populace or a selected person and doubtlessly assist to save people breakers and pandemics, remedy disease, reduce down prices, etc. For many decades, it's been high-priced and time-eating to accumulate large quantities of facts for clinical use. With enhancing technology, it's been less difficult to gather such facts and to develop complete healthcare reviews and to supply applicable important understandings with the aid of using changing those reviews to offer higher care. And to summarize, healthcare facts analytics makes use of facts-pushed conclusions are expecting and remedy a trouble earlier than its miles too delayed. It additionally measures techniques and remedies quicker, hold right path of inventory and inventory, inspire affected person contribution and affected person authorization with its numerous tools (Pramanik, P. K. D. & Choudhury, P, 2018).

The cap probable of healthcare enterprises to apply large facts in healthcare may be demonstrated helpful finished tele-medicine as they illustrate thru and social disease. The get admission to applicable facts thru tele-medicine is beneficial because it gives more possibilities for active interference and a correct review of the patients with combined real-time data.

Role of Artificial Intelligence in Healthcare Industry

- **Unifying focus and mechanism via brain-computer system interfaces:** The use of laptop machine to speak is neve a brand new idea, however producing direct obstacles among generation and the human thoughts without using a keyboard, mouse, and reveal is a contemporary place of studies that has big packages for a few sufferers. Nervous machine trauma can deprive a few sufferers of the capacity to speak, move, and have interaction in significant approaches with humans and their surroundings. Artificial intelligence-assisted brain-laptop interfaces (BCIs) should deliver those essential stories returned to people who feared they might be misplaced forever. "If the person is with inside the neurological extensive care unit on a Monday and it is noticed that the person has all of sudden misplaced the capability to transport or speak, it needs to repair that capability to speak via way of means of Tuesday," stated Leigh Hochberg, MD, PhD, director of the centre for neuro technology and nonrecovery on the MGH. By the usage of a BCI and synthetic intelligence, it will decipher the neural activations related to the meant motion of the hand, and also wants to permit that man or woman to do the equal component as minimum number of humans on this room have communicated 5instanceswithinside the route of the morning with ubiquitous conversation generation including drugs or phones for sufferers with ALS, stroke, or locked-in syndrome and for the 500,000 humans global who are suffering spinal twine accidents every year.
- **Developing the following era of radiology equipment:** Radiological pictures acquired with MRI machines, CT scanners and X-ray machines offer non-invasive insights into the internal workings of the human body, however

many diagnostic approaches are none the less primarily based totally on bodily tissue samples acquired via biopsies, which consists of dangers inclusive of the opportunity for infection. Artificial Intelligence will permit the following era of radiology equipment which might be specific and certain sufficient updating needs for tissue samples in a few cases, professionals predict. The system needs to deliver the imaging group collectively with the interventional healthcare professional or radiologist and the pathologist, " stated Alexandra Golby, MD, director of image-guided neurosurgery at Brigham and Women's Hospital (BWH). "Bringing different teams together and coordinating goals is a great challenge." If the system needs to get information from the images that they are currently getting from tissue samples, it have to achieve a very precise registration so that the basic truth is known for each pixel. Succeeding in the questions can allow clinicians to develop a more accurate understanding of the behaviour of tumours as a whole, rather than basing treatment decisions on the characteristics of a small segment of the malignancy. Providers can also better define the aggressiveness of cancer and use treatments in a more targeted manner. Artificial intelligence helps enable "virtual biopsies" and advance the innovative field of radio mics, which focuses on the use of image-based algorithms to characterize the phenotypes and genetic properties of tumours.

- **Increasing admission to care in underserved or evolving areas:** The lack of trained health care providers, including ultrasound technicians and radiologists, can severely limit access to life-saving care in developing countries around the world. The half-dozen hospitals along Boston's famous Longwood Avenue have more radiologists than anywhere in West Africa, the meeting said. Artificial intelligence could help alleviate the consequences of this severe shortage of qualified clinical staff by taking on some of the diagnostic tasks that are normally assigned to humans. This capability could be implemented through an app available to providers in areas with limited resources, reducing the need for a trained on-site diagnostic radiologist. "The potential of this technology to improve access to health care is enormous," said Jayashree Kalpathy Cramer, PhD, neuroscience assistant at MGH and associate professor of radiology at HMS. Algorithm developers must always be aware that different ethnic groups or residents of different regions may have unique physiologists and environmental factors that affect the presentation of the disease. "The course of the disease and the population impacted by the disease can look very different in India than, for example, in the USA," he said. In developing these algorithms, it is very important to ensure that the data represent a variety of diseases and populations –It might not able to enhance an algorithm based on a single population and hope it will work for others too.

- **Dropping the weights of electronic health record usage:** EHRs have played a pivotal role in the journey to digitize healthcare, but change has brought a myriad of problems associated with cognitive overload, endless documentation, and user burnout. EHR developers are now using Artificial Intelligence to create more intuitive interfaces and automate some difficulties. Routine processes that consume a majority of the time of a user who spends the most time on three tasks: clinical documentation, order entry, and basket sorting, said Adam Landman, MD, vice president and CIO of Brigham Health. Voice recognition and dictation help improve the clinical documentation process, but natural language processing (NLP) tools may not go far enough. Like the applications of Siri and Alexa, doctors are going to be virtual bedside assistants with built-in intelligence for input. Artificial intelligence can also help handle routine inquiries from your inbox, such as medication refills and result notifications. It can also help prioritize tasks that really require the doctor's attention.

- **Covering the hazards of antibiotic struggle:** Antibiotic resistance poses a growing threat to populations around the world, as the overuse of these critical drugs encourages the development of super bacteria that no longer respond to treatments. Multiseriate organisms can have devastating effects in the hospital environment, claiming thousands of lives every year. It costs the US healthcare system approximately $5 billion annually and kills more than 30,000 people. Electronic health record data can help identify patterns of infection and identify at-risk patients before they show symptoms. These analyse can improve your accuracy and produce faster, more accurate alerts for healthcare providers. "Artificial intelligence tools can meet expectations for infection control and antibiotic resistance," said Erica Shenoy, MD, PhD, assistant director of the infection control unit at MGH. "If they don't, then it really is a failure of all of our parts. For the hospitals that are in the mountains of EHR data and not exploiting it to the full, for the industry that isn't doing smarter clinical trials design and faster, and it would be a mistake for the EHRs that create this data not to use it.

- **Generating more exact analytics for pathology pictures:** Pathologists provide one of the primary sources of diagnostic data for providers across the spectrum of care, says Jeffrey Golden, MD, chairman of the BWH department of pathology and professor of pathology at HMS. The reporting analysed that "Seventy percent of all healthcare decisions are based on a pathological finding". Approximately between 70 and 75 percent of all data in an EHR come from a pathological result. Hence, specifically the optimal and also accurate diagnosis report can be achieved. This is exactly what digital pathology and artificial intelligence offer analysis that can break down to the pixel level in extremely large digital images can enable providers to spot nuances that the human eye may miss. Finally, people can analyse proper outcome like whether cancer is progressing quickly or slowly, and how that could change the way patients are treated, based on an algorithm rather than clinical staging or histopathological analysis,", said Golden. Artificial intelligence can also improve productivity by identifying features of interest on slides before a human doctor reviews the data, he added. The AI can filter the slides and guide us to the right topic, so people can judge what is important and what is not. This increases the efficiency of the pathologist's work and increases the value of the time he spends on each case.

- **Transporting intellect to medical devices and machineries:** Smart devices are taking over the consumer environment, offering everything from real-time video from inside a refrigerator to cars that can tell when the driver is distracted. In the medical environment, intelligent devices are critical to monitoring patients in the intensive care unit and elsewhere. Artificial intelligence to improve the ability to detect deterioration, suggest sepsis is prevalent, or believe that developing complications can significantly improve outcomes and reduce costs associated with penalties for hospital-acquired illness. "Integrate the health system and generate an alert urging an intensive care doctor to intervene from the start; Aggregating this data is not something a human is very good at, "said Mark Michalski, MD, executive director of the MGH and BWH Centre for Clinical Data Science. Putting intelligent algorithms into these devices can reduce the cognitive burden on clinicians while at the same time ensuring that patient care is as prompt as possible.

- **Progressing the usage of immunotherapy for cancer handling:** Immunotherapy is one of the most promising ways to treat cancer. By using the body's immune system to fight malignancy, patients can defeat stubborn tumours. However, few patients respond to current immunotherapy options, and oncologists still do. The system doesn't have an accurate and reliable way to determine which patients will benefit from this option. Machine learning algorithms and their ability to synthesize highly complex data sets can open up new options for tailoring therapies to an individual's unique genetic makeup. "One exciting development has been checkpoint inhibitors, which block some proteins sometimes made by immune cells, " said Long Le, MD, PhD, director of Computational Pathology and Technology Development at the MGH Centre for Integrated Diagnostics. It could not understand the whole biology of the disease. This is a very complex problem. This system definitely need more patient data. Because it is relatively new, not many patients have received these drugs. Therefore, if the system need to integrate data within a facility or between multiple facilities, this will be a key factor in increasing the patient population to drive the modelling process forward.

- **Revolving the electronic health record into a dependable risk forecaster:** Electronic health records are a gold mine for patient data, but extracting and analysing this vast amount of data accurately, timely and reliably is a constant challenge for vendors and developers. Unstructured records and incomplete records have made it very difficult to understand exactly how to perform meaningful risk stratification, predictive analysis and clinical decision support. "Part of the hard work is getting the data in one place," noted Dr. Ziad Obermeyer, assistant professor for emergency medicine at BWH and assistant professor at HMS. But another problem is understanding what the diseases are predicting in an EHR. "An algorithm can predict depression or stroke, but if people can scratch the surface, also find that what they actually predict is a stroke billing code, offering a more specific set of data," like the clinician continued . But now it's time to think about who can and can't pay for MRI. It can predict the billing of a stroke in humans, which can pay for a diagnosis instead of a kind of cerebral ischemia.

- **Auditing health through wearables and individual devices:** Almost all consumers now have access to devices with sensors that can collect valuable data about their health. From smartphones with pedometers to portable devices that can track heartbeats throughout the day, an increasing amount of health-related data is generated on the go. This data, supplemented with information provided by the patient through apps and other home monitoring devices, can offer a unique perspective on the health of individuals and the public. Artificial intelligence will play an important role in extracting usable information from this vast and diverse wealth of data. Helping patients become comfortable sharing data from this intimate and ongoing monitoring may require a little extra work, says Omar Arnaout, MD, co-director of the Computation Neuroscience Outcomes Centre and assistant neurosurgeon at BWH. But when things like Cambridge Analytica and Facebook invade the collective consciousness, people become more and more cautious about who they share what type of data with. Because the people attention is very episodic and the data. By continuously collecting granular data, there is a greater chance that the data will help us better care for patients.

- **Manufacturing smartphone selfies into powerful analytic tools:** Continuing the topic of harnessing the power of wearable devices, experts believe that consumer-grade images from smartphones and other sources will be an important addition to obtaining clinical-quality images, especially in underserved populations or in developing countries and can generate images suitable for analysis with artificial intelligence algorithms. Dermatology and ophthalmology are the first to benefit from this trend. Researchers in the UK have even developed a tool that identifies developmental diseases by analysing images of a child's face. Detect normal features such as a child's jaw line, the position of the eyes and nose, and other features that could indicate a craniofacial abnormality. Currently, the tool can match common images to more than 90 disturbances to aid clinical decision-making. The population is armed with powerful, pocket-sized devices that have many built-in sensors, said HadiShafiee, PhD, director of the Laboratory for Micro / Nanomedicine and Digital Health at BWH. This is a great opportunity for us. Almost everyone is great, A player in the industry has started developing artificial intelligence software and hardware on its devices, and it's no coincidence. Every day in our digital world, we create more than 2.5 million data terabytes.

- **Transforming clinical decision construction with artificial intelligence at the bedside:** As the healthcare industry moves away from charging for services, it moves further away from reactive care. Staying one step ahead of chronic illness, costly acute events, and sudden deterioration is the goal of all providers, and the reimbursement structures ultimately enable them to be successful. The processes that enable proactive and predictive interventions Artificial intelligence will form much of the foundation for this evolution by driving predictive analytics and clinical decision support tools that cause providers to pose problems long before they realize the need. Above are the warnings for conditions like seizures or sepsis, which often require intensive analysis of highly complex data sets. Machine learning can also help support decisions about whether to continue caring for critically ill patients, such as those who have fallen into a coma after cardiac arrest, says Brandon Westover, MD, PhD, director of the MGH Clinical Data Animation Centre in General these patients' EEG data will be checked visually, he explained. The procedure is time-consuming and particular, and the results may vary depending on the skills and understanding of the specific practitioner. "With these patients, trends can develop slowly. Sometimes when we see someone is recovering, we take data from ten seconds of monitoring at a time. But trying to see if they changed from data from ten seconds to 24 hours is like seeing if they have changed "Your hair will grow longer." However, if the AI algorithm and many and many data from many patients, it's easier to match long-term patterns and subtle improvements that affect clinical care decisions.

APPLICATIONS OF BIG DATA IN HEALTHCARE INDUSTRY

Fighting the Flu

The flu is an widespread which can break out at any time and spread in a rapid period of time. Each year the flu kills millions around the world. "Centres for Disease Control and Prevention" (CDC), an operational element of the US Health Department, combats disease, controls and prevents it. CDC receives 700,000 big data medical patient reports with flu indications every week. Health care providers, hospitals and laboratories transmit a bulky amount of information to the CDC. The reports embrace where and what category of treatment the doctor received. Big data analysis has been hugely useful in extracting scientific information from data which has been accumulated over time. CDC published the evidence on Flu View, an application enhanced and implemented at CDC . Flu View descriptions in real time how the influenza is scattering and in what way vaccines and antivirals can help patients, etc. It offers clinicians answers they need to effectually fight the outbreak, such as expressive which vaccine is effective for which straining of the virus, and whether antiviral drugs are effective in retrieval. The pandemic data is "FluNearYou" and "GermTracker". FluNearYou prompts the person to enter data on their symptoms; According to the symptoms, the application creates a map which allows consumers to make and take protective measures against infection. Germ Tracker yields statistics from social media posts and analyses it to detect the onset of the disease. The enormous amount of data acquired offers a vision of a pandemic, which the doctors may have overlooked.

Diabetes Associated with Big Data

Recently Diabetes are one of the biggest health problems in the globe. Utmost people are diagnosed with type 2 diabetes, a condition in which the body might not use insulin efficiently. Like these cases, patients are given insulin injections monitoring the blood sugar levels. By regularly observing the patient's sugar levels along with giving more insulin depending on the situation. To control diabetes and improve patient health, Common Sensing established the smart insulin pen cap technology called GoCap. Injection needle from a typical insulin pen and units the insulin volume in the pen. Go Cap records the time, sum and category of insulin in the logbook and directs the statistics to the mobile devices of clinicians and relatives via the Internet. Moreover it is displayed and registered in the mobile device application. The Go Cap mobile app helps patients enter information about their food intake and glucose levels at different times of the day. This collected data about patients assists doctors to suggest their patients personalized medical care.

Fight Cancer

Cancer treatment in big data is a collection of data gathered from cancer patients at numerous medical treatment stages such as "pre-detection, pre-treatment and end-stage". These facts can be utilized effectively in predicting cancer for new cases. The learning procedure can perceive cancer. Flatiron health has enhanced an oncology cloud service called OncoCloud, which aims to collect statistics at the time of diagnosis and treatment and make it obtainable to the investigator for further studies. The treatment program is the Cancer Moonshot Program. Cancer is caused by genetic changes, and genomic information is often required for threptic treatment, and its background. The valuable information which can be gleaned from this data will assistance to recognize the genetic changes which have caused cancer in a patient and the method of treatment. Big data, made up of millions of comprehensible and serviceable samples, would enable scientists around the globe to analyse and manipulate the data. Data sharing is essential for the medical investigator to have a wealth of data on cancer patient recovery and treatment plans.

Improved Diagnosis and Treatment

Big data plays a fundamental vital role in the healthcare industry. The big data application includes the analysis of the clinical picture and expects outbreaks. In addition, it enables public health surveillance and epidemic pursuing, and assists doctors and health policymakers avoid imminent outbreaks. The data enables the physician to efficiently record the patient's medical history, thus enabling physicians to provide adequate healthcare to their patients. In addition, the data information enables doctors to carry out diagnoses and patient treatments remotely via the Internet. Contact the doctors, and they will advise you in a minute. Activating the IoT helps monitor the patient and generate alerts in real time. Big data assists together with sick as well as healthy patients join doctors to enhance health and treatment.

Handling Opioid Abuse

Opioid exploitation is frequently described as a novel "epidemic" in the globe. More than 15,000 patients die each year from pain medicine and numerous thousand dies from drug overdose or abuse. Pain relievers are a sensitive area for doctors; Based on the individual's capability, doctors proscribe the prescription of opioids above specific threshold. By overlooking the given medicine and its dosages, patients abuse their medication intake and often abuse it in what is known as substance abuse. The abuse is shared between the patient himself and the health system. To stop this, surveillance programs have been instituted in the United States which include maintaining a central database of data analysis and a decision-making system which detects prescription irregularities, monitors drug delivery patterns, and prevents the patient from taking dangerous levels of opioids, "Electronic Prescription for Controlled Substances" (EPCS) is a standard practice which has supported contain the opioid epidemic by allowing doctors to electronically prescribe drugs which can be shared and observed anywhere.

Precision Medicine

The EHR is an important prevention in clinical field, that generates more big data. The EHR includes details about socio demographic, medical, and genetic treatments which enable scientists and doctors to more precisely predict a patient's suffering and other causes for precision medicine. Approaches based on the patient's genetic makeup, lifestyle and environmental features which work successfully for a person. Doctors are often misinformed with immediate diagnosis (for emergencies) and symptomatic treatment. It can get the context of the patient. This information would be used to make precise inflexible decisions.

Evidence-Based Medicine

"Evidence-based medicine" (EBM) is a standard form of medication worldwide. Clinical studies on diseases or methods of treating complaints involve rigorous experiments on patients and involve risks. Evidence of drugs is frequently problematic to generalize. Clinical study procedures and regularly the positive assessment result. In a trivial group of people, it may not effort in the external world. Big data assists EBM classify and categorize actual clinical methods which are used on real patients. By extracting clinical data based on actual patient practice, it is easy to determine which patient received which treatment, how well the treatment worked, or had side effects. The statistics can be analysed at the discrete level to generate a patient model which can be amassed across the population to provide broader knowledge of disease prevalence, treatment patterns, etc. Clinicians relate the symptoms to a larger patient database and identify the exact sickness earlier and more efficiently.

Genomic Analytics

With advances in big data analysis, researchers are gaining a fascinating new perspective on the human genome. Since genes are about statistics, big data is a faultless fit for genetics. Researchers can take a closer look at mankind genes and apply big data. Data analysis in this problem, A distinctive human genome comprises more than 20,000 genes and mapping a genome requires 100 gigabytes of data. Multiple genome sequencing and gene interaction tracking multiplies the number many times over. Plentiful of the work with the human genome and Big Data Analytics is closely related to health and medicine. One of the breakthrough applications of genetics and big data is in the development of personalized drugs and new drugs. Genetic analysis could help find heritable traits which can be transferred on to the next generation. This is especially significant for people who are prone to transmitting diseases such as diabetes, anaemia, heart disease, cancer, obesity, etc. to their children. Bigdata analytics assist the researchers understand the human genome and can provide insights into future diseases.

Clinical Operations

Big data, which accumulates a huge quantity of clinical statistics from numerous environments, can support operate in clinical processes. Its assistances improve health facility operations, the quality of clinical trials, and research. Big data has transformed the way investigators think from hypothesis-based health-care to research-based analysis of a huge quantity of data, subsequent in an accurate technique of treatment.

Patient Monitoring

The widespread implementation of EPAs in hospitals and health centre has supplemented big data. The big data offers in-depth clinical information and understanding of diseases and conditions. Numerous sensors are used for patient monitoring in demand to record vital patient statistics such as blood pressure, heartbeat, breathing, blood oxygen, sugar level, etc. All changes to the data pattern are analysed together with big data, and additional warnings for preventive procedures are generated. Big data uses the patient's previous medical knowledge, analyses current statistics in order to predict upcoming medical complications and complaints.

Medical Device and Pharma Supply-Chain Management

The proper operational of hospitals and clinics is of the utmost importance The availability of medical devices and drugs in sufficient quantities Many hospitals fail to implement the right strategies for the supply chain, which costs hospitals in terms of poor service Non-standard assembling methods and unnecessary products can affect the supply chain it's not just about the product, but also about the persons who buy, change and use it The implementation of automation tools and big data analysis makes managing the supply chain much easier. Apply more time providing quality care and less time looking for product availability. Technologies like RFID (Radio Frequency Identification) have been used to track products. The date and date it was shipped so which suppliers can track the item throughout its lifecycle. The prediction of the number and type of patient and the needed consumables make it possible to keep the inventory at an optimal level. In the case of stocks, the fill level reduces the automatic warehouse gathering is done.

Drug Discovery and Development Analysis

Drug research necessitates the dispensation and analysis of structured and unstructured biomedical data gained from numerous surveys and experimentations, including gene sequencing data, protein communication data, drug data, electronic health records and clinical studies, data from self-reports, etc. A variety of different domains has emerged throughout the Time, enriches the medical information base. The pharmaceutical company uses analysis of this data as it develops a new drug or conducts a clinical trial to derive knowledge and create a predictive model for the design of new drugs. Previous data have accelerated drug discovery and development compared to the traditional method.

Big Data for Personalised Healthcare

Genomic technologies are developing rapidly. With large domain of data, it is easier for healthcare professionals to comprehend the mechanisms underlying disease which lead to better treatment for patients. Many diseases have avoidable risk influences. The doctor takes the patient's medical history, performs the physical exam, and laboratory tests to identify future disease risk, and applying big data in this direction makes the process quick and easy. The patient's health and medical profile provides a personalized medical vision that is specific to a patient. The personalized treatment profile is derived not only from the individual patient's electronic medical report, but also from other similar types of patient records. Profiling, Disease Management Plans, and Health Plan for an Individual Patient.

Infection Prevention, Prediction, and Control

According to the European Centre for Disease Prevention and Control, an assessed 100,000 people become diseased with hospital infections (HAIs) each year and an estimated 37,000 persons die each year as a direct result of infection. Guiding principle which can minimalize the risk of dispersal infection. Some guidelines are easy to follow and others are difficult to implement due to limited technology. In this direction, big data technology integrates genomics with epidemiological data in order not only to control, but also to prevent and consider the possibility of infections spreading within hospitals and clinics.

Health Insurance Fraud Detection

Health care fraud is a major problematic around the world. Over the past decade, the healthcare industry has consumed billions of dollars on improper claims. Supplementary than 1.5 million people have been victims. These information signify stoppable health care costs. The health industry uses analytical controls throughout the treatment process and also includes the damage review process. The review process includes rule-based data analysis and predictive modelling. The treatment process performed and the patient's medication administered are analysed for symptom cases to determine whether the treatment and drug used are legitimate based on the context or to a vague one (Flores, 2013).

LIMITATIONS AND SOLUTIONS

Every entity has its own challenges and limitations. These limitations are the obstacle of the efficiency of those entities. To improve the efficiency of an enterprise or an organisation or a company one need to find out the remedies and the solutions for these limits. The below figure - 5 illustrates some limitations.

Figure 5. Illustration of the major limitations faced in AI and Big data in the healthcare industry

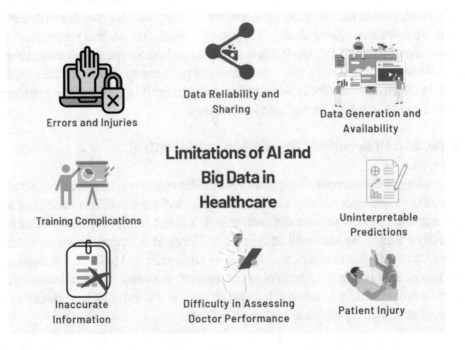

1. **Errors and injuries**: The major issue which the AI systems is it might give be incorrect healthcare solutions which intern lead to patient injury. When errors occur in the system, the system may recommend wrong precautions and remedies to the patients. When this error occurs in the system, it creates an injury to the patients. The main reason of error occurrence is lack of cross checking and inaccuracy. Thus the errors and injuries can be reduced by cross checking the systems and also one can get approval from a doctor before using the drugs or following the remedies.

2. **Data reliability and sharing**: Data reliability is one of the most severe problems experienced in healthcare industry while implementing big data. The healthcare industry will definitely have a huge amount of data, simultaneously this data must be reliable and must be capable of sharing. At the time of sharing the data must possess confidentiality. All person cannot access the data, there should be a proper surveillance on authentication if not those data will be vulnerable to everyone. To overcome this problematic scenario, one need to implement strong authentication methods.

3. **Data generation and availability**: In healthcare dataset there will be lots and lots of electronic health records. As the dataset involves it is another issue in big data in healthcare industry, which is the confidentiality of the patients. Guaranteeing active confidentiality protections for these bulky measured datasets will be expected to be crucial to ensure the patient belief and contribution.

4. **Uninterpretable predictions**:It is not possible to understand the predictions is one of the core problems in the healthcare industry in AI systems. Analysing a predictive data is very important because "Prevention is better than cure". Without a prediction the analysis is incomplete. And the health providers must be in a position which one should be able to identify the problems. Providing medical education for healthcare providers is an apt solution for the uninterpretable predictions.

5. **Patient injury**: The AI system and big data is implemented for the ease of the patients. What if these patients are getting hurt by these technologies? it will definitely make a drastic change in the efficiency of the AI system. The patient injury is caused due to the least performance in the quality checking. One must check the quality of the services available in the AI systems. To overcome the issue of patient injury is to oversight the quality.

6. **Difficulty in assessing doctor performance**: These AI systems are meant to ease the patients and to predict the diseases and treat them as soon as possible. For the AI system it is not easy to assess the performance of the doctor. Although assessing the doctor performance is an essential procedure in healthcare industry because only these assessments can help the efficiency

of the AI systems and the human welfare. There exist a solution to assess the performance is to carefully track the performance of the healthcare providers.

7. **Inaccurate information**:Information plays a vital role in healthcare industry. When the provided information goes wrong the healthcare services also reduces the effectiveness. The information is provided by the patients and there might occur duplication of data, approximate values, wrong prediction of diseases etc., These kinds of issues can be rectified by double checking every bit of data. The checking is not quite simple work because is really very hard to find the faults from a huge set of data. It is better to enter accurate data before every implementation.

8. **Training complications**: There are numerous initial issues which give a scope to arise training complications such as less amount of training data, poor quality of data, inaccuracy in data etc., Before performing any procedures with AI system, those must be trained properly else it will become a dangerous boon to the healthcare systems. Many algorithms are used to train the AI systems if the trainers did not use an appropriate algorithm, it becomes complicated. To avoid training complications one must improve the strength of training algorithms.

CONCLUSION

The healthcare industry is very essential field for every human being. The healthcare industry will be having a huge amount of data in connection with patient records such as patient age, gender, disease, symptoms, remedies, medicines, dosage, doctor details, period of the disease, cause of disease etc. There are lots and lots of data related to the patient as well as diseases. These data must be kept safe somewhere. Not only keeping it safe but also it must be in a state which if an indusial need certain information about any disease or the analysis reports, those data must possess the feature of availability.

There are many applications available for big data analytics like Apache spark, Cassandra, Talend, Hadoop, Mango DB etc., Although there are lot more ways to handle this bulk quantity of data, still there arises the challenges and threat to the tools. Some of the threats are errors and injuries, data sharing, data generation, training complications, Uninterruptable predictions, Inaccurate information, patient injury, Difficulty in assessing doctor performance etc., These issues can solved to an extend with some more procedures and algorithms(Shah, S, 2016).

The main issue with the AI system is going to arise when the AI system performs surgeries and if a small error occurs the whole procedure might go wrong. The failure of these system might also lead to the death of a patient because AI systems are trained by humans and it does not have a capability to change the decisions according to the changing situations.

REFERENCES

Chadwick, R. (2017). What's in a Name: Conceptions of Personalized Medicine and Their Ethical Implications. *LatoSensu. Revue de La Société de Philosophie Des Sciences*, *4*(2), 5–11. doi:10.20416/lsrsps.v4i2.893

Committee on the Review of Omics-Based Tests for Predicting Patient Outcomes in Clinical Trials, Board on Health Care Services, Board on Health Sciences Policy, and Institute of Medicine. (2012). *Evolution of Translational Omics: Lessons Learned and the Path Forward* (C. M. Micheel, S. J. Nass, & G. S. Omenn, Eds.). National Academies Press. doi:10.17226/13297

Flores, Glusman, & Brogaard, Price, & Hood. (2013). P4 Medicine: How Systems Medicine Will Transform the Healthcare Sector and Society. *Personalized Medicine*, *10*(6), 565–576. doi:10.2217/pme.13.57

Haynes, R. B., & Goodman, S. N. (2015). An Interview with David Sackett, 2014–2015. *Clinical Trials. Journal of the Society for Clinical Trials*, *12*(5), 540–551. doi:10.1177/1740774515597895

Jorland, G., Opinel, A., & Weisz, G. (Eds.). (2005). Body Counts: Medical Quantification in Historical and Sociological Perspective [La Quantification Medicale, Perspectives Historiques et Sociologiques]. McGill Queen's University Press.

Latonero, M. (2018, Oct.). Governing artificial intelligence: Upholding human rights & dignity. *Data & Society*.

Marks, H. M. (2000). The Progress of Experiment: Science and Therapeutic Reform in the United States, 1900–1990. In Cambridge History of Medicine. Cambridge Univ. Press.

Mian, M., Teredesai, A., Hazel, D., Pokuri, S., & Uppala, K. (2014). In-Memory Analysis for Healthcare Big Data. *IEEE International Congress on Big Data*.

NITRD (Networking and Information Technology Research and Development), National Coordination Office (NC), & National Science Foundation. (2019). Notice of Workshop on Artificial Intelligence & Wireless Spectrum: Opportunities and Challenges. Notice of workshop. *Federal Register*, *84*(145), 36625–36626.

Pramanik, P. K. D., & Choudhury, P. (2018). IoT Data Processing: The Different Archetypes and their Security & Privacy Assessments. In *Internet of Things (IoT) Security: Fundamentals, Techniques and Applications*. River Publishers. doi:10.4018/978-1-5225-4044-1.ch007

Shah, S. (2016, February 18). *Why patient engagement is so challenging to achieve*. Retrieved August 2, 2018, from https://www.ibmbigdatahub.com/blog/why-patient-engagement-so-challenging-achieve

United Healthcare uses Hadoop to Detect Health Care Fraud, Waste and Abuse. (2018). Retrieved April 20, 2018, from https://mapr.com/customers/unitedhealthcare/

White House. (2019). Executive Order on Maintaining American Leadership in Artificial Intelligence. *Executive Orders: Infrastructure & Technology*. https://www.whitehouse.gov/presidential-actions/executive-order-maintaining-american-leadership-a

Wilkinson, M. D., Dumontier, M., Aalbersberg, I. J., Appleton, G., Axton, M., Baak, A., Blomberg, N., Boiten, J. W., da Silva Santos, L. B., Bpeoplene, P. E., & Bouwman, J. (2016). The FAIR Guiding Principles for scientific data management and stewardship. *Scientific Data*, 3.

Chapter 4
A Systematic Review of Fuzzy Logic Applications for the COVID–19 Pandemic

Erman Çakıt

Department of Industrial Engineering, Gazi University, Ankara, Turkey

ABSTRACT

A variety of fuzzy logic approaches have been employed in order to handle uncertainty by examining the capability of fuzzy logic techniques and improve effectiveness in various aspects of the COVID-19 pandemic. After an inclusion-exclusion procedure, a total of 52 articles were chosen from a set of 399 articles. The objectives of this study were 1) to introduce briefly the fuzzy logic concepts, 2) to review the literature, 3) to classify the literature based on the applications of fuzzy logic to COVID-19 pandemic, 4) to emphasize future developments and trends. The application of fuzzy logic includes screening, diagnostics, and forecasting the COVID-19 outbreak. ANFIS approach and its modified models were revealed to be the most commonly employed for estimation of COVID-19 pandemic. Furthermore, the study found that fuzzy decision-making approaches have mostly been used for detection and diagnosis. In this regard, it is anticipated that the findings of this study will provide decison makers with new tools and ideas for combating the COVID-19 epidemic using fuzzy logic.

INTRODUCTION

The severe respiratory illness coronavirus type 2 causes a new coronavirus disease 19, commonly known as COVID-19 (SARS-CoV-2) (Manigandan et al., 2020). Dry

DOI: 10.4018/978-1-7998-9172-7.ch004

cough, loss of smell and taste, fever, exhaustion, and respiratory disease such as shortness of breath are the most typical symptoms of COVID-19 infection (Jalaber et al., 2020). For the identification of coronavirus disease, two types of standard testing are being used: diagnostic tests and antibody tests. These methods are expensive, time-consuming, need particular materials and tools, and are ineffective in providing real positive rates. As a result, established methods for diagnosing and tracking coronavirus disease are ineffective (Pham et al., 2020). Recent research has revealed that fuzzy logic is a viable technique that may be used in a variety of industries, including process industries, agriculture, finance, computing, and healthcare (Liu et al., 2020; Wirtz et al., 2019).

Many issues in real-world applications might be tackled theoretically rather than analytically. However, owing to the complexity, uncertainty, and vast time required for computing, it is not possible to answer some issues theoretically. Different types of uncertainty may be discovered depending on the variable nature of the uncertainty, such as randomness, fuzziness, indistinguishability, and incompleteness. The Covid-19 pandemic is progressing, but concerns among individuals and policymakers continue to grow. This is because Covid-19 is a challenging task in a complicated system. By definition, complex systems are made up of many interconnected parts (Thurner et al., 2018). Such systems are open, dynamically evolving, unpredictable and self-organising (Thurner et al., 2018). Only through understanding complex systems in their totality can they be adequately understood; isolating a component of the system to "solve" it does not result in a solution that works across the system in the long run. Uncertainty, tension, and conflict are inevitable and must be accepted rather than addressed (Greenhalgh and Papoutsi, 2018). In the field of soft computing, many techniques, such as fuzzy logic, have been developed to deal with this ambiguity.

Eddy (1984) suggested about the global Covid 19 pandemic, "Uncertainty creeps into medical practice through every pore. Whether a physician is defining a disease, making a diagnosis, selecting a procedure, observing outcomes, assessing probabilities, assigning preferences, or putting it all together, he (or she) is walking on very slippery terrain". COVID-19 has quickly become a disease associated with unfettered ambiguity in its aetiology and management, for healthcare systems and health professionals who provide care, as well as for patients and their families, who are its ultimate victims. Under these circumstances, conventional approaches may not be able for modeling these relationships effectively and efficiently. A variety of fuzzy logic approaches have been employed in order to handle these circumstances by examining the capability of fuzzy logic techniques and improve effectiveness and efficiency in various aspects of Covid 19 pandemic. Recently, there have been successful applications of fuzzy logic techniques in the area of Covid 19 pandemic. These application areas can be classified as more specifically: disease detection, disease diagnosis and epidemic forecasting. In this framework, this paper aims to: i) to introduce briefly the fuzzy logic concepts, ii) to review the literature, iii) to classify the literature based on the applications of fuzzy logic to COVID-19 pandemic, iv) to emphasize future developments and trends.

The remainder of this article is divided into the following sections. Subsequent to the introduction in Section 1, the research approach and procedure of this study are described in Section 2. The third section gives a quick review of fuzzy logic. The outcomes of this review are presented in Section 4 based on the study objectives and questions. The results based on the study questions are discussed in Section 5. Section 6 concludes with a summary of the findings, limitations, and recommendations for further study.

METHODOLOGY

The research methodology involves reviewing papers for fuzzy logic approaches in the battle against the COVID- 19 outbreak.

Research Questions

The following study questions were extracted based on the aims of this systematic review listed in the abstract and form the basis of this literature review:

- RQ1:What are the published fuzzy logic studies in the domain of COVID- 19 pandemic and how can these be categorized?
- RQ2: What are the existing research gaps and future research opportunities for using fuzzy logic in the battle against the COVID-19 pandemic?

Protocol

The Preferred Reporting Items for Systematic Reviews and Meta-analyses (PRISMA) standards (Moher et al., 2009) were followed during the present literature evaluation. The procedure was developed based on the above-mentioned research topics and the search method given below.

Figure 1. Flowchart for PRISMA (Moher et al., 2009)

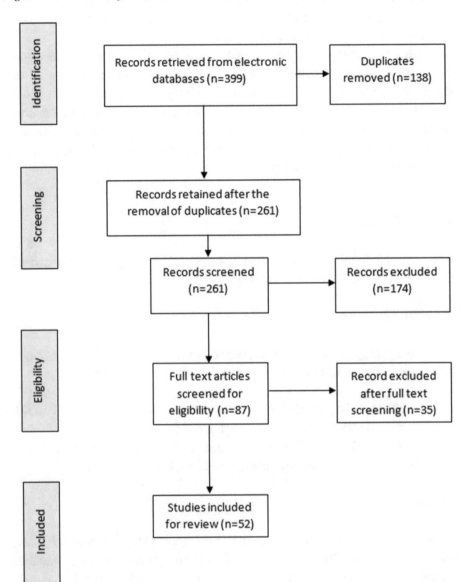

Sources and Search Methods

The literature was searched utilizing different repositories using Boolean operators and defined search phrases, such as ("fuzzy logic" OR "COVID-19") AND ("fuzzy" OR "COVID-19" OR "fuzzy sets" OR "COVID-19"). "Web of Science", "Scopus",

"Engineering Village Compendex", "EBSCO Host", "ProQuest", "PsychINFO", and "Google Scholar" were among the databases examined in this study.

Inclusion and Exclusion Criteria

The following criteria were used to filter identified sources: i) papers were only available in English language, ii) they appeared in peer-reviewed journal publications, iii) they were published until 25ᵗʰ November, 2021 (last search date). Books, book chapters,conference proccedings, and review articles unrelated to the study issues were not included. Visualization of the reviewing procedure is shown in Figure 1.

Study Selection

The search results included 399 articles from the specified databases. The Prisma flowchart in Fig. 1 depicts the article selection process as it progresses through the exclusion-inclusion criteria. The research selection procedure began with the removal of duplicated articles from 399 publications, and a total of 138 were excluded during the first round of screening. Following that, English-language papers were reviewed based on their abstracts and, in certain cases, introductions to determine their compatibility with the exclusion criteria. A total of 174 articles were eliminated at the completion of the second round of the selection process. Thirty-five papers were rejected in round three because more current versions of these publications had been published on the same set of data and addressed the same aim. A total of 52 articles were included in the evaluation after performing the indicated exclusion criteria in three steps. Original research and peer-reviewed journal papers are included in the final selection of articles.

SOFT-COMPUTING TECHNIQUES

Many issues in real-world applications can be solved conceptually rather than analytically. However, because to the complexity, uncertainty, and vast time required for computing, certain issues cannot be solved theoretically. Methods inspired by nature are typically incredibly efficient and successful for these types of challenges. Although the answers obtained by these approaches may not always correspond to mathematically exact solutions, an estimated optimal solution is sometimes sufficient for most practical purposes. Soft computing refers to these biologically inspired approaches.

Zadeh (1994) defined the term soft computing as follows: "Basically, soft computing is not a homogeneous body of concepts and techniques. Rather, it is a partnership of distinct methods that in one way or another conform to its guiding principle. At this juncture, the dominant aim of soft computing is to exploit the tolerance for imprecision, uncertainty, partial truth, and approximation to achieve tractability, robustness, and low solution cost. The principal constituents of soft computing are fuzzy logic, neurocomputing, and probabilistic reasoning, with the latter subsuming genetic algorithms, belief networks, chaotic systems, and parts of learning theory. In the partnership of fuzzy logic, neurocomputing, and probabilistic reasoning, fuzzy logic is mainly concerned with imprecision and approximate reasoning; neurocomputing with learning and curve-fitting; and probabilistic reasoning with uncertainty and belief propagation."

Soft computing techniques basically use numerical data that characterize input-output relationships that support decision making. With these kinds of techniques it is possible to handle imprecision, uncertainty, and complexity in data. These techniques are usually preferred while other traditional approaches may not produce acceptable predicted results. Furthermore, these techniques have some attributes that allow identifying cause and affect relationships in terms of verbal statements and if-then rules. Fuzzy inference systems, evolutionary computation, artificial neural networks, machine learning, and probabilistic reasoning are the fundamental components of soft computing (Figure 2).

Figure 2. Hybrid approaches and the main components of Soft Computing (Adapted from Cordon et al., 2001)

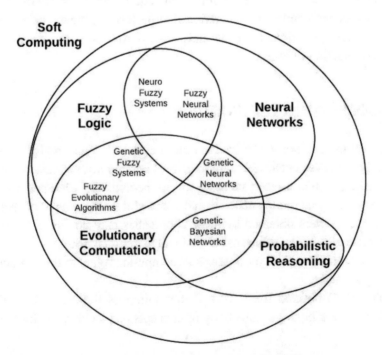

Overview of Fuzzy Set Theory

Lukasiewicz (1920) presented a systematic alternative to Aristotle's bi-valued logic when he developed a three valued logic that may be interpreted as the term "possible" and assigned it a numeric value between "True" and "False" (Fullér, 2000). The notion of infinite-values logic, "fuzzy sets" were introduced by Zadeh (1965) that represent imprecise data and a generalization of classical (crisp) set theory. A fuzzy set is defined by a function that assigns degrees of membership to each element in the set by using a number between 0 and 1 (Ammar and Wright, 2000). Zadeh proposed a language explanation of human thinking (Zadeh, 1968) and a linguistic technique to model complicated and ill-defined systems linked to fuzzy systems (Zadeh, 1973) after publishing the first paper in fuzzy set theory in 1965. (Zadeh, 1965).

Table 1. Comparison of fuzzy sets and crisp sets

Fuzzy Sets	Crisp Sets
The set A can be represented by its membership function: $\mu A : X \rightarrow [0,1]$	The set A can be represented by its characteristic function: $m_A : X \rightarrow \{0,1\}$

As stated in Table 1, the membership of elements in regard to a set is evaluated in binary terms according to a crisp condition in classical set theory. Fuzzy set theory, on the other hand, allows for a progressive assessment of an element's membership in respect to a set, which is represented by a membership function with a real unit interval of [0, 1]. Crisp sets are thus particular instances of fuzzy sets; crisp sets are, in other words, subsets of fuzzy sets.

Fuzzification, database, rulebase, fuzzy inference systems (inference operations), and defuzzification are the five functional blocks of a fuzzy system (Figure 3). In addition, variables for input and output can be provided. Actual numbers are converted into fuzzy sets with linguistic values such as low, medium, and high using a fuzzification interface. A fuzzy rule base is a collection of fuzzy if-then rules that cover all conceivable fuzzy connections between inputs and outputs, as well as a database that describes the membership functions of the fuzzy sets utilized in the fuzzy rules.

Figure 3. Fuzzy system framework

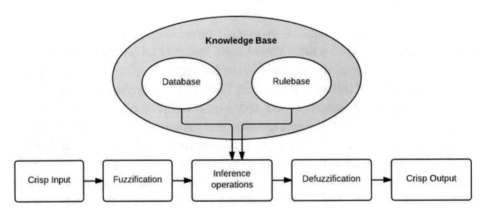

Fuzzy inference systems perform the inference operations through a set of fuzzy rules. This unit performs decision making, which is a critical aspect of the overall system, by constructing appropriate IF-THEN rules. Takagi-Sugeno-Kang (TSK) and Mamdani fuzzy inference systems are two types of fuzzy inference systems that have been widely employed to address issues in a number of applications. For each type of model, the rule aggregation and defuzzification technique differs.

Adaptive Neuro-Fuzzy Inference Systems (ANFIS)

Integrating neural networks with fuzzy systems, sometimes known as neuro-fuzzy systems, is a strong design technique for having both learning and interpretability capabilities in a single system (Zaheeruddun and Garima, 2006). The advantages and characteristics of both systems are combined in this approach (Çakıt and Karwowski, 2017a; Çakıt et al. 2020) (Table 2).

Table 2. Main properties of neural network and fuzzy systems (Adapted from Nauck et al. 1997)

Neural Network	Fuzzy System
"Rule-based knowledge cannot be used"	"Rule-based knowledge can be used"
"Different learning algorithms available"	"Cannot learn"
COMPLEMENTARY	

A neuro-fuzzy system's aim is to identify the parameters of a fuzzy system using learning methods acquired from neural networks, and depending on the application type, there are numerous approaches to integrating ANNs and Fuzzy Inference Systems (FISs) (Nauck et al., 1997). For example, Jang's ANFIS model may be used to build a set of fuzzy if-then rules with appropriate membership functions to generate the input-output pairs needed (Jang, 1993). ANFIS has been applied by several authors in different areas, especially for prediction purpose. The results of most of the studies demonstrate that ANFIS is an alternative method to traditional statistical methods for the estimation purpose. ANFIS can handle complicated, ill-defined, and nonlinear problems because it combines neural networks and fuzzy logic (Çakıt et al., 2014; Çakıt and Karwowski, 2017b). Even if the objectives aren't specified, ANFIS may be able to achieve the best outcome quickly. number of rules. The architecture of ANFIS is made up of five layers, each with the same number of neurons as the number of rules.

Figure 4. ANFIS architecture

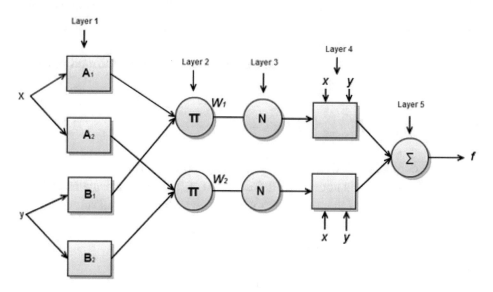

The number of rules is equal to the number of neurons in each layer of ANFIS' design (Figure 4). For simplicity, a FIS with two inputs and one output is used as an example. Rule sets can be defined using the first-order Sugeno fuzzy model as follows:

Rule 1: If "x" is "A_1" and "y" is "B_1" then $z_1 = p_1 x + q_1 y + r_1$
Rule 2: If "x" is "A_2" and "y" is "B_2" then $z_2 = p_2 x + q_2 y + r_2$

Where x and y are non-fuzzy inputs, A_i and B_i are fuzzy sets, z_i is the output value; p_i, q_i and r_i are the consequent parameters that are determined during the training process. As illustrated in Figure 1, ANFIS structure has five layers and each layer is described as follows (Jang, 1993):

Layer 1: This layer is the fuzzification layer which contains membership functions. $O_{1,i}$ represents the output of node i in layer l (Eq. 1). Every node i in layer 1 is an adaptive unit with a function given by:

$$O_{1,i} = \mu_{A_i}(x), \text{ for } i = 1, 2, \text{ or} \tag{1}$$

$$O_{1,i} = \mu_{B_{i-2}}(y), \text{ for } i = 3, 4,$$

where x and y are input values to node i and A_i and B_{i-2} are linguistic variables (such as old, young) associated with this node. Any fuzzy membership function can be used for A and B in this case.

Layer 2: Every node in this layer is labeled Đ which indicates the multiplication of incoming inputs (Eq. 2):

$$O_{2,i} = w_i = \mu_{A_i}(x) \times \mu_{B_i}(y), i = 1, 2. \tag{2}$$

Each node output is called firing strengths (weights) of the rules.

Layer 3: This layer's nodes are all designated N. This layer calculates the ratio of the firing strength of the ith rule to the total firing strength of all rules (Eq. 3):

$$O_{3,i} = \bar{w}_i = \frac{w_i}{w_1 + w_2}, i = 1, 2 \tag{3}$$

Layer 4: This layer has linear functions in each node (Eq. 4):

$$O_{4,i} = \bar{w}_i f_i = \bar{w}_i (p_i x + q_i y + r_i) \tag{4}$$

where $\bar{w}_i$ is an output from layer 3 and $\{p_i, q_i, r_i\}$ are the consequent parameters set.

Layer 5: There is a single node designated å in this layer that combines the entire output as the sum of all incoming signals (Eq. 5):

$$O_{5,i} = overall \ output = \sum_i \overline{w}_i f_i = \frac{\sum_i w_i f_i}{\sum_i w_i} \tag{5}$$

PREDICTING THE SPREAD OF THE INFECTION

The capacity to foresee the progress of the COVID-19 pandemic is a key strategy for limiting the transmission of virus. This would guarantee that specific preventative steps are implemented. Using fuzzy logic, researchers from many nations have developed models and recommendations to anticipate the spread of COVID-19. We found 22 papers that attempted to forecast the COVID-19 pandemic trend (Table 3). Twelve of these research employed the ANFIS model in combination with other models to forecast COVID-19 incidence, confirmed cases, fatalities and recoveries, development trend, and likely stopping time.

Based on previously confirmed cases, Al-qaness et al. (2020a) developed a flower pollination method utilizing the salp swarm algorithm (FPASSA) with ANFIS to estimate the number of confirmed cases of COVID-19 in the next ten days. The authors compared the FPASSA-ANFIS model with several existing models, and it showed better accuracy in terms of performance metrics. Similarly, Al-qaness et al. (2020b) used an enhanced version of the ANFIS model to estimate the number of persons infected in four countries: Italy, Iran, Korea, and the United States. The suggested model's evaluation was carried out by comparing it to several existing forecasting models. The results revealed that using time-series data, the suggested ANFIS model could predict the number of instances.

Alsayed et al. (2020) used the Genetic Algorithm with ANFIS model to offer short-term forecasting of the number of infected patients, and the authors concluded with a high prediction accuracy. Saif et al. (2021) suggested a mutation-based Bees Algorithm (mBA) with an ANFIS model for the COVID-19 epidemic dataset for India and the United States, and anticipated the number of confirmed cases in India over the following ten days. Pinter et al. (2020) used ANFIS and a multi-layered perceptron-imperialist competitive algorithm (MLP-ICA) to forecast infected persons and death rates in Hungary. To investigate the death rate of the highly contagious COVID-19, Mangla et al. (2021) used a rule-based model under the Mamdani-based fuzzy expert system (FES). The findings obtained by the proposed model were encouraging, implying that the proposed approach is effective. In Wuhan, Hubei Province, China, Hao et al. (2020) conducted a trend analysis of cumulative confirmed cases, cumulative deaths, and cumulative cured cases. The growth range of confirmed cases, fatalities, and cured patients was forecasted using an SVM with fuzzy granulation.

Ardabili et al. (2020) used soft computing techniques to estimate the COVID-19 pandemic in addition to SIR and SEIR models. ANFIS outperformed a wide range of soft-computing approaches in terms of performance. Vedaei et al. (2020) performed the Fuzzy Mamdani system to estimate the risk of infection spreading in real time by taking into account environmental risk and user health status. Aabed and Lashin (2021) performed a fuzzy logic model to forecast the impact of factors on the pace of COVID-19 viral spread in Italy, Spain, and China.

To forecast COVID-19 cases, Zivkovic et al. (2020) suggested a hybrid technique combining machine learning, ANFIS, and augmented beetle antennae search swarm intelligence metaheuristics. According to the comparison study, the suggested hybrid technique outperformed more advanced algorithms evaluated on the same datasets and proved to be a helpful tool for time-series prediction. Chowdhury et al. (2021) used ANFIS and LSTM to forecast newly infected patients in Bangladesh. The authors concluded that LSTM achieved more accurate results. Melin et al. (2021) introduced the firefly algorithm for ensemble neural network optimization in a weighted average integration technique for COVID-19 time series prediction with type-2 fuzzy logic.

Castillo and Melin (2020) suggested a hybrid intelligent technique that integrates fractal theory and fuzzy logic to estimate COVID-19 time series. Al-Qaness et al. (2021) suggested a novel short-term forecasting model based on an improved ANFIS. To improve the ANFIS and prevent its shortcomings, the authors used an upgraded marine predators algorithm (MPA) termed chaoticMPA (CMPA). Kumar and Susan (2021) used the Particle Swarm Optimization (PSO) technique to optimize the number and duration of intervals, as well as the fuzzy order, for fuzzy time series forecasting of the COVID-19. Ly (2021) developed an ANFIS model to predict the number of COVID-19 cases in the UK. The author recommended that policymakers use the ANFIS model to estimate the COVID-19 pandemic's spreading effect. Mydukuri et al. (2021) proposed a new technique termed least square regressive Gaussian neuro-fuzzy multi-layered data classification (LSRGNFM-LDC) technique to estimate the COVID prediction with better accuracy. For both short- and long-term projections of the experimental data, Alkhammash et al. (2021) used compartmental models such as SIR and SEIRD, as well as ANFIS models. According to the results, ANFIS-based models outperformed compartmental models.

According to the criteria for COVID-19 patients from diverse areas of India, Sharma et al. (2021) performed a mediative fuzzy correlation approach. The proposed prediction approach showed promising results in India for continuous conflicting prediction. Razavi-Termeh et al. (2021) monitored the COVID-19 disease in Iran by using geographic information system (GIS) and applied ANFIS model to predict vulnerability in the next two months. Dos Santos Gomes et al. (2021) used interval type-2 fuzzy systems to anticipate the dynamic spread behavior of the COVID-19 epidemic in Brazil in real time. The findings of these investigations may have much further implications by assisting in the control and prevention of COVID-19.

Table 3. Application of fuzzy logic for estimating the epidemic trend and prognosis of COVID-19

References	Methodology	Aim	Country
Al-qaness et al. (2020a)	FPASSA- ANFIS	Estimate the number of confirmed cases	China
Al-qaness et al. (2020b)	ANFIS	Estimate the number of infected people	Italy, Iran, Korea, and the USA
Alsayed et al. (2020)	GA with ANFIS	Predict the infection rate	Malaysia
Saif et al. (2021)	(mBA) with ANFIS	Forecast the number of confirmed cases	India and USA
Pinter et al. (2020)	ANFIS, MLP-ICA	Predict the infection rate	Hungary
Mangla et al. (2021)	FES	Analyze the mortality rate of the highly contagious COVID-19	India
Hao et al. (2020)	SVM with fuzzy granulation	Estimate the number of confirmed cases	China
Ardabili et al. (2020)	ANFIS	Estimate the COVID-19 outbreak	Five countries
Zivkovic et al. (2020)	ANFIS	Predict COVID-19 cases	China
Chowdhury et al. (2021)	ANFIS, LSTM	Predict the newly infected cases	Bangladesh
Castillo and Melin (2020)	Fractal theory and fuzzy logic	Estimate COVID-19 time series	Ten countries
Al-Qaness et al. (2021)	CMPA to enhance the ANFIS	Forecast COVID-19cases in hotspot regions	Russia and Brazil
Kumar and Susan (2021)	FTS, PSO	Forecasting of the COVID-19	Ten countries
Ly (2021)	ANFIS	Forecast the number of COVID-19 cases	United Kingdom
Mydukuri et al. (2021)	LSRGNFM-LDC	Perform the COVID prediction	Worldwide
Alkhammash et al. (2021)	ANFIS	Predict the COVID-19 spread	Saudi Arabia
Sharma et al. (2021)	Mediative fuzzy correlation technique	Estimate the COVID-19 outbreak	India

Continued on following page

Table 3. Continued

References	Methodology	Aim	Country
Razavi-Termeh et al. (2021)	ANFIS	Predict COVID-19 vulnerability	Iran
dos Santos Gomes et al. (2021)	interval type-2 fuzzy systems	Forecast the dynamic spread behavior of COVID-19	Brazil
Vedaei et al. (2020)	Fuzzy Mamdani system	Estimate the risk of infection spreading	Worldwide
Aabed and Lashin (2021)	fuzzy logic	Predict the COVID-19 spread	Italy,Spain, and China.
Melin et al. (2021)	type-2 fuzzy logic	COVID-19 time series prediction	Twenty-six countries

GA, "Genetic Algorithm"; ANFIS, "Adaptive Neuro-Fuzzy Inference System"; LSTM, "Linear regression and long short-term memory"; SVM, "Support Vector Machine"; MLP, "Multilayer perceptron"; FTS, "Fuzzy Time Series"; FPASSA, "Flower Pollination Algorithm Using The Salp Swarm Algorithm"; MLP-ICA, "Multi-Layered Perceptron-Imperialist Competitive Algorithm"; PSO, "Particle Swarm Optimization"; CMPA, "ChaoticMPA"; LSRGNFM-LDC, "Least Square Regressive Gaussian Neuro-Fuzzy Multi-Layered Data Classification"; FES, "Fuzzy Expert System"; mBA, "Mutation-Based Bees Algorithm"

DETECTION AND DIAGNOSIS OF COVID-19

Fuzzy Decision Making Approaches

The number of papers published recently on the identification and diagnosis of COVID-19 using computed tomography scans has increased dramatically. Fourteen papers were found for detection and diaognosis of COVID-19 (Table 4). Adaptive Fuzzy C-means (AFCM) and enhanced Slime Mould Algorithm based on L'evy distribution, specifically AFCM-LSMA, were developed by Anter et al. (2021) to extract high-level characteristics of COVID-19 from chest X-ray images to aid in quick diagnosis. Tuncer et al. (2021) detected COVID- 19 using a novel fuzzy tree classification approach. COVID-19, pneumonia, and normal chest x-ray images were among the datasets used by the researchers. SuFMoFP algorithm was suggested by Chakraborty and Mali (2021a) to segment radiological images for improved explanation of COVID-19 radiological images. The findings obtained are highly good and outperform some of the traditional methodologies, which is encouraging for the practical applications of the suggested methodology to screening COVID-19 patients. Similarly, Chakraborty and Mali (2021b) introduced SUFMACS, a novel unsupervised machine learning-based technique for rapidly interpreting and segmenting COVID-19 radiological images.

Asadi et al. (2021) investigated the factors that might be used to respond to the COVID-19 epidemic in Malaysia, restricting the disease's spread. The authors used a collection of questionnaires filled by health care experts to examine the variables using the DEMATEL and Fuzzy Rule-Based methods. The most critical factors in avoiding the spread of COVID-19 infections, according to the data analysis, were movement control orders, foreign travel restrictions, and mass gathering cancellations.

Global health agencies have suggested a variety of social and physical interventions such as social and physical distancing, outdoor usage of face masks, refraining from excessive travel, sanitation, adequate diet, health monitoring, and so on (Coronavirus Disease situation report, 2020). Researchers from many countries have propsed models and suggestions to prioritize those interventions that are more effective in controlling the spread over others that have less impact. Several preventive strategies impact decision making in this circumstance. For instance, Sayan et al. (2020) used multi-criteria decision-making approaches to assess the COVID-19 diagnostic tests, namely the fuzzy PROMETHEE and the fuzzy TOPSIS. Samanlioglu and Kaya (2020) used a hesitant fuzzy AHP technique to help decision makers, particularly decision makers assess the value of COVID-19 pandemic intervention plan choices used by different nations. Baz and Alhakami (2021) applied Fuzzy Analytic Hierarchy Process (AHP) technique to assess the severity of COVID-19 pandemic in Saudi Arabia. Dutta and Borah (2021) proposed a novel SM for generalized trapezoidal fuzzy numbers. In light of the current COVID-19 epidemic, the authors proved the usefulness and applicability of recommended method by selecting the suitable anti-virus mask.

The q-rung orthopair fuzzy TOPSIS approach was performed by Alkan and Kahraman (2021) to identify government strategies against the COVID-19 pandemic. "Mandatory quarantine and rigorous isolation policy" was the most critical technique that countries should undertake. The integrated fuzzy-based ANP-TOPSIS approach was applied by Ahmed and Alhumam (2021) to assess the impact of COVID-19 on various aspects of human life in Saudi Arabia. Using the fuzzy-analytical hierarchical process (AHP) technique, Upadhyay et al. (2021) identified the major obstacles to social isolation in India during the COVID-19 pandemic. The most significant barrier in social isolation was recognized as dense population.

Using hesitant fuzzy sets, Mishra et al. (2021) looked at the treatment selection dilemma for moderate COVID-19 illness symptoms. The work was separated into two parts: first, the authors developed a novel divergence measure and its features to assess the discrimination for hesitant fuzzy sets. Second, the HF-ARAS technique was proposed, which is a modified hesitant fuzzy ARAS approach. As the COVID-19 outbreak spreads, the incidence of risk factors among healthcare professionals grows at work, posing a major health threat to the vulnerable population. Rathore and Gupta (2020) developed a fuzzy-based hybrid decision-making framework for ranking Indian hospitals based on the incidence of safety risk indicators among health-care employees.

Table 4. Fuzzy decision making approaches for detection and diaognosis of COVID-19

References	Methodology	Aim
Anter et al. (2021)	AFCM-LSMA	Extract high-level characteristics of COVID-19 from chest X-ray images
Tuncer et al. (2021)	Fuzzy tree classification approach	Detect COVID-19
Chakraborty and Mali (2021a)	SuFMoFP algorithm	Segment radiological images
Chakraborty and Mali (2021b)	SUFMACS	Interpret and segment COVID-19 radiological images
Asadi et al. (2021)	DEMATEL and Fuzzy Rule-Based methods	Investigate the factors to avoid the spread of COVID-19
Sayan et al. (2020)	Fuzzy PROMETHEE and the fuzzy TOPSIS	Assess the COVID-19 diagnostic tests
Samanlioglu and Kaya (2020)	Hesitant fuzzy AHP	Assess the value of COVID-19 pandemic intervention plan choices
Baz and Alhakami (2021)	Fuzzy AHP	Assess the severity of COVID-19
Dutta and Borah (2021)	A novel SM approach	Select the suitable anti-virus mask
Alkan and Kahraman (2021)	q-rung orthopair fuzzy TOPSIS	Identify government strategies against the COVID-19 pandemic
Ahmed and Alhumam (2021)	Fuzzy-based ANP-TOPSIS	Assess the impact of COVID-19
Upadhyay et al. (2021)	Fuzzy AHP	Identify the major obstacles to social isolation
Mishra et al. (2021)	Hesitant fuzzy ARAS	Focus on treatment selection dilemma for moderate COVID-19 illness symptoms
Rathore and Gupta (2020)	Hybrid decision-making framework	Rank hospitals based on the incidence of safety risk indicators

AFCM-LSMA, "Adaptive Fuzzy C-means (AFCM) and enhanced Slime Mould Algorithm based on L'evy distribution"; SuFMoFP, "Superpixel based Fuzzy Modified Flower Pollination Algorithm"; SUFMACS, "SUperpixel based Fuzzy Memetic Advanced Cuckoo Search"; DEMATEL, "Decision making trial and evaluation laboratory"; PROMETHEE, "Preference Ranking Organization Method for Enrichment. Evaluation"; TOPSIS, "Technique for Order of Preference by Similarity to Ideal Solution"; AHP, "Analytic Hierarchy Process"; ARAS, "The Additive Ratio ASsessment"

Other Approaches

Sixteen papers were found based on the applications of fuzzy logic techniques in the area of Covid 19 pandemic (Table 5). The impacts of several climate-related parameters and population density on the spread of the COVID-19 were explored by Behnood et al. (2020) by using a combination of the virus optimization algorithm (VOA) and ANFIS. Based on the obtained results, the importance of social distancing was highlighted in reducing the infection rate. Mahmoudi et al. (2020) applied the fuzzy clustering approach to examine the distributions of Covid-19 distributed in the USA, Spain, Italy, Germany, the UK, France, and Iran. The distribution of spreading in Spain and Italy was roughly comparable and different from other nations, according to the clustering data.

The generalized fuzzy weighted assessment approach was presented by Wu et al. (2020) to assess the overall success of an intervention plan for combating the COVID-19 pandemic. To combat the COVID-19 pandemic, the suggested technique was used to compare 15 current intervention options. Majumder et al. (2020) proposed a probabilistic rough fuzzy hybrid model with linguistic information of a COVID-19 susceptible person. Using this method, the authors assessed who was infected and who should be sent for self-isolation, home quarantine, and medical care in an emergency. Chen et al. (2020) suggested a fuzzy collaborative intelligence technique for evaluating a factory's vulnerability to the COVID-19 pandemic. The authors performed the suggested approach to analyze the COVID-19 pandemic resilience of a wafer manufacturing plant in Taiwan. In a fuzzy context, Alderremy et al. (2021) offered a numerical investigation of a fractional mathematical model of COVID-19. Graphs were used by the authors to demonstrate the influence of fractional order on the suspected, exposed, infected, and asymptotic carrier.

Wang et al. (2021) used multi-fuzzy regression discontinuity to investigate data from 212 nations between December 31, 2019 and May 21, 2020. The authors observed that while industrialized nations were less sensitive to the policy stringency index, policy control measures had a substantial impact on epidemic control. With a fuzzy fractional differential equation constructed in Caputo's sense, Ahmad et al.

(2020) developed a new coronavirus infection system. The authors concluded that the proposed approach was successful for addressing the uncertainty condition in the pandemic situation. Rallapalli et al. (2021) suggested a unique fuzzy-based Bayesian model to select targeted people and optimal places with the highest likelihood of detecting the COVID-19 pandemic in wastewater networks. Hassan et al. (2021) used c-FACS to model and analyze daily Covid-19 instances in Malaysia in order to observe the trend and severity of the condition in Malaysia. In addition, the authors classified the severity of zones. The behavior of new daily cases of COVID-19 in Brazil was described using a fuzzy model by Stiegelmeier and Bressan (2021). The infected population and environmental action were the input variables, and the level of infestation was the output variable. The authors concluded that intervention measures played an important role in determining the success of COVID- 19 eradication programs.

Ghosh and Biswas (2021) used a fuzzy inference technique to evaluate the current condition of states and provinces affected by COVID-19. Population density, the number of COVID-19 tests done, verified COVID-19 cases, recovery rate, and death rate are all parameters included in the suggested methodology. Kumar and Kumar (2021) used a modified fuzzy C-means clustering approach to develop a hybrid fuzzy time series model for predicting forthcoming COVID-19 infected cases and fatalities in India. Prabakaran et al. (2021) investigated the process of the outbreak of the COVID-19 epidemic and made recommendations using a fuzzy logic system. According to the key factors associated to the COVID-19 pandemic, D'Urso et al. (2021) suggested a fuzzy clustering model for the 20 Italian regions. Fan et al. (2021) used fuzzy-set Qualitative Comparative Analysis (fsQCA) to determine a different taxonomy of four equally successful configurations of urban acts in stopping COVID-19 transmission in China.

Table 5. Other applications related to fuzzy logic in COVID-19

References	Methodology	Aim
Behnood et al. (2020)	VOA and ANFIS	Explore density on the spread of the COVID-19
Mahmoudi et al. (2020)	Fuzzy clustering approach	Examine the distributions of Covid-19
Wu et al. (2020)	Fuzzy weighted assessment approach	Combat the COVID-19 pandemic
Majumder et al. (2020)	Fuzzy hybrid model	Assess the infection rate

Continued on following page

Table 5. Continued

References	Methodology	Aim
Chen et al. (2020)	Fuzzy collaborative intelligence technique	Evaluate a factory's vulnerability to the COVID-19 pandemic
Alderremy et al. (2021)	Fractional mathematical model	Demonstrate the influence of fractional order on the suspected, exposed, infected, and asymptotic carrier
Wang et al. (2021)	Multi-fuzzy regression	Investigate COVID-19 data from 212 nations
Ahmad et al. (2020)	Fuzzy fractional differential equation	Develop a new coronavirus infection system
Rallapalli et al. (2021)	Fuzzy-based Bayesian model	Select targeted people and optimal places with the highest likelihood of detecting the COVID-19 pandemic
Hassan et al. (2021)	c-FACS	Model and analyze daily Covid-19 instances
Stiegelmeier and Bressan (2021)	A fuzzy model	Describe the behavior of new daily cases of COVID-19
Ghosh and Biswas (2021)	Fuzzy inference technique	Evaluate the current condition of states and provinces affected by COVID-19
Kumar and Kumar (2021)	Fuzzy C-means clustering approach	Predict COVID-19 infected cases and fatalities
Prabakaran et al. (2021)	Fuzzy logic system	Investigate the process of the outbreak of the COVID-19 epidemic
D'Urso et al. (2021)	Fuzzy clustering model	Determine the key factors associated to the COVID-19 pandemic
Fan et al. (2021)	Fuzzy-set Qualitative Comparative Analysis	Determine a different taxonomy of four equally successful configurations of urban acts in stopping COVID-19 transmission

VOA, "Virus optimization algorithm"; c-FACS, "chemometrics fuzzy autocatalytic set"

CONCLUSION

Fuzzy logic is a promising approach that is widely employed in a variety of sectors, including healthcare. This paper has discussed an extensive literature review and applications of fuzzy logic in the domain of COVID-19 pandemic. It was revealed over the course of this study that fuzzy logic applications have been applied to the majority of traditional areas of COVID-19 pandemic, and research in the domain of COVID-19 pandemic has developed in recent years. The application of fuzzy logic includes screening, diagnostics, and forecasting the COVID-19 outbreak.

ANFIS approach and its modified models were revealed to be the most commonly employed for estimation of COVID-19 pandemic. However, several obstacles and limitations are encountered while developing ANFIS -based models due to a lack of huge data and poor data quality. In this context, research groups are working day and night to collect and extract more valuable data from existing sources. Furthermore, our study found that fuzzy decision-making approaches have mostly been used for detection and diagnosis.

The main advantage of the use of the fuzzy logic techniques in the COVID-19 pandemic context is able to accommodate several types of inputs including vague, distorted or imprecise COVID-19 pandemic data. A major drawback of fuzzy logic techniques in the Covid 19 pandemic context is that they are completely dependent on human knowledge and expertise. Another drawback is to regularly update the rules of a fuzzy logic techniques. One significant problem is to bridge the gap between research and effect. There is a lot of study and fresh ideas around establishing new fuzzy logic systems, but seeing them implemented in the real world is another issue. More close collaboration between researchers and practitioners is required. In this regard, it is anticipated that the findings of this study will provide researchers, healthcare organizations, government officials, policymakers, and decison makers with new tools and ideas for combating the COVID-19 epidemic using fuzzy logic. It would be a fundamental review for fuzzy logic researchers to expand on the toolset for the COVID-19 epidemic in future studies.

REFERENCES

Aabed, K., & Lashin, M. M. (2021). An analytical study of the factors that influence COVID-19 spread. *Saudi Journal of Biological Sciences*, *28*(2), 1177–1195. doi:10.1016/j.sjbs.2020.11.067 PMID:33262677

Ahmad, S., Ullah, A., Shah, K., Salahshour, S., Ahmadian, A., & Ciano, T. (2020). Fuzzy fractional-order model of the novel coronavirus. *Advances in Difference Equations*, *2020*(1), 1–17. doi:10.118613662-020-02934-0 PMID:32922446

Ahmed, S., & Alhumam, A. (2021). Analyzing the Implications of COVID-19 Pandemic: Saudi Arabian Perspective. *Intelligent Automation and Soft Computing*, *27*(3), 835–851. doi:10.32604/iasc.2021.015789

Al-Qaness, M. A., Ewees, A. A., Fan, H., & Abd El Aziz, M. (2020a). Optimization method for forecasting confirmed cases of COVID-19 in China. *Journal of Clinical Medicine*, *9*(3), 674. doi:10.3390/jcm9030674 PMID:32131537

Al-Qaness, M. A., Ewees, A. A., Fan, H., Abualigah, L., & Abd Elaziz, M. (2020b). Marine predators algorithm for forecasting confirmed cases of COVID-19 in Italy, USA, Iran and Korea. *International Journal of Environmental Research and Public Health*, *17*(10), 3520. doi:10.3390/ijerph17103520 PMID:32443476

Al-Qaness, M. A., Saba, A. I., Elsheikh, A. H., Abd Elaziz, M., Ibrahim, R. A., Lu, S., ... Ewees, A. A. (2021). Efficient artificial intelligence forecasting models for COVID-19 outbreak in Russia and Brazil. *Process Safety and Environmental Protection*, *149*, 399–409. doi:10.1016/j.psep.2020.11.007 PMID:33204052

Alderremy, A. A., Gómez-Aguilar, J. F., Aly, S., & Saad, K. M. (2021). A fuzzy fractional model of coronavirus (COVID-19) and its study with Legendre spectral method. *Results in Physics*, *21*, 103773. doi:10.1016/j.rinp.2020.103773 PMID:33391986

Alkan, N., & Kahraman, C. (2021). Evaluation of government strategies against COVID-19 pandemic using q-rung orthopair fuzzy TOPSIS method. *Applied Soft Computing*, *110*, 107653. doi:10.1016/j.asoc.2021.107653 PMID:34226821

Alkhammash, H. I., Otaibi, S. A., & Ullah, N. (2021). Short-and long-term predictions of novel corona virus using mathematical modeling and artificial intelligence methods. *International Journal of Modeling, Simulation, and Scientific Computing*, 2150028.

Alsayed, A., Sadir, H., Kamil, R., & Sari, H. (2020). Prediction of epidemic peak and infected cases for COVID-19 disease in Malaysia, 2020. *International Journal of Environmental Research and Public Health*, *17*(11), 4076. doi:10.3390/ijerph17114076 PMID:32521641

Ammar, S., & Wright, R. (2000). Applying fuzzy-set theory to performance evaluation. *Socio-Economic Planning Sciences*, *34*(4), 285–302. doi:10.1016/S0038-0121(00)00004-5

Anter, A. M., Oliva, D., Thakare, A., & Zhang, Z. (2021). AFCM-LSMA: New intelligent model based on Lévy slime mould algorithm and adaptive fuzzy C-means for identification of COVID-19 infection from chest X-ray images. *Advanced Engineering Informatics*, *49*, 101317. doi:10.1016/j.aei.2021.101317

Ardabili, S. F., Mosavi, A., Ghamisi, P., Ferdinand, F., Varkonyi-Koczy, A. R., Reuter, U., Rabczuk, T., & Atkinson, P. M. (2020). Covid-19 outbreak prediction with machine learning. *Algorithms*, *13*(10), 249. doi:10.3390/a13100249

Asadi, S., Nilashi, M., Abumalloh, R. A., Samad, S., Ahani, A., Ghabban, F., ... Supriyanto, E. (2021). Evaluation of Factors to Respond to the COVID-19 Pandemic Using DEMATEL and Fuzzy Rule-Based Techniques. *International Journal of Fuzzy Systems*, 1–17.

Baz, A., & Alhakami, H. (2021). Fuzzy based decision making approach for evaluating the severity of COVID-19 pandemic in cities of kingdom of saudi arabia. *Computers, Materials, & Continua*, 1155-1174.

Behnood, A., Golafshani, E. M., & Hosseini, S. M. (2020). Determinants of the infection rate of the COVID-19 in the US using ANFIS and virus optimization algorithm (VOA). *Chaos, Solitons, and Fractals*, *139*, 110051. doi:10.1016/j.chaos.2020.110051 PMID:32834605

Çakıt, E., & Karwowski, W. (2017). Predicting the occurrence of adverse events using an adaptive neuro-fuzzy inference system (ANFIS) approach with the help of ANFIS input selection. *Artificial Intelligence Review*, *48*(2), 139–155. doi:10.100710462-016-9497-3

Çakıt, E., & Karwowski, W. (2017b). Estimating electromyography responses using an adaptive neuro-fuzzy inference system with subtractive clustering. *Human Factors and Ergonomics in Manufacturing & Service Industries*, *27*(4), 177–186. doi:10.1002/hfm.20701

Çakıt, E., Karwowski, W., Bozkurt, H., Ahram, T., Thompson, W., Mikusinski, P., & Lee, G. (2014). Investigating the relationship between adverse events and infrastructure development in an active war theater using soft computing techniques. *Applied Soft Computing*, *25*, 204–214. doi:10.1016/j.asoc.2014.09.028

Çakıt, E., Karwowski, W., & Servi, L. (2020). Application of soft computing techniques for estimating emotional states expressed in Twitter® time series data. *Neural Computing & Applications*, *32*(8), 3535–3548. doi:10.100700521-019-04048-5

Castillo, O., & Melin, P. (2020). Forecasting of COVID-19 time series for countries in the world based on a hybrid approach combining the fractal dimension and fuzzy logic. *Chaos, Solitons, and Fractals*, *140*, 110242. doi:10.1016/j.chaos.2020.110242 PMID:32863616

Chakraborty, S., & Mali, K. (2021a). SuFMoFPA: A superpixel and meta-heuristic based fuzzy image segmentation approach to explicate COVID-19 radiological images. *Expert Systems with Applications*, *167*, 114142. doi:10.1016/j.eswa.2020.114142 PMID:34924697

Chakraborty, S., & Mali, K. (2021b). SUFMACS: A machine learning-based robust image segmentation framework for covid-19 radiological image interpretation. *Expert Systems with Applications*, *178*, 115069. doi:10.1016/j.eswa.2021.115069 PMID:33897121

Chen, T., Wang, Y. C., & Chiu, M. C. (2020, December). Assessing the robustness of a factory amid the COVID-19 pandemic: A fuzzy collaborative intelligence approach. In Healthcare (Vol. 8, No. 4, p. 481). Multidisciplinary Digital Publishing Institute.

Chowdhury, A. A., Hasan, K. T., & Hoque, K. K. S. (2021). Analysis and Prediction of COVID-19 Pandemic in Bangladesh by Using ANFIS and LSTM Network. *Cognitive Computation*, *13*(3), 761–770. doi:10.100712559-021-09859-0 PMID:33868501

Cordon, O., Herrera, F., Hoffmann, F., & Magdalena, L. (2001). *Genetic Fuzzy Systems: Evolutionary Tuning and Learning of Fuzzy Knowledge Bases. In Advances in Fuzzy Systems - Applications and Theory* (Vol. 19). World Scientific. doi:10.1142/4177

Coronavirus Disease. (COVID-19) situation report – 43. (2020). *World Health Organization*. Available from: https://www.who.int/docs/default-source/coronaviruse/situation-reports/20200303-sitrep-43-covid-19.pdf?sfvrsn=76e425ed_2

D'Urso, P., De Giovanni, L., & Vitale, V. (2021). Spatial robust fuzzy clustering of COVID 19 time series based on B-splines. *Spatial Statistics*, 100518. doi:10.1016/j.spasta.2021.100518 PMID:34026473

dos Santos Gomes, D. C., & de Oliveira Serra, G. L. (2021). Machine Learning Model for Computational Tracking and Forecasting the COVID-19 Dynamic Propagation. *IEEE Journal of Biomedical and Health Informatics*, *25*(3), 615–622. doi:10.1109/JBHI.2021.3052134 PMID:33449891

Dutta, P., & Borah, G. (2021). Multicriteria decision making approach using an efficient novel similarity measure for generalized trapezoidal fuzzy numbers. *Journal of Ambient Intelligence and Humanized Computing*, 1–23. doi:10.100712652-021-03347-x PMID:34178177

Eddy, D. M. (1984). Variations in physician practice: The role of uncertainty. *Health Affairs*, *3*(2), 74–89. doi:10.1377/hlthaff.3.2.74 PMID:6469198

Fan, D., Li, Y., Liu, W., Yue, X. G., & Boustras, G. (2021). Weaving public health and safety nets to respond the COVID-19 pandemic. *Safety Science*, *134*, 105058. doi:10.1016/j.ssci.2020.105058 PMID:33110294

Fullér, R. (1999). *Introduction to Neuro-Fuzzy Systems*. Physica-Verlag.

Ghosh, B., & Biswas, A. (2021). Status evaluation of provinces affected by COVID-19: A qualitative assessment using fuzzy system. *Applied Soft Computing*, *109*, 107540. doi:10.1016/j.asoc.2021.107540 PMID:34093096

Greenhalgh, T., & Papoutsi, C. (2018). *Studying complexity in health services research: Desperately seeking an overdue paradigm shift*. Academic Press.

Hao, Y., Xu, T., Hu, H., Wang, P., & Bai, Y. (2020). Prediction and analysis of corona virus disease 2019. *PLoS One*, *15*(10), e0239960. doi:10.1371/journal.pone.0239960 PMID:33017421

Hassan, N., Ahmad, T., Ashaari, A., Awang, S. R., Mamat, S. S., Mohamad, W. M. W., & Fuad, A. A. A. (2021). A fuzzy graph approach analysis for COVID-19 outbreak. *Results in Physics*, *25*, 104267. doi:10.1016/j.rinp.2021.104267 PMID:33968605

Jalaber, C., Lapotre, T., Morcet-Delattre, T., Ribet, F., Jouneau, S., & Lederlin, M. (2020). Chest CT in COVID-19 pneumonia: A review of current knowledge. *Diagnostic and Interventional Imaging*, *101*(7-8), 431–437. doi:10.1016/j.diii.2020.06.001 PMID:32571748

Jang, J. S. R. (1993). ANFIS: Adaptive-network-based fuzzy inference system. *IEEE Transactions on Systems, Man, and Cybernetics*, *23*(5), 665–685. doi:10.1109/21.256541

Kumar, N., & Kumar, H. (2021). A novel hybrid fuzzy time series model for prediction of COVID-19 infected cases and deaths in India. *ISA Transactions*. Advance online publication. doi:10.1016/j.isatra.2021.07.003 PMID:34253340

Kumar, N., & Susan, S. (2021). Particle swarm optimization of partitions and fuzzy order for fuzzy time series forecasting of COVID-19. *Applied Soft Computing*, *110*, 107611. doi:10.1016/j.asoc.2021.107611 PMID:34518764

Liu, J., Chang, H., Forrest, J. Y. L., & Yang, B. (2020). Influence of artificial intelligence on technological innovation: Evidence from the panel data of china's manufacturing sectors. *Technological Forecasting and Social Change*, *158*, 120142. doi:10.1016/j.techfore.2020.120142

Lukasiewicz, J. (1920). On 3-valued Logic. In Polish Logic. Oxford U.P.

Ly, K. T. (2021). A COVID-19 forecasting system using adaptive neuro-fuzzy inference. *Finance Research Letters*, *41*, 101844. doi:10.1016/j.frl.2020.101844 PMID:34131413

Mahmoudi, M. R., Baleanu, D., Mansor, Z., Tuan, B. A., & Pho, K. H. (2020). Fuzzy clustering method to compare the spread rate of Covid-19 in the high risks countries. *Chaos, Solitons, and Fractals*, *140*, 110230. doi:10.1016/j.chaos.2020.110230 PMID:32863611

Majumder, S., Kar, S., & Samanta, E. (2020). A fuzzy rough hybrid decision making technique for identifying the infected population of COVID-19. *Soft Computing*, 1–11. PMID:33250663

Mamdani, E. H., & Assilian, S. (1975). An experiment in linguistic synthesis with a fuzzy logic controller. *International Journal of Man-Machine Studies*, *7*(1), 1–13. doi:10.1016/S0020-7373(75)80002-2

Mangla, M., Sharma, N., & Mittal, P. (2021). A fuzzy expert system for predicting the mortality of COVID'19. *Turkish Journal of Electrical Engineering and Computer Sciences*, *29*(3), 1628–1642. doi:10.3906/elk-2008-27

Manigandan, S., Wu, M. T., Ponnusamy, V. K., Raghavendra, V. B., Pugazhendhi, A., & Brindhadevi, K. (2020). A systematic review on recent trends in transmission, diagnosis, prevention and imaging features of COVID-19. *Process Biochemistry*.

Melin, P., Sánchez, D., Monica, J. C., & Castillo, O. (2021). Optimization using the firefly algorithm of ensemble neural networks with type-2 fuzzy integration for COVID-19 time series prediction. *Soft Computing*, 1–38. doi:10.100700500-020-05549-5 PMID:33456340

Mishra, A. R., Rani, P., Krishankumar, R., Ravichandran, K. S., & Kar, S. (2021). An extended fuzzy decision-making framework using hesitant fuzzy sets for the drug selection to treat the mild symptoms of Coronavirus Disease 2019 (COVID-19). *Applied Soft Computing*, *103*, 107155. doi:10.1016/j.asoc.2021.107155 PMID:33568967

Moher, D., Liberati, A., Tetzlaff, J., & Altman, D. G. (2009). Preferred reporting items for systematic reviews and meta-analyses: The PRISMA statement. *PLoS Medicine*, *6*(7), e1000097. doi:10.1371/journal.pmed.1000097 PMID:19621072

Mydukuri, R. V., Kallam, S., Patan, R., Al-Turjman, F., & Ramachandran, M. (2021). Deming least square regressed feature selection and Gaussian neuro-fuzzy multi-layered data classifier for early COVID prediction. *Expert Systems: International Journal of Knowledge Engineering and Neural Networks*, 12694. doi:10.1111/exsy.12694 PMID:34230740

Nauck, D., Klawonn, F., & Kruse, R. (1997). *Foundations of Neuro-Fuzzy Systems*. John Wiley & Sons, Inc.

Pham, Q. V., Nguyen, D. C., Huynh-The, T., Hwang, W. J., & Pathirana, P. N. (2020). *Artificial intelligence (AI) and big data for coronavirus (COVID-19) pandemic: A survey on the state-of-the-arts*. Academic Press.

Pinter, G., Felde, I., Mosavi, A., Ghamisi, P., & Gloaguen, R. (2020). COVID-19 pandemic prediction for Hungary; a hybrid machine learning approach. *Mathematics*, 8(6), 890. doi:10.3390/math8060890

Prabakaran, G., Vaithiyanathan, D., & Kumar, H. (2021). *Fuzzy Decision Support System for the Outbreak of COVID-19 and Improving the People Livelihood*. Academic Press.

Rallapalli, S., Aggarwal, S., & Singh, A. P. (2021). Detecting SARS-CoV-2 RNA prone clusters in a municipal wastewater network using fuzzy-Bayesian optimization model to facilitate wastewater-based epidemiology. *The Science of the Total Environment*, 778, 146294. doi:10.1016/j.scitotenv.2021.146294 PMID:33714094

Rathore, B., & Gupta, R. (2021). A fuzzy based hybrid decision-making framework to examine the safety risk factors of healthcare workers during COVID-19 outbreak. *Journal of Decision Systems*, 1–34.

Razavi-Termeh, S. V., Sadeghi-Niaraki, A., & Choi, S. M. (2021). Coronavirus disease vulnerability map using a geographic information system (GIS) from 16 April to 16 May 2020. *Physics and Chemistry of the Earth, Parts A/B/C*, 103043.

Saif, S., Das, P., & Biswas, S. (2021). *A Hybrid Model based on mBA-ANFIS for COVID-19 Confirmed Cases Prediction and Forecast. Journal of The Institution of Engineers. Series B.*

Samanlioglu, F., & Kaya, B. E. (2020). Evaluation of the COVID-19 pandemic intervention strategies with hesitant F-AHP. *Journal of Healthcare Engineering*. doi:10.1155/2020/8835258 PMID:32850105

Sayan, M., Sarigul Yildirim, F., Sanlidag, T., Uzun, B., Uzun Ozsahin, D., & Ozsahin, I. (2020). Capacity evaluation of diagnostic tests for COVID-19 using multicriteria decision-making techniques. *Computational and Mathematical Methods in Medicine*. doi:10.1155/2020/1560250 PMID:32802146

Sharma, M. K., Dhiman, N., & Mishra, V. N. (2021). Mediative fuzzy logic mathematical model: A contradictory management prediction in COVID-19 pandemic. *Applied Soft Computing*, 105, 107285. doi:10.1016/j.asoc.2021.107285 PMID:33723486

Stiegelmeier, E. W., & Bressan, G. M. (2021). A fuzzy approach in the study of COVID-19 pandemic in Brazil. *Research on Biomedical Engineering, 37*(2), 263–271. doi:10.100742600-021-00144-5

Thurner, S., Hanel, R., & Klimek, P. (2018). *Introduction to the theory of complex systems.* Oxford University Press. doi:10.1093/oso/9780198821939.001.0001

Tuncer, T., Ozyurt, F., Dogan, S., & Subasi, A. (2021). A novel Covid-19 and pneumonia classification method based on F-transform. *Chemometrics and Intelligent Laboratory Systems, 210,* 104256. doi:10.1016/j.chemolab.2021.104256 PMID:33531722

Upadhyay, H. K., Juneja, S., Maggu, S., Dhingra, G., & Juneja, A. (2021). Multi-criteria analysis of social isolation barriers amid COVID-19 using fuzzy AHP. *World Journal of Engineering.*

Vedaei, S. S., Fotovvat, A., Mohebbian, M. R., Rahman, G. M., Wahid, K. A., Babyn, P., Marateb, H. R., Mansourian, M., & Sami, R. (2020). COVID-SAFE: An IoT-based system for automated health monitoring and surveillance in post-pandemic life. *IEEE Access: Practical Innovations, Open Solutions, 8,* 188538–188551. doi:10.1109/ACCESS.2020.3030194 PMID:34812362

Wang, X., Chen, C., Du, Y., Zhang, Y., & Wu, C. (2021, February). Analysis of Policies Based on the Multi-Fuzzy Regression Discontinuity, in Terms of the Number of Deaths in the Coronavirus Epidemic. In Healthcare (Vol. 9, No. 2, p. 116). Multidisciplinary Digital Publishing Institute.

Wirtz, B. W., Weyerer, J. C., & Geyer, C. (2019). Artificial intelligence and the public sector—Applications and challenges. *International Journal of Public Administration, 42*(7), 596–615. doi:10.1080/01900692.2018.1498103

Wu, H. C., Wang, Y. C., & Chen, T. C. T. (2020). Assessing and comparing COVID-19 intervention strategies using a varying partial consensus fuzzy collaborative intelligence approach. *Mathematics, 8*(10), 1725. doi:10.3390/math8101725

Zadeh, L. A. (1965). Fuzzy Sets. *Information and Control, 8*(3), 338–353. doi:10.1016/S0019-9958(65)90241-X

Zadeh, L. A. (1968). Fuzzy algorithm. *Information and Control, 12*(2), 94–102. doi:10.1016/S0019-9958(68)90211-8

Zadeh, L. A. (1973). Outline of a new approach to the analysis of complex systems and decision processes. *IEEE Transactions on Systems, Man, and Cybernetics, 3*(1), 28–44. doi:10.1109/TSMC.1973.5408575

Zadeh, L. A. (1994). Soft computing and fuzzy logic. *IEEE Software*, *11*(6), 48–56. doi:10.1109/52.329401

Zaheeruddin & Garima. (2006). A neuro-fuzzy approach for prediction of human work efficiency in noisy environment. *Applied Soft Computing, 6*(3), 283-294.

Zivkovic, M., Bacanin, N., Venkatachalam, K., Nayyar, A., Djordjevic, A., Strumberger, I., & Al-Turjman, F. (2021). COVID-19 cases prediction by using hybrid machine learning and beetle antennae search approach. *Sustainable Cities and Society*, *66*, 102669. doi:10.1016/j.scs.2020.102669 PMID:33520607

Chapter 5
Knowledge Extraction From ICU Data Using Data Visualization

Tiago Guimarães
Centro ALGORITMI, Universidade do Minho, Portugal

Inês Afonso Quesado
Centro ALGORITMI, Universidade do Minho, Portugal

Inês Tavares
Centro ALGORITMI, Universidade do Minho, Portugal

Maria Passos
Centro ALGORITMI, Universidade do Minho, Portugal

Júlio Duarte
https://orcid.org/0000-0002-5458-3390
Centro ALGORITMI, Universidade do Minho, Portugal

Manuel Filipe Santos
https://orcid.org/0000-0002-5441-3316
Centro ALGORITMI, Universidade do Minho, Portugal

Álvaro Silva
Centro Hospitalar, Universitário do Porto, Portugal

ABSTRACT

Due to ICU critical environment, where seriously ill patients must be constantly monitored, it is imperative to make quick but assertive decisions. Several studies have shown that continuous monitorization of ICU patients result in large amounts of data, from which knowledge can be extracted and better decisions made. This chapter aims to analyse and visualize the data obtained by an ICU, so that conclusions can be deduced regarding patients' outcome, clinical errors, as well as healthcare service quality. To achieve the objective, initially, the data was acquired and collected

DOI: 10.4018/978-1-7998-9172-7.ch005

from several data sources such as bedside monitors and electronic nursing records. Secondly, the raw data was transformed so that it could be used in visualization. Finally, interactive charts were built so that data could be forecasted and patterns discovered. The results allow one to draw conclusions such as the source of data gaps, the correlation between medication and vital signs, as well as the importance of SAPS regarding patient outcomes.

INTRODUCTION

Intensive Medicine is an area of medicine that focuses on the prevention, diagnosis, and treatment of patients with critical health problems (Gramacho, 1971). This medicine is fundamentally applied in Intensive Care Units (ICUs), as they are prepared to continuously monitor the vital functions and organ systems of patients. (Braga et al., 2015) Therefore, it is crucial for ICUs to have access to data on any patient at any time and place, so that healthcare professionals can make decisions as accurately as possible. (Veloso et al., 2014) All of this is possible through the use of Information Systems (IS), which in recent years has seen exponential growth in these units. IS increase the satisfaction of intensivists, the quality of data and services provided, as well as saving time, supporting decisions, and improving research. (Ehteshami et al., 2013) As a result, every day large amounts of data are generated in the ICUs that need to be processed and transformed in order to extract knowledge. (Santos et al., 2009)

The present study aims to draw conclusions about the source of data gaps, the correlation between medication and vital signs, as well as the importance of Simplified Acute Physiology Score (SAPS) regarding patients' outcome. For this purpose, the team used python programming for the whole process of data cleaning and processing and, at last, used the tableau tool to visualise the data and thus be able to draw conclusions about the analyses carried out. All the work was performed using real data provided by Centro Hospitalar Universitário do Porto and always with the help of Dr. Álvaro Silva who guided the team to the crucial points of the analysis. The results obtained showed that the errors in the data occurred mostly on the night shift; noradrenaline administration has indeed an impact on vital signs; and there is a correlation between the expected mortality rate and the recorded values of the vital signs.

This article is divided in four chapters. The first section is the Introduction, that describes a general introduction to the problem and the topics that will be discussed during the paper. The second section is called Background in which it is defined the problem and the theory and concepts of the work presented. The third section is the Main Focus of the Chapter, where it is described all the work carried out in order to achieve the intended objectives. The fourth and last section concerns the conclusion, in which the results achieved with this work are presented.

BACKGROUND

Intensive Medicine and ICUs

In the field of medicine there is one particular area, Intensive Care Medicine, whose main goal is to diagnose and treat patients with serious illnesses and restore their previous health condition (Veloso et al., 2017).

Intensive Care Medicine is recognized as a multidisciplinary field of medical sciences that deals with the prevention, diagnosis, and treatment of potentially reversible acute situations in patients with failure in one or more vital functions. These can be grouped into 6 organ systems: neurological, respiratory, hepatic, haematological, cardiovascular, and renal (Santos et al., 2009).

The process of reversing a patient's condition is conducted in qualified facilities called ICUs. These units provide specialized care for patients in complex health conditions, usually in organ failure and, consequently, in severe life-threatening conditions (Ramon et al., 2007).

In the ICU, the patient's vital signs are continuously monitored, and its vital functions can be supported by medication or mechanical devices, until the patient is able to do it autonomously (Santos et al., 2009).

Healthcare Quality in the ICUs

An ICU is usually characterized as a restricted area of the hospital, responsible for continuously monitoring the vital signs of severely ill patients. Multiple teams and healthcare processes operate simultaneously in an extremely complex and high-risk environment for inpatients.

Due to the significant increase in demand for intensive care, there has also been a greater difficulty for doctors, in providing care that consistently complies with quality and safety standards.

Healthcare providers analyse hundreds of data to make decisions, since, in most cases, it carries the patient's life. The choices of medications, procedures and therapies often arise in emergency conditions, affecting not only the health status of the patient at risk, but also the availability of drugs that could be used in other patients (Marty, 1996).

Information and Communication Technologies have revolutionized society's everyday lives, through the development of applications and systems, designed to improve, in some extent, quality of life.

In the healthcare field, specifically in ICUs, such technologies have allowed resource optimization, service improvement and remote health monitoring, which is essential for its patients whose health conditions are severe and, consequently, require continuous surveillance and vital sign monitorization (Bhatia & Sood, 2016).

The data is collected through numerous devices that constantly provide detailed data regarding each patient in real-time, allowing doctors to have accurate information and provide curative and diagnostic services in a timelier manner. Despite that, only a small fraction of the data collected is utilized, due to the overwhelming amount of existing information, compared to the availability of resources and time. Furthermore, the data format is inevitably heterogeneous due to the different monitors and devices used for data collection (Portela et al., 2013).

Information Systems in Healthcare

Over the past decades, the world has seen the rapid evolution of collecting and accessing information, as well as the escalation of its importance in businesses and organizations. The growth of communication has majorly impacted the way Information Systems (IS) are perceived. Nowadays IS are involved throughout all levels of an organization, from operations to management, in order to provide strategic elements that can help businesses become more efficient and, perhaps, gain a competitive advantage. (Kadry, 2014)

Healthcare being a global industry noted for using the latest technology and support new scientific discoveries to help combat and prevent threatening diseases, is now facing a scenario in which healthcare providers have introduced Information Technologies in their workflow with some level of independence. Researchers affirm that this might be making it difficult for IS to interoperate, since the acquirement of this systems is done over the years, with heterogenous developments. Moreover, besides hospitals, healthcare systems include patients, nurses, doctors, pharmacists, medications, and specialists, each one with unique needs and specific goals, different types of data and various services. That said, the adoption of standards is indicated as a possible solution to improve interoperability. (Barbarito et al., 2012)

Healthcare has been greatly impacted by the vast amount of information available, using IT to automate processes such as transaction, inventory, record management and repetitive task reduction. At the same time, as has happened in other areas, consumers of healthcare have become more demanding on having access to relevant information, as well as to be informed of their health options. That said, the question lies on how to use Information Systems effectively to improve healthcare and support decision-making. (Beaver, 2002)

The diagnosis of an illness begins with the patient description, physical and psychological exams, and laboratory tests. Then, treatment and therapy are prescribed, after acknowledging medication reactions and allergies. However, in most cases, access to patients' history is limited, resulting mostly in information coming from the patient or from a recent entry in the hospital. Such lack of data can result in unexpected drug reactions or allergies and may lead to life threatening situations. An IT System that is usually utilized in medical diagnosis is the DSS (Decision Support System). (Rajalakshmi et al., 2011)

Clinical Decision Support Systems are "computer systems designed to impact clinical decision making about patients at the point in time that decisions are made" (Sadegh-Zadeh, 2015) in which the "characteristics of an individual patient are matched to a computerized clinical knowledge base and patient-specific assessment, or recommendations are then presented to the clinical for a decision". (Ammenwerth et al., 2003)

Over the years, this system has improved patient care and healthcare providers' efficiency, through its electronic health record systems, screen recommendations, web-based personal health record systems and remote patient care. With barriers falling to digital health care acceptance and its ability to improve patient outcomes and provide correct diagnosis, the future will likely witness the need for more technology tools such as artificial intelligence and machine learning for decision support.

Medication Errors in ICU

Medication errors are one of the main concerns of the healthcare systems and are seen as an indicator to determine patients' security level in hospitals, since they represent a risk factor for patients' lives (Cheraghi et al., 2011). Therefore, are defined by any adverse, unwelcome, or preventable event which can lead to an inappropriate use of medication. These errors may occur at any stage of the medication management process: prescription, transmission of the prescription, labelling, packing or denomination, distribution, administration, or monitoring. However, most of them happen at the administration stage (di Muzio et al., 2017).

According to Wilmer et al. (2010), the occurrence of medication errors is significantly higher in patients admitted to the ICUs in comparison with other general medical wards. This may happen as a result of patients' clinical complexity, the amount of medication administered, the frequency with which prescriptions are changed, the need to adjust the drug dose to the patients' weight, or the potential incompatibility among intravenous medication and the speed of its administration (di Muzio et al., 2017).

133

In agreement with Cheraghi et al. (2011), the most common type of medication errors relates to the flow rate of drugs and the dose that is administered, which is usually due to abbreviations of medications or similarities between their names.

Finally, and according to estimates, ICU patients undergo an average of 1.7 errors per day which in most cases can be fatal. Therefore, this demonstrates that the use of strategies to minimise its occurrence is crucial to improve ICU service quality (di Muzio et al., 2017).

Data Collection and Errors

As previously mentioned, the health condition of ICU's patients is likely to change often and in an unpredictable way. This implies that data collection from monitors and other devices must be done continuously, so that both nurses and doctors may detect adverse events and promptly respond (Reid & Kenny, 1984).

Despite having access to timely detection of changes, nurses are usually overwhelmed with significant cognitive demands, such as evaluating all the patient's physiologic parameters and having to interpret it in the context of its history, dealing with documents, communicating with other healthcare professionals and, in case of an expected event occurs, quickly analyse the available data and act promptly. This gives rise to errors and bad practices when providing healthcare (Drews, 2008).

Several studies also show a strong correlation between chronical tiredness and medical errors, usually more frequently during night or long shifts. Chronical tiredness is defined as a reduction of the capacity in performing mental and physical tasks, which in the context of ICUs may impact drastically patient's safety.

A study (Landrigan et al., 2004) has shown that medical professionals make 36% more mistakes when working 24h shifts compared to shorter shifts. Moreover, another study conducted by (Maltese et al., 2016) reported that the cognitive abilities of ICU physicians decreased after a night shift.

Among several medical errors, the two most found in studies were medication errors and vital signs recording. Regarding medication errors, it was shown that the conditions influencing medication administration errors (MAEs) included inadequate prescription, documentation and transcription, medicine supply and storage issues, high workload, equipment problems and tiredness and fatigue (Wang et al., 2015). With regard to vital signs recording, a study conducted by (Reid & Kenny, 1984) that analysed about 48000 ICU stays, has shown that approximately 30% of vital sign days included at least one gap greater than 70 minutes between measurements and that roughly 27% of them contained at least one statistical outlier.

This information corroborates the necessity for continuous improvement in decreasing medical errors to enhance patient safety and, consequently, increase the quality of critical healthcare.

Data Quality Defects in ICUs

The ref. (Cruz-Correia et al., 2009) describe information as "the interpretation of data and knowledge that intelligent systems perform to support their decisions", which in medical care is critical, since data is essential to assist decision-making processes. Moreover, it helps physicians to have a greater understanding of patients' health conditions, to diagnose and then prescribe the most appropriate treatment.

In order to transform raw health data in information, informatic experts go through several processes such as Data Cleaning, Data Integration and Data Quality. Unfortunately, it has been shown that quite frequently data items are inaccurately recorded or simply omitted, which makes the work of these professionals utterly more difficult.

A study conducted by Oregon Health and Science University, indicated that, a large fraction of data of several ICU rounds, were either omitted or incorrectly presented, with the majority of errors unknown (A. Gold et al., 2017). Moreover, (Cruz-Correia et al., 2009) stated that the quality of patient data in computer-based patient records is considered low in several health Information Systems, the main reasons being human error and bad system design.

That being said, it is important that healthcare professionals and IT professionals make an effort to increase the availability of data and increase the quality of the resulting information, respectively, so that can be used by professionals in a much more efficient manner and, consequently, improve patient's health condition and service quality.

Impact of Noradrenaline on Mean Arterial Pressure

Among the vast amount of data that is collected in ICUs, vital signs are one of the most common and relevant variables to evaluate the patient's health status, as they are objective measures of physiological functions (Kaieski et al., 2020).

With the aim of regulating vital signs, there are several medicaments that can be administered according to the intended purpose. Vasopressors, for example, are a type of medication whose main function is to increase blood pressure (Braga et al., 2016). They are commonly used to recover organ perfusion pressure when there is an inadequate response to intravascular volume in ICU's patients (Sviri et al., 2014). Pharmaceuticals such as adrenaline, noradrenaline, and dopamine may be found in this group. Noradrenaline can be used to treat hypotension, cardiac arrest, or septic shock (Braga et al., 2016).

According to Genay et al. (2013), noradrenaline is the primary choice, among all vasopressors, to obtain and maintain the Mean Arterial Pressure (MAP) higher than 65 mmHg, since when noradrenaline is administered, there is a quick stabilisation of the MAP. Similarly, a study carried out by Monge García et al. (2018) proved that MAP increased in the group of patients in whom noradrenaline was initiated or there was an increase in its inflow, and that MAP decreased in the group of patients in whom noradrenaline administration was withdrawn or there was a decrease in its inflow.

Finally, Sviri et al. (2014) stated that the need of high-dose vasopressor therapy at any time during the patient's admission to the ICU was related to a high mortality rate.

SAPS II

Over the years, intensive care physicians and clinical researchers have developed several scoring systems to address issues such as efficiency, effectiveness, equity, and quality of intensive care as well as to improve the clinical experience in ICUs (Suter et al., 1994).

In the context of intensive care medicine, some of these systems have been developed to assess the severity of illness and organ dysfunction in a critical environment such as in ICUs, allowing patients to be stratified based on the risk of their clinical condition, patient data, and physiological variables obtained in the first 24 hours after ICU admission (Silva et al., 2008).

One of these systems is the Simplified Acute Physiology Score (SAPS). SAPS is a classification system of disease severity to predict mortality using logistic regression.

The Simplified Acute Physiology Score II (SAPS II), the most used indicator in the ICUs of the Centro Hospitalar Universitário do Porto, is an evolution of SAPS and provides an estimate of the risk of death without the need to specify a primary diagnosis. SAPS II lead to a prediction of the patients' expected mortality rate (Gall et al., 1993) (Pereira, 2005).

This score is determined based on 17 variables that can be calculated one or more times during the first 24 hours of ICU admission, although only the worst values are considered. The system considers the following parameters for evaluating the probability of mortality: age, heart rate, systolic blood pressure, body temperature, oxygenation and respiration rates, urinary output, amount of urea, potassium and sodium, white blood cell count, bilirubin level, Glasgow coma scale, type of admission, HIV carrier, carrier of haematological pathology and existence of metastatic cancer (Gall et al., 1993).

Although SAPSII is widely used in ICUs, it suffers the disadvantage of being static, since it is only calculated once and with values obtained in a short time window, not considering any events recorded during the period in which the patient is in the ICU. These events may change the health status or the initial prognosis and may also put into question the initially calculated probability of death (Pereira, 2005).

MAIN FOCUS OF THE CHAPTER

The purpose of the study was to draw conclusions about the origin of the missing data, the correlation between drug administration and vital signs, as well as the importance of SAPS to predict patient outcome.

Data Understanding

The study began with the data extraction from the ICU of the Centro Hospitalar Universitário do Porto, specifically the reading of vital signs of patients whose hospitalisation was between 2020 and 2021, as well as the administration of medication to them.

These data were organised into two datasets: Vital Signs, which contained information about the vital signs of patients coming from the ICU; and Medications, which contained all the data about the prescription and administration of medications to patients.

Initially, it was necessary to carry out a prior study of the data provided so that the work team would become familiar with the subject of datasets and thus be able to understand which analyses would be most relevant for the project.

Finally, all relevant variables of the datasets were defined in order to understand the meaning of each one, as explained in the following tables.

Table 1. Vital signs dataset

Variable	Definition
NUM_SEQUENCIAL	Sequential admission number
TSTAMP	Data collection timestamp (2 minutes interval)
NUM_CAMA	Patient bed number
SEXO	Patient gender
IDADE	Patient Age
DATAHORA_ENTRADA	Date and time of admission
COD_ESPECIALIDADE	Medical speciality code
COD_PATOLOGIA	Patient pathology code
ESTADO	Patient's condition (pre- or post-operative)
MNDRY_BLD_PULS_RATE_ART_ABP	Pulse rate
MDC_PRESS_BLD_ART_ABP_SYS	Systolic arterial pressure
MDC_PRESS_BLD_ART_ABP_MEAN	Mean arterial pressure
MDC_PRESS_BLD_ART_ABP_DIA	Diastolic arterial pressure
MDC_TEMP	Body temperature
MDC_PULS_OXIM_SAT_O2	Oxygen saturation

Table 2. Medications dataset

Variable	Definition
FMP_DATA	Date of administration of medication
NUM_SEQUENCIAL	Sequential admission number
FHC_NEPISODIO	Patient episode number
MED_DESIGNACAO	Name of drug administered

Visualization: Evolution of the Hospitalisation

Initially, it was not possible to compare the patients' stay throughout their hospitalisation due to the format of the data, which was organised by date. In order to generate patterns, make comparisons and establish correlations in the Data Mining phase, the column "Dia de Internamento" (day of hospitalisation) was added so that the evolution of patients in equivalent days of hospitalisation could be compared. In the various 24h periods, the behaviours were typical, so, regardless of the length of stay, equal time windows could be compared.

Figure 1. Analysis of the 1st day of hospitalisation and comparison between patients and vital signs

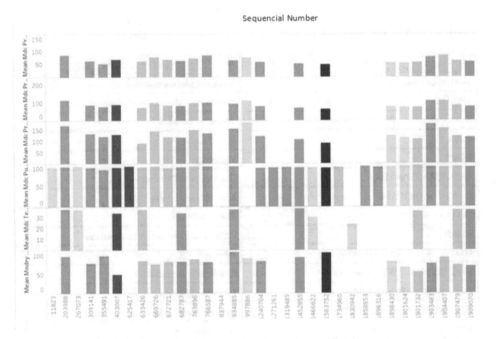

The first day of hospitalization was initially compared, as described in figure 1, and then it was suggested to add other variables, as well as to extend the time window to the first four days of hospitalization. This was due to the fact that after this period, complications might occur as a consequence of the hospital environment, and therefore medication is administered to prevent the aggravation of the patients' state of health. Such phenomena made the analysis of the change in vital signs values impractical, as the team is not aware of how they might affect each patient.

Medication and Vital Signs

In order to investigate the possibility of effectively extracting information from the reading of vital signs, the team added, to the visualization software Tableau, a new dataset with the description of the medication administered to patients during hospitalisation. After cleaning and processing the data, two charts were built: "Evolution of mean blood pressure values over the first days of hospitalisation" and "Follow-up of medication administered throughout hospitalisation". Afterwards, to draw conclusions, both charts were integrated into a single panel, and the respective dates and patients were associated.

As requested by the medical team, the vital sign "Mdc Press Bld Art Abp Mean", the medicine "Noradrenaline" and the patients, filtered one by one, were used for visualization purposes. The result obtained is shown in the figure 2.

Figure 2. Evolution of MAP values over time and medication monitoring

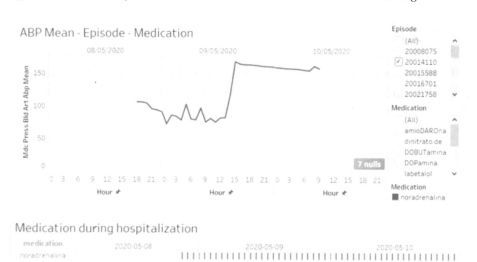

According to figure 2, there is an effective relationship between taking noradrenaline and the Mean Arterial Pressure (MAP) readings, with a stabilisation approximately 24 hours after the treatment started.

SAPS II: Simplified Acute Physiology Score

In order to obtain more information about patients' health condition and consequently perform a more accurate analysis, a new column called "INTERVALO_SAPS" was added to the dataset, and the score was divided between percentage ranges of expected mortality. The conversion was carried out according to the correlation between SAPS II and the established probability of hospital mortality in a study conducted by (Gall et al., 1993). The correlation is explained in table 1.

Table 3. SAPS II and Expected Mortality Ratio (Gall et al., 1993)

SAPS Interval	Expected Mortality
29 points	Equal or less than 10%
40 points	Between 11% and 25%
52 points	Between 26% and 50%
64 points	Between 51% and 75%
77 points	Between 76% and 90%
Equal or greater than 78 points	Equal or greater than 91%

SAPS Data Visualization

After associating a SAPS interval to each one of the 36 patients in the dataset, a graph was built with the distribution of patients by expected mortality range, as described in the figure 3.

Figure 3. Percentage distribution of patients in each expected mortality range

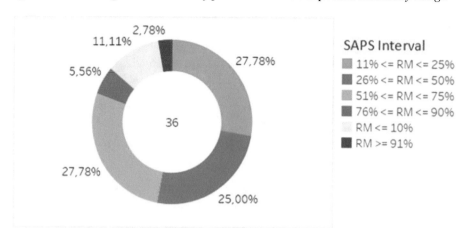

As it is shown, in the sample of 36 patients, there are 4 with expected mortality equal or less than 10%, 10 between 11% and 25%, 9 between 26% and 50%, 10 between 51% and 75%, 2 between 76% and 90% and 1 with expected mortality equal or greater than 91%.

Aiming to find trends and establish relationships between the previously treated data and SAPS II, the team proceeded to visualize the distribution in Box Plot, as well as to identify the expected mortality range. As described in the figures below, it was possible to trace trends regarding the severity of patients' health condition and the dispersion of values over the shifts.

For an expected mortality range between 11% and 25%, it was verified that the quartiles Q2 and Q3 were close and equally divided, which meant that the median was a good indicator of the central tendency, and the variance of the data was not very significant, since only three whiskers appeared to have a greater dispersion of values in the night and morning shifts.

Figure 4. Distribution of diastolic pressure values with RM between 11% and 25%.

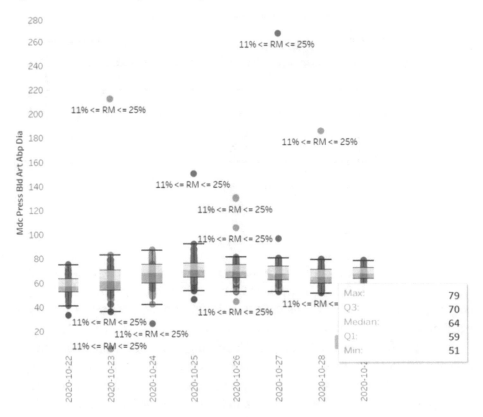

In Figure 5 it is shown that the situation changed towards an expected mortality of between 26% and 50%, demonstrating greater bias in the data and generally longer whiskers. The Q2 and Q3 quartiles also became less balanced, which corroborated the observation of more dispersed values of diastolic pressure. The median did not divide the quartiles in half, which was an indicator that it was not an accurate reflection of the central tendency. Regarding shifts, the night shift continued to be the shift with the highest dispersion of data.

Figure 5. Distribution of diastolic pressure values with RM between 26% and 50%.

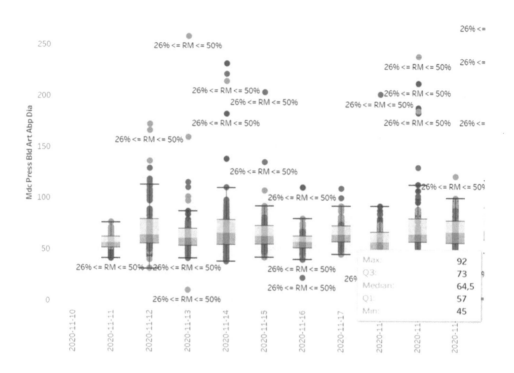

In figure 6, the expected mortality rate varied between 76% and 90%, with a significantly higher dispersion in the data and a notable discrepancy between shifts. The team concluded that there was apparently a visible relationship between the expected mortality rate, the variation of the values read on the devices responsible for collecting vital signs, and the shifts. The night shift, in addition to having the highest percentage of nulls, was also the time when greater changes in the values took place, relating to vital signs.

Figure 6. Distribution of diastolic pressure values with RM between 76% and 90%.

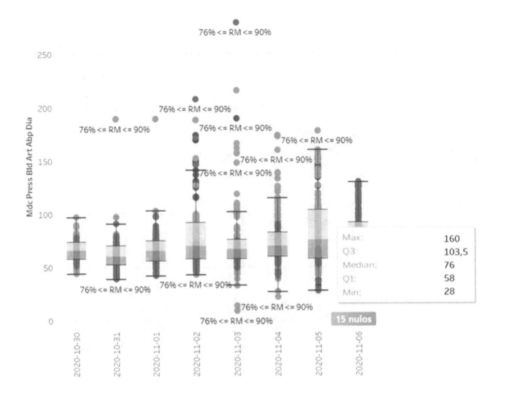

RESULTS AND FUTURE WORK

In regard to future work, the research carried out proved to be quite relevant to draw conclusions about the day-to-day in the ICUs and, consequently, how tasks can be performed more efficiently. The goals initially established are considered met, as the team managed to understand the origin of the data gaps, as well as establish correlations between medication and vital signs. The relationships established between each patient's vital signs and the result of norepinephrine administrations allowed to conclude how this drug and the different associated dosages can produce an effect on improving the patient's health condition. In the future, it would be interesting to extend this analysis to other medications, in order to prevent "peaks" of values that could negatively influence the patient's condition and, consequently, shorten the period of stay in the ICU. In addition to this, the investigation allowed to arouse the importance of the Simplified Acute Physiology Score II for predicting the health status of patients in the short term. That said, the team believes that in the future it might be quite interesting to explore this classification system and its predictive capacities.

CONCLUSION

The large amount of data generated daily in an ICU is particularly interesting for the knowledge that can be extracted by analysing it to help health professionals in the decision-making process.

As a result of our study, it was possible to draw several conclusions that met the objectives initially set. Regarding the origin of missing data, it was found that most of the nulls were identified during the night shift, as well as a greater discrepancy in the values related to vital signs. Regarding the possible existence of a correlation between the administration of medication and vital signs, it was possible to conclude that there is indeed an impact on vital signs when taking noradrenaline, with a stabilisation of vital signs 24 hours after the start of treatment. Finally, in regard to SAPS, it was found that there is a correlation between the expected mortality rate and the recorded values of the vital signs.

Such conclusions could be interesting for the hospital staff to evaluate the inconsistent quality of intensive care that it is being provided at various times, as well as to take steps to improve its general performance, so that medical errors can be severely reduced.

Further work will encompass collecting more data, using real time data, or even having access to other types of data that will give us more insight into what we want to analyse. In addition, the work may also include the use of other monitors and an improvement in the problems and settings.

ACKNOWLEDGMENT

The work has been supported by FCT – Fundação para a Ciência e Tecnologia within the Project Scope: DSAIPA/ DS/ 0084/ 2018.

REFERENCES

Ammenwerth, E., Gräber, S., Herrmann, G., Bürkle, T., & König, J. (2003). Evaluation of health information systems - Problems and challenges. *International Journal of Medical Informatics*, *71*(2–3), 125–135. doi:10.1016/S1386-5056(03)00131-X PMID:14519405

Barbarito, F., Pinciroli, F., Mason, J., Marceglia, S., Mazzola, L., & Bonacina, S. (2012). Implementing standards for the interoperability among healthcare providers in the public regionalized Healthcare Information System of the Lombardy Region. *Journal of Biomedical Informatics*, *45*(4), 736–745. doi:10.1016/j.jbi.2012.01.006 PMID:22285983

Beaver, K. (2002). *Healthcare Information Systems*. CRC Press. doi:10.1201/9781420031409

Bhatia, M., & Sood, S. K. (2016). Temporal Informative Analysis in Smart-ICU Monitoring: M-HealthCare Perspective. *Journal of Medical Systems*, *40*(8), 190. Advance online publication. doi:10.100710916-016-0547-9 PMID:27388507

Braga, A., Portela, F., Santos, M. F., Abelha, A., Machado, J., Silva, Á., & Rua, F. (2016). Data mining to predict the use of vasopressors in intensive medicine patients. *Jurnal Teknologi*, *78*(6–7), 1–6. doi:10.11113/jt.v78.9075

Braga, A., Portela, F., Santos, M. F., Machado, J., Abelha, A., Silva, Á., & Rua, F. (2015). Step Towards a Patient Timeline in Intensive Care Units. *Procedia Computer Science*, *64*, 618–625. doi:10.1016/j.procs.2015.08.575

Cheraghi, M. A., Reza, A., Nasrabadi, N., Nejad, E. M., Salari, A., Ehsani, S. R., & Kheyli, K. (2011). *Medication Errors Among Nurses in Intensive Care Units*. ICU.

Cruz-Correia, R. J., Rodrigues, P. P., Freitas, A., Almeida, F. C., Chen, R., & Costa-Pereira, A. (2009). Data quality and integration issues in electronic health records. In *Information Discovery on Electronic Health Records*. doi:10.1201/9781420090413-c4

di Muzio, M., de Vito, C., Tartaglini, D., & Villari, P. (2017). Knowledge, behaviours, training and attitudes of nurses during preparation and administration of intravenous medications in intensive care units (ICU). A multicenter Italian study. *Applied Nursing Research*, *38*, 129–133. doi:10.1016/j.apnr.2017.10.002 PMID:29241505

Drews, F. A. (2008). *Patient Monitors in Critical Care: Lessons for Improvement. In Advances in Patient Safety: New Directions and Alternative Approaches* (Vol. 3). Performance and Tools.

Ehteshami, A., Sadoughi, F., Ahmadi, M., & Kashefi, P. (2013). Intensive care information system impacts. *Acta Informatica Medica*, *21*(3), 185–191. doi:10.5455/aim.2013.21.185-191 PMID:24167389

Genay, S., Décaudin, B., Ethgen, S., Barthélémy, C., Odou, P., & Lebuffe, G. (2013). Impact of noradrenaline infusion set on mean arterial pressure: A retrospective clinical study. *Annales Francaises d'Anesthesie et de Reanimation, 32*(11), e159–e162. Advance online publication. doi:10.1016/j.annfar.2013.08.011 PMID:24138772

Gold, J., McGrath, K., & Mohan, V. (2017). *Perceptions of Data Quality and Accuracy During ICU Round*. Academic Press.

Gramacho, M. (1971). Cuidados intensivos. *Revista de Enfermagem, 18*(1). PMID:5211521

Kadry, S. (2014). On the Evolution of Information Systems. Academic Press.

Kaieski, N., da Costa, C. A., da Rosa Righi, R., Lora, P. S., & Eskofier, B. (2020). Application of artificial intelligence methods in vital signs analysis of hospitalized patients: A systematic literature review. In *Applied Soft Computing Journal* (Vol. 96). Elsevier Ltd. doi:10.1016/j.asoc.2020.106612

Landrigan, C. P., Rothschild, J. M., Cronin, J. W., Kaushal, R., Burdick, E., Katz, J. T., Lilly, C. M., Stone, P. H., Lockley, S. W., Bates, D. W., & Czeisler, C. A. (2004). Effect of reducing interns' work hours on serious medical errors in intensive care units. *The New England Journal of Medicine, 351*(18), 1838–1848. doi:10.1056/NEJMoa041406 PMID:15509817

Le Gall, J.-R., Lemeshow, S., & Saulnier, F. (1993). A new Simplified Acute Physiology Score (SAPS II) based on a European/North American multicenter study. *Journal of the American Medical Association, 270*(24), 2957–2963. doi:10.1001/jama.1993.03510240069035 PMID:8254858

Maltese, F., Adda, M., Bablon, A., Hraeich, S., Guervilly, C., Lehingue, S., Wiramus, S., Leone, M., Martin, C., Vialet, R., Thirion, X., Roch, A., Forel, J. M., & Papazian, L. (2016). Night shift decreases cognitive performance of ICU physicians. *Intensive Care Medicine, 42*(3), 393–400. doi:10.100700134-015-4115-4 PMID:26556616

Marty, A. T. (1996). Textbook of Critical Care. *Critical Care Medicine, 24*(5), 901–902. doi:10.1097/00003246-199605000-00039

Monge García, M. I., Santos, A., Diez Del Corral, B., Guijo González, P., Gracia Romero, M., Gil Cano, A., & Cecconi, M. (2018). Noradrenaline modifies arterial reflection phenomena and left ventricular efficiency in septic shock patients: A prospective observational study. *Journal of Critical Care, 47*, 280–286. doi:10.1016/j.jcrc.2018.07.027 PMID:30096635

Pereira, J. (2005). *Modelos de Data Mining para multi-previsão: aplicação à medicina intensiva*. Academic Press.

Portela, F., Gago, P., Santos, M. F., Machado, J., Abelha, A., Silva, Á., & Rua, F. (2013). Implementing a pervasive real-time intelligent system for tracking critical events with intensive care patients. *International Journal of Healthcare Information Systems and Informatics*, 8(4), 1–16. doi:10.4018/ijhisi.2013100101

Rajalakshmi, K., Chandra Mohan, S., & Babu, S. D. (2011). Decision Support System in Healthcare Industry. *International Journal of Computers and Applications*, 26(9), 42–44. doi:10.5120/3129-4310

Ramon, J., Fierens, D., Güiza, F., Meyfroidt, G., Blockeel, H., Bruynooghe, M., & Van Den Berghe, G. (2007). Mining data from intensive care patients. *Advanced Engineering Informatics*, 21(3), 243–256. doi:10.1016/j.aei.2006.12.002

Reid, J. A., & Kenny, G. N. C. (1984). Data collection in the intensive care unit. *Journal of Microcomputer Applications*, 7(3), 257–269. doi:10.1016/0745-7138(84)90058-7

Sadegh-Zadeh, K. (2015). Clinical Decision Support Systems. In Philosophy and Medicine (Vol. 119). doi:10.1007/978-94-017-9579-1_20

Santos, M. F., Portela, F., Vilas-Boas, M., Machado, J., Abelha, A., Neves, J., Silva, A., & Rua, F. (2009). Information architecture for intelligent decision support in intensive medicine. *WSEAS Transactions on Computers*, 8(5), 810–819.

Silva, Á., Cortez, P., Santos, M. F., Gomes, L., & Neves, J. (2008). Rating organ failure via adverse events using data mining in the intensive care unit. *Artificial Intelligence in Medicine*, 43(3), 179–193. doi:10.1016/j.artmed.2008.03.010 PMID:18486459

Suter, P., Armaganidis, A., Beaufils, F., Bonfill, X., Burchardi, H., Cook, D., Fagot-Largeault, A., Thijs, L., Vesconi, S., Williams, A., Le Gall, J. R., & Chang, R. (1994). Predicting outcome in ICU patients. *Intensive Care Medicine*, 20(5), 390–397. doi:10.1007/BF01720917 PMID:7930037

Sviri, S., Hashoul, J., Stav, I., & van Heerden, P. (2014). Does high-dose vasopressor therapy in medical intensive care patients indicate what we already suspect? *Journal of Critical Care*, 29(1), 157–160. doi:10.1016/j.jcrc.2013.09.004 PMID:24140297

Veloso, R., Portela, F., Santos, M. F., Machado, J., da Silva Abelha, A., Rua, F., & Silva, Á. (2017). Categorize readmitted patients in intensive medicine by means of clustering data mining. *International Journal of E-Health and Medical Communications*, 8(3), 22–37. doi:10.4018/IJEHMC.2017070102

Veloso, R., Portela, F., Santos, M. F., Silva, Á., Rua, F., Abelha, A., & Machado, J. (2014). A Clustering Approach for Predicting Readmissions in Intensive Medicine. *Procedia Technology*, *16*, 1307–1316. doi:10.1016/j.protcy.2014.10.147

Wang, H. F., Jin, J. F., Feng, X. Q., Huang, X., Zhu, L. L., Zhao, X. Y., & Zhou, Q. (2015). Quality improvements in decreasing medication administration errors made by nursing staff in an academic medical center hospital: A trend analysis during the journey to Joint Commission International accreditation and in the post-accreditation era. *Therapeutics and Clinical Risk Management*, *11*, 393–406. doi:10.2147/TCRM. S79238 PMID:25767393

Wilmer, A., Louie, K., Dodek, P., Wong, H., & Ayas, N. (2010). Incidence of medication errors and adverse drug events in the ICU: A systematic review. In Quality and Safety in Health Care (Vol. 19, Issue 5). doi:10.1136/qshc.2008.030783

KEY TERMS AND DEFINITIONS

Data Visualization: Is the graphical representation of information and data, through charts, graphs, and maps.

Intensive Care Unit: An area where care is provided to patients with a critical health condition or who present a potential risk, requiring continuous and intensive surveillance.

Intensive Medicine: An area of medicine that is dedicated to the diagnosis and treatment of potentially reversible acute illness in patients who have impending or established failure of one or more vital functions.

Knowledge Extraction: Consists in the process of gathering and analysing significant volumes of data and compiling it into useful information. This process of identifying valuable information can be extremely useful to organizations that are interested in improving efficiency and gain competitive advantage, due to its capacity to identify patterns and support decision making.

MAP: Mean Arterial Pressure throughout one cardiac cycle, systole, and diastole.

Noradrenaline: Is a chemical compound involved in several important processes in the body. One of its best-known effects is vasopressor, which means, it causes an increase in blood pressure.

Simplified Acute Physiology Score (SAPS): Disease severity classification system, with the aim of predicting patient mortality using logistic regression techniques. This indicator is estimated based on 17 variables.

Vital Signs: Set of physiological variables that physicians analyse for the valuation of elementary organic functions.

Chapter 6

Classification of Polycystic Ovary Syndrome Based on Correlation Weight Using Machine Learning

Marcelo Marreiros
Centro ALGORITMI, Universidade do Minho, Portugal

Diana Ferreira
Centro ALGORITMI, Universidade do Minho, Portugal

Cristiana Neto
Universidade do Minho, Portugal

Deden Witarsyah
Telkom University, Indonesia

José Machado
https://orcid.org/0000-0003-4121-6169
Centro ALGORITMI, Universidade do Minho, Portugal

ABSTRACT

Polycystic ovarian syndrome (PCOS) is the most common endocrine pathology in reproductive-age women worldwide. Research has shown that the application of machine learning (ML) and data mining (DM) can have a positive impact in this condition's diagnosis. This study aims to develop a model to identify patients with PCOS using different scenarios based on correlation weights. Five DM techniques were applied, namely random forest (RF), decision tree (DT), naive bayes (NB), logistic regression (LR), and artificial neural network (ANN), to determine the best model, which was the RF classifier. Additionally, the results show that the model was able to predict PCOS with 93.06% of accuracy, 92.66% of precision, 93.52% of sensitivity, and 92.59% of specificity. Compared with a previous work conducted by the authors, the feature selection-based solo on the correlation weight decreased the accuracy values by 1.9%, precision by 3.7%, sensitivity by 0.3%, and specificity by 3.6%.

DOI: 10.4018/978-1-7998-9172-7.ch006

INTRODUCTION

Nowadays, the Stein-Leventhal syndrome currently known as Polycystic Ovary Syndrome (PCOS) is the most common endocrine pathology in reproductive-age women around the world (Leon & Mayrin, 2020; Balen & Rajkowha, 2003). PCOS is a hormonal disorder that represents a condition in which about 10 small cysts ranging in diameter between 2 and 9 mm develop in one or both ovaries and/or the ovarian volume in at least one ovary surpasses 10 ml (El Hayek et al., 2016). Its major features include menstrual dysfunction, anovulation, and signs of hyperandrogenism (Witchel et al., 2019). Consequently, the population of women at greater risk involve reproductive age females with clinical evidence of hyperandrogenism (i.e., hirsutism, acne, or alopecia), menstrual and/or ovulatory dysfunction, polycystic ovary morphology, insulin resistance and metabolic abnormalities or obesity (ESHRE & ASRM-Sponsored PCOS Consensus Workshop Group, 2004). PCOS affects about 5 to 15% of women worldwide depending on the diagnostic criteria used (Leon & Mayrin, 2020). In spite of having such a high prevalence, many cases remain undiagnosed and even when they are correctly diagnosed, the process usually is lengthy (Gibson-Helm et al., 2017).

In general, it is widely accepted that the diagnosis of PCOS should be based in the presence of two of the following three criteria: chronic anovulation, hyperandrogenism (clinical or biological), and polycystic ovaries (Leon & Mayrin, 2020). Nonetheless, consistent with the fact of being a syndrome, no single test is available to establish its diagnosis, and various disorders may present in a similar way. This leads to the necessity of extensive workup if clinical features suggest other causes (Azziz et al., 2009; El Hayek et al., 2016).

In today's world, more than ever before, it is progressively easier to create and store data from many fields which is accumulating at a dramatic pace (Ferreira et al., 2020). Consequently, there is an increasing gap between the generation of data and human understanding of it. In the growing pool of data lies hidden, potentially useful information, that is rarely made explicit or taken advantage of. Thus, one of the grand challenges of the information age is turning data into information and turning information into knowledge (Witten et al., 2005). This can be achieved through the use of Machine Learning (ML) (Zhang, 2020) and Data Mining (DM) (Hand & Adams 2014) since the first is used to extract information from the raw data in databases and the second is the application of specific algorithms for extracting patterns from data (Silva et al., 2018).

As health organizations generate and store large volumes of data every day, clinical decisions could be made not only based on doctor's intuition and experience but also based on hidden knowledge stored over time in healthcare databases (Silva et al., 2018). In this sense, the aim of this study is to predict if a patient has POCS by applying classification techniques such as Random Forest (RF), Decision Tree (DT), Naive Bayes (NB), Logistic Regression (LR), and Artificial Neural Network (ANN). This application of DM may improve operating efficiency in healthcare organizations since the diagnosis of this syndrome can be hard to achieve. Out of the array of DM methodologies, Cross Industry Standard Process for Data Mining (CRISP-DM) was the one applied to the problem at hand, since this is a popular methodology used for improving the efficiency and the scalability of DM projects.

The paper is organized as follows: the next section presents information about previous studies made on PCOS classification; following, the CRISP-DM methodology and a detailed description of each stage is presented; then, the discussion of the results is made and lastly, the paper is concluded and some ideas for future work are outlined.

RELATED WORK

A wide range of work is being done regarding the use of ML and DM in the medical field, specifically some studies have dedicated to its use for PCOS diagnosis. In this section, studies with different approaches for the classification of PCOS will be presented and later discussed.

Bindha et al. (2019) used *Python* and *Jupyter Notebooks* in order to apply classification algorithms to a dataset obtained from a survey of 119 females with ages ranging from 18 to 22 years. The dataset is comprised by 14 binary attributes and 3 categorical attributes. It was concluded that from the six classification algorithms used, namely Logistic Regression (LR), Support Vector Machine (SVM), Decision Tree (DT), k Nearest Neighbours (k-NN), Linear Discriminant Analysis (LDA), and Naïve Bayes (NB), the DT classifier was the best suited for predicting the occurrence of PCOS. The DT classifier had the best accuracy $96.6 \pm 0.033\%$, followed by the k-NN algorithm, which reached an accuracy of $93.3 \pm 0.066\%$. On the other hand, the classifiers with the worst performance were NB and LDA with an accuracy of $76.6 \pm 0.233\%$ and $36.6 \pm 0.633\%$, respectively. However, some limitations can be highlighted from the study. The first limitation is related to the small number of instances of the dataset (only 119 entries). In addition, the dataset presents an unbalanced distribution of classes. Finally, the study did not include data preparation steps (for example, the dataset contains some missing values, but the authors did not mention its treatment), representing a drawback for the reliability of the results achieved in this paper (Bindha et al., 2019).

Satish et al. (2020) used Python-Scikit Learn package and RapidMiner to predict cases of PCOS, using the same dataset of this study (Kottarathil, 2020). Despite using different tools, the highest accuracy - 93.12% - was shown by the Random

Forest (RF) algorithm using the RapidMiner and the dataset with all features. On the other hand, k-NN and SVM show similar accuracy performances - 90.83% - also using RapidMiner but with the dataset that contains 10 selected features, namely *Marriage Status, BMI, Follicle R, FSH, Hip, Weight, Fast food, Hair growth, Skin Darkening*, and *BPDiastolic*. The feature selection was based on the removal of highly correlated attributes (Satish et al., 2020).

Denny et al. (2019) proposed a system for early detection and prediction of PCOS from clinical and metabolic parameters, which act as an early marker for this disease. The techniques employed in this study were: LR, LDA, k-NN, Classification and regression Trees (CART), RF, NB, and SVM. The authors used the same dataset used in this study (Kottarathil, 2020). Using *SPSS V 22.0*, 8 features were selected from the 23 present in the clinical and metabolic test results. For the application of ML techniques, the environment chosen was *Spyder Python IDE*. Additionally, the results show that the system was able to predict PCOS with 89.02% Accuracy when the RF classifier was used. The second-best classifier was k-NN with an Accuracy of 86.58% (Denny et al., 2019).

Neto et al. (2021) used *Python* and the same dataset used in this study (Kottarathil, 2020) to forecast PCOS cases. The study used five different classifiers, namely, LR, RF, SVM, Gaussian Näive Bayes (GNB), and Multilayer Perceptron (MLP). It also used normalization and the outliers were removed based on the Interquartile Range. The missing values and the highly correlated attributes (with the target and between themselves) were also removed. The dataset was balanced using Oversampling (replication of cases of the minority class) and Undersampling (removal of cases of the majority class). In the end, it was found that the RF classifier provides the best classification, allowing to achieve a sensitivity of 0.94, an accuracy of 0.95, a precision of 0.96 and a specificity of 0.96 (Neto et al., 2021). In order to try to improve the results obtained in this paper, some of the authors decided to conduct the present study taking some different approaches which will later be described in detail. Hence, this is a key study for the present work, since a direct comparison is going to be established in Section 4.

MATERIALS AND METHODS

The dataset used in this work is publicly available in the Kaggle repository, the world's largest data science community (Kaggle.com, 2021), and has been collected from 10 different hospitals in Kerala, India, and has information on 541 patients (Kottarathil, 2020). As already mentioned, the goal of this study was to apply a DM process in order to develop different models capable of making an effective prediction of PCOS cases. The RapidMiner software was the tool chosen to conduct this DM process. RapidMiner supports the design and documentation of overall DM process, offering not only an almost comprehensive of operators, but also structures that express the control flow of the process (Hofmann & Klinkenberg, 2016).

DT is a classifier that works by greedily selecting the best split point to make forecasts and reiterate the mechanism until the tree reaches a fixed depth. Once the tree is built, it is pruned to enhance the model's generalization capacity (Myles et al., 2004; Neto et al., 2017).

RF offers an advantage towards DT since the latter one tends to overfit the training data. RF is basically a set of DTs where, initially, a bootstrap sample is selected from the training data (random sample obtained with replacement) for the purpose of inducing a DT. This process is repeated until a set of DTs is generated, each with its own predictive value. Thus, the final prediction is obtained by integrating the output of all trees, which corresponds to the most frequent output of the ensemble (Cutler et al., 2012; Neto et al., 2019).

LR is a fast and simple classification technique which assumes that the input variables are numeric and have a Gaussian (bell curve) distribution. Basically, algorithms learn a coefficient for each input value that is linearly combined into a regression function and transformed using a logistic (s-shaped) function (Neto et al., 2017). Eq. 1 represents the mathematical expression for calculating P, which is the probability of the outcome of interest, i.e., PCOS (Peng et al., 2002).

$$P = \frac{e^{a+bX}}{1+e^{a+bX}} \tag{1}$$

The NB classifier is based on the Bayes Theorem, which is a probabilistic theorem that is used to find out the probability of something happening (A) by knowing that (B) has occurred, as mathematically described in Eq. 2 (Neto et al., 2017). Hence, in the context of the problem at hand, the A variable can be considered the label/target, the attribute *PCOS* and the B variable can be extended and seen as the rest of the features of the dataset (Rish, 2001).

$$P(A|B) = \frac{P(B|A) \times P(A)}{P(B)} \tag{2}$$

Finally, the Artificial Neural Network (ANN) used in this study was implemented through the Deep Learning operator of the RapidMiner software, which is based on a multi-layer feed-forward ANN that is trained with stochastic gradient descent using back-propagation (GmbH, 2021; Graupe, 2013).

A comparative analysis of the advantages and disadvantages of each data mining technique are presented in Table 1.

Table 1. Comparative analysis of each data mining technique

ML Algorithm	Advantages	Disadvantages
Decision Tree (Bhatt, H. et al., 2015; Dhiraj, K. (2019); Pranckevičius, T. and Marcinkevičius, V., 2017)	- Behooves less effort during pre-processing, more specifically in the data preparation, comparing to other algorithms; - Does not need neither data normalization nor data scaling; - It is a very intuitive model.	- Its calculation can be much more complex than other algorithms; - Often requires higher training times; - Unsuitable for regression and predicting continuous values.
Random Forest (Wang, Q. et al., 2019; Pranckevičius, T. and Marcinkevičius, V., 2017)	- Suitable for both categorical and continuous variables; - Automatically handles missing values; - Does not require feature scaling (standardization and normalization).	- Presents higher complexity as it creates a large number of trees and combines their outputs. - It requires more training time than decision trees because it generates a large number of trees and makes decisions based on the majority of votes.
Logistic Regression (Pranckevičius, T. and Marcinkevičius, V., 2017)	- It is easier to implement, interpret, and train; - It can easily be extended to multinomial regression; - It is very fast at classifying unknown records.	- It is sensitive to outliers; - It assumes linearity between the dependent and independent variables; - It can only be used to predicts discrete functions.
Naïve Bayes (Wang, Q. et al., 2019; Pranckevičius, T. and Marcinkevičius, V., 2017)	- It is simple to implement since the conditional probabilities are easy to evaluate; - It requires a small amount of training data. So, the training period is less; - It is extremely fast and can save a significant amount of time.	- It is most fitting for categorical input variables than numerical variables. - It assumes that all features are independent, which in real life does not always stand, as features usually have some form of dependency.
Artificial Neural Network (Mijwel, M. M., 2018)	- It is fault tolerant; - It has the capability of working with incomplete knowledge; - It is able to provide the data to be processed in parallel.	- The functioning of the network is not possible to explain; - It is dependent on hardware since it requires processors with parallel processing power; - Its duration is not known.

During the DM process, the CRISP-DM methodology was followed, which is a popular methodology used for increasing the success of DM projects and allowing the implementation of DM models in real environments (Martins et al., 2021). CRISP-DM is a hierarchical process model that divides the DM process into six different stages, namely Business Understanding, Data Understanding, Data Preparation,

Modeling, Evaluation, and Deployment (Ferreira et al., 2020). Figure 1 represents the lifecycle of this methodology.

Figure 1. CRISP-DM operational cycle

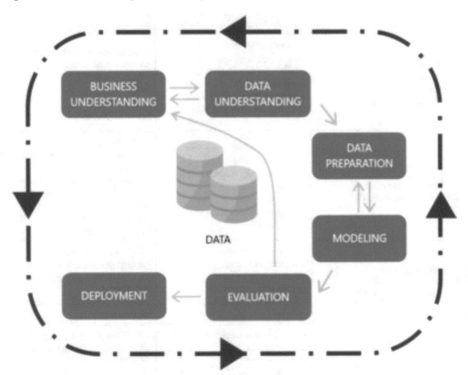

Next, each stage of the CRISP-DM methodology will be described in detail.

Business Understanding

PCOS is a heterogeneous condition hard to diagnose given the variety of features, symptoms, complications and the fact that the causes are unknown, which makes it impossible to diagnose with only one type of test since a specific one for this heterogeneous condition does not exist. Because of this, the presence of POCS is confirmed by the analysis of the clinical history and a few laboratory tests that exclude other entities that may present in the same way (ESHRE & ASRM-Sponsored PCOS Consensus Workshop Group, 2004). The business goal of the work presented in this paper is the prediction of cases of PCOS, considering demographic data, clinical history and laboratory test results through different scenarios based on the correlation weight analysis of the different features. After defining the goal of the study from a business perspective, it is necessary to transform this goal into a DM problem. Hence, the present study fits in the scope of a binary classification problem for predicting if female patients have PCOS (labeled as 1) or not (labeled as 0). Figure 2 shows the research plan made to conduct the present study.

Figure 2. CRISP-DM operational cycle

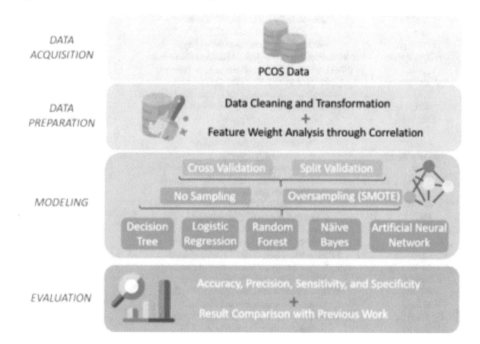

Data Understanding

The dataset provided relates to the detection of cases of PCOS, including 541 patients (instances) and 40 features considered important to diagnose the disease (Kottarathil, 2020). Table 2 contains the description of the attributes of the dataset.

The target variable is the *PCOS* attribute, which is binomial and represents whether an individual has the syndrome or not. Furthermore, 0 represents a healthy individual in what concerns PCOS and 1 represents a patient with PCOS. Figure 3 shows the data distribution of the target variable on the dataset used and as it can be observed, only 32.7% of the instances correspond to individuals with the disease, which represents an imbalanced dataset.

Table 2. Description of the attributes of the dataset under study

Attribute	Description	Type
Sl No	Serial number	Integer
Patient File No	Patient file number	Integer (role: id)
PCOS	Polycystic Ovary Syndrome (PCOS)	Binomial (role:target)
Age	Patient's age in years	Integer
Weight	Patient's weight in kg	Real
Height	Patient's height in cm	Real
BMI	Patient's Body Mass Index (BMI)	Real
Pulse rate	Patient's pulse rate in bpm	Integer
RR	Respiratory rate in breaths/min	Integer
Hb	Hemoglobin in g/dl	Real
Cycle length	The length of fertile period in days	Integer
Marriage Status	Number of years the patient has been married	Binomial
Pregnant	Whether the patient has been pregnant before	Binomial
No of aborptions	Number of abortions the patient had	Real
FSH	Follicle-stimulating hormone (FSH) value in mIU/mL	Real
LH	Luteinizing Hormone (LH) value in mIU/mL	Real
FSH/LH	FSH/LH ratio	Real
Hip	Patient's hip size in inches	Integer
Waist	Patient's waist size in inches	Integer
Waist/Hip Ratio	Waist/Hip ratio	Real
TSH	Thyroid Stimulating Hormone (TSH) in mIU/L	Real
AMH	Anti-Mullerian Hormone (AMH) in ng/mL	Real
PRL	Prolactin (PRL) in ng/mL	Real
Vit D3	Vitamin D3 in ng/mL	Real
PRG	Progesterone (PRG) in ng/mL	Real
RBS	Random Blood Sugar Test (RBS) in mg/dl	Integer
Weight gain	Whether the patient has gained weight	Binomial
Hair growth	Whether the patient has felt hair growth	Binomial
Skin darkening	Whether the patient's skin tone has darkened	Binomial
Hair loss	Whether the patient has hair loss	Binomial
Pimples	Whether the patient has gained pimples	Binomial
Fast food	Whether the patient eats fast food	Binomial
Reg Exercise	Whether the patient practices regular exercise	Binomial
BP Systolic	Systolic blood pressure in mmHg	Integer
BP Diastolic	Diastolic blood pressure in mmHg	Integer
Follicle No (L)	Number of left follicles	Integer
Follicle No (R)	Number of right follicles	Integer
Avg F size (L)	Average size of left follicles in mm	Real
Avg F size (R)	Average size of right follicles in mm	Real
Insulin levels	Insulin levels in μIU/mL	Integer
Endometrium	Endometrial thickness in mm	Real

Figure 3. Data distribution of the target variable PCOS

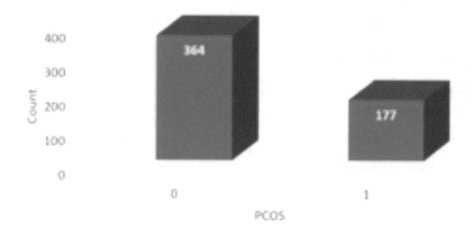

Figures 4 and 5 show the data distribution of PCOS cases according to the attributes such as *hair growth* and *skin darkening*, respectively. The analysis of these figures suggests that these attributes have an influence in identifying PCOS cases, where patients with PCOS (PCOS=1) seem to be associated with skin darkening and hair growth symptoms, meaning that these two attributes may be strong predictors in the forecast of this disease.

Figure 4. Distribution of PCOS cases according to hair growth

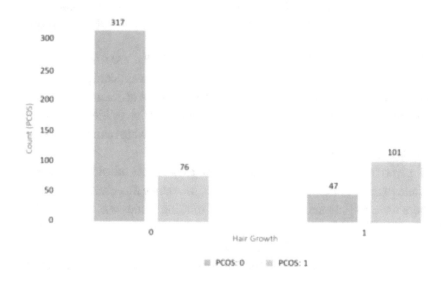

Figure 5. Distribution of PCOS cases according to skin darkening

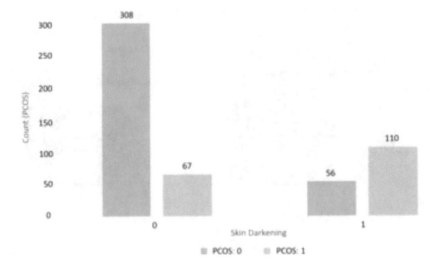

Data Preparation

Data preparation can be the most time demanding phase in the DM process. This step is of great importance because real world data can be incomplete (missing values), noisy (errors or outliers) and incoherent (Martins et al., 2021). In order to achieve effective models and quality standards it is essential to feed quality data into the high-performance DM systems. This phase is comprised by several steps that aim to increase the quality of the dataset, namely data integration, data cleaning, data transformation, data reduction and data sampling. However, their application must be in accordance to the needs of each specific dataset and with this in mind the following actions were taken.

First, since there were two features, *Serial number* and *Patient file number*, that acted as IDs, they were removed from the dataset. This action was taken because these features have no predictive value and maintaining both is not efficient. Afterwards, when importing data to the *RapidMiner*, it automatically tries to identify the type of data, which does not always go perfectly. So, some fields were manually tweaked to correspond to the ones mentioned in Table 2.

There were no duplicated instances in the data. However, 3 missing values were identified, one in each of the following attributes: *Marriage Status*, *AMH* and *Fast food*. As there were 541 instances, the number of missing values was relatively low, which led to their elimination. Additionally, to check for outliers, i.e., observations that are far away from most or all other observations (Ghosh & Vogt, 2012), the *Detect Outlier (LOF)* operator was used. This operator is based on a concept of a local density, where locality is given by the k nearest neighbours, whose distance is used to estimate the density. This results in a new column *outlier* containing Outlier Scores that helped to quickly summarize and find outliers as well as to carefully check for natural aberrant values. The larger the number in this new column, the further away that data point is relative to the dataset. So, to achieve better performance, only the instances with Outlier Scores below 2 were chosen. This was done with the *Filter Examples* operator and resulted in the elimination of 19 instances, bringing the total number of instances down to 519. The treatment of outliers was the first significant difference between this work and the study performed in (Neto et al., 2021), in which the outliers were detected based on the Interquartile Range.

On top of that, in the data reduction step the weights were analyzed using the operator *Weights by Correlation*, which provides a correlation of each feature with the target attribute (*PCOS*) in which very high correlation values could be damaging to the results. The results of this analysis are shown in Table 3. This information was important to the definition of the scenarios in the next phase (Modeling). Since the attribute Insulin levels presented a very high correlation, 0.894, it was removed from the selected features as to not negatively impact the results, as performed in (Neto et al., 2021).

Table 3. Distribution of feature weights using the correlation criteria

Feature	Weight	Feature	Weight	Feature	Weight	Feature	Weight
Insulin levels	0.894	Age	0.188	LH	0.094	RR	0.049
Follicle No (R)	0.647	BMI	0.186	Avg F. size (R)	0.091	TSH	0.023
Follicle No (L)	0.598	Cycle length	0.177	Hb	0.086	BP Diastolic	0.022
Skin darkening	0.478	Hair Loss	0.169	Reg Exercise	0.083	Pregnant	0.020
Hair Growth	0.459	Hip	0.157	FSH/LH	0.079	RBS	0.017
Weight gain	0.434	Waist	0.155	Height	0.079	BP systolic	0.014
Fast food	0.374	Marriage status	0.131	FSH	0.067	PRL	0.010
Pimples	0.290	Avg F. size (L)	0.127	Vit D3	0.064	Waist/Hip Ratio	0.005
AMH	0.256	Pulse rate	0.103	No of abortions	0.060	SI No	0.000
Weight	0.204	Endometrium	0.102	PRG	0.050	Patient File No	0.000

Last but not least, as seen in Figure 3 the data was not balanced - 67.3% PCOS(0) and 32,7% PCOS(1). This disparity in classes can, in this case, lead the algorithm to learn more from the healthy individuals and not identify what makes the individuals with the PCOS syndrome different or even underlying patterns that allow the distinction between these two classes. The operator selected to balance the data was the *SMOTE Upsampling*, which implements the Synthethic Minority Over-Sampling Technique as proposed in (Chawla et al., 2002). This technique, which creates the new examples based on the k nearest neighbors, has proven over time to achieve good performances. This is another distinguishing aspect from the work done in (Neto et al., 2021), in which the data balancing was done using Oversampling (replication of cases from the minority class) and Undersampling (removal of cases from the majority class). Since the best result was obtained with Oversampling, it was decided to study in this paper another Oversampling technique, the SMOTE, which instead of replicating cases, consists in the creation of synthetic data.

Modeling

This phase consisted in the preparation of different Data Mining Models (DMM) using the *RapidMiner* with the dataset resulting from the Data Preparation stage. Each DMM can be described as belonging to an Approach (A), being composed by a Scenario (S), a Data Mining Technique (DMT), a Sampling Method (SM), a Data Approach (DA) and a Target (T), as expressed in Eq. 3.

$$DMM = \{A, S, DMT, SM, DA, T\} \tag{3}$$

As mentioned, there was only one target (T) variable, which was the *PCOS* variable.

Since Classification was the chosen Approach (A), there were five different classifiers selected to be used as DMTs, namely RF, DT, ANN, LR, and NB, the description of which was given in the Materials and Methods section.

For each DMT, two Sampling Methods (SM) were tested: *Split Validation*, with 70% of the data used for training and the remaining amount for testing and *Cross Validation*, using 10 folds (Chui et al., 2020; Alqahtani et al., 2019) and where all data is used for testing as it can be seen in Figure 6.

Figure 6. Comparison between Split and Cross Validation functioning

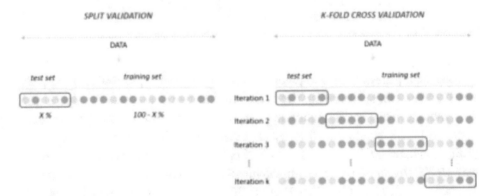

In addition, given the imbalanced distribution of the target variable shown in Figure 3, there were two Data Approaches (DA) tested: Without Sampling and With Oversampling, more specifically using the SMOTE Upsampling technique.

The considered scenarios, in order to evaluate which attributes were the most relevant to predict the diagnosis of PCOS, were defined according to the weights obtained with the operator *Weights by Correlation* (Table 3). The first scenario (S1) contains all attributes except the ones removed in the Data Preparation stage. The second scenario (S2) contains all attributes except the ones with a weight inferior to 0.1. The last scenario (S3) contains the same attributes as S2, except *Follicle No (R)* and *Follicle No (L)* since a maximum threshold of 0.55 was also established for this scenario.

- S1: {All attributes except Insulin levels, Serial Number, and Patient File Number};
- S2: {Follicle No (L), Follicle No (R), Skin darkening, Hair growth, Weight gain, Fast food, Pimples, AMH, Weight, Age, BMI, Cycle length, Hair loss, Hip, Waist, Marriage status, Avg F size (L), Pulse Rate, Endometrium};
- S3: {Skin darkening, Hair growth, Weight gain, Fast food, Pimples, AMH, Weight, Age, BMI, Cycle length, Hair loss, Hip, Waist, Marriage status, Avg F size (L), Pulse Rate, Endometrium}.

Hence, for the context of this work, the DMMs are described as:

- A = {Classification}
- S = {S1, S2, S3}
- DMT = {RF, DL, LR, NB, DT}
- SM = {Split Validation (70% for training) and Cross Validation (10 folds)}
- DA = {Without Sampling, With Oversampling (SMOTE Upsampling)}
- T = {PCOS}

In total, 60 models were induced according to Eq. 4.

$$DMM = \{1(A) \times 3(S) \times 5(DMT) \times 2(SM) \times (DA) \times 1(T)\} \qquad (4)$$

Evaluation

Since the approach is of the Classification type, for each model the evaluation was derived from the confusion matrix, shown in Figure 7, which represents the number of False Positives (FP), False Negatives (FN), True Positives (TP) and True Negatives

(TN) (Visa et al., 2011). From these values various metrics can be derived. In this case, the evaluation was supported by accuracy (Eq. 5), precision (Eq. 6), sensitivity (Eq. 7) and specificity (Eq. 8).

Figure 7. Confusion matrix structure of a binary classification problem

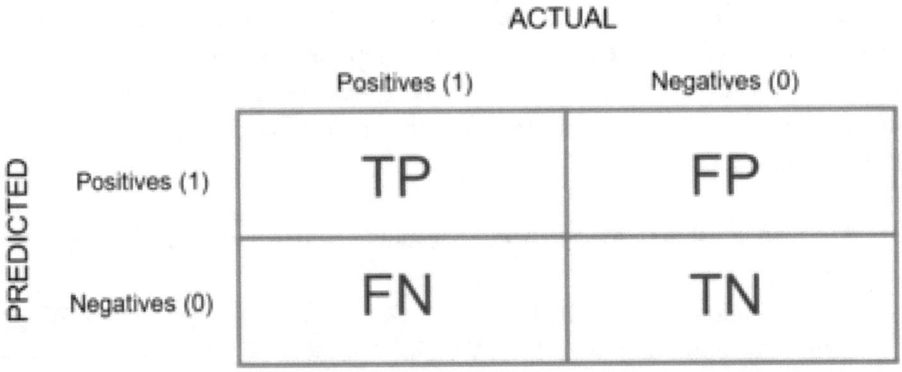

Accuracy concerns the correctly TP classified instances, as mathematically expressed in Eq. 5. It calculates the ratio between the instances correctly classified by the model and all the classified instances. In this study, this metric refers to the number of patients that were correctly classified either as having PCOS or not out of all the patients. Hence, this metric answers to the question: Out of all the patients, how many were correctly labeled?

$$Accuracy = \frac{TP + TN}{TP + FP + TN + FN} \tag{5}$$

Precision measures the exactness of a classifier and is calculated through Eq. 6. This metric calculates the ratio between the number of positive instances correctly classified by the model and the total number of instances classified as being positive. Hence, in the context of this study, Precision evaluates the ability of the model to identify patients with PCOS, i.e. the fraction of patients who were classified as having PCOS and that actually have the disease. This metric provides the answer to the following question: How many of those labeled has having PCOS actually had PCOS?

$$Precision = \frac{TP}{TP + FP} \tag{6}$$

Sensitivity, also known as Recall, measures the completeness of a classifier and is calculated using Eq. 7. This metric calculates the ratio between the number of positive instances correctly classified by the model and all the positive instances of the dataset (Martins et al., 2021). In this study, sensitivity assesses the ability of the model to correctly identify patients with PCOS, i.e. the fraction of patients classified as having PCOS, labeled as 1, who actually have the disease among all patients with PCOS.

Thus, sensitivity is an efficient evaluation metric for assessing the performance of models in the field of clinical diagnosis, where the cost associated with FN is high. A higher FN value is harmful because it means that the model predicted that a patient did not had PCOS when, in fact, she had the disease, leading physicians to neglect treatments that could save her life. In this sense, Sensitivity provides answer to the question: Of all the patients with PCOS, how many of those were correctly predicted?

$$Sensitivity = \frac{TP}{TP + FN} \tag{7}$$

Specificity gives information on the correctly TN classified instances as mathematically expressed in Eq. 8. It calculates the ratio between the number of negative instances correctly classified by the model and all the negative instances. In this study, specificity is determined by the proportion of patients who did not have PCOS that the model was able to correctly classify, i.e. the fraction of patients who were classified as not having PCOS and who actually did not have the disease. Specificity answers to the question: Of all the healthy people, how many of those were correctly predicted?

$$Specificity = \frac{TN}{TN + FP} \tag{8}$$

RESULTS AND DISCUSSION

Table 4, Table 5, Table 6, and Table 7 concern the best results, for each DMT, in what regards accuracy, precision, sensitivity, and specificity, respectively.

Table 4. DMMs with the best accuracy for each DMT

DMM	DMT	S	SM	DA	Accuracy
1	RF	S2	Split validation	SMOTE	93.06%
2	ANN	S2	Cross validation	SMOTE	90.25%
3	LR	S2	Split validation	SMOTE	90.74%
4	NB	S2	Split validation	Without oversampling	88.75%
5	DT	S2	Split validation	SMOTE	85.19%

Table 5. DMMs with the best precision for each DMT

DMM	DMT	S	SM	DA	Precision
1	RF	S2	Split validation	SMOTE	92.66%
6	ANN	S2	Split validation	SMOTE	92.86%
3	LR	S2	Split validation	SMOTE	91.51%
7	NB	S2	Cross validation	SMOTE	89.76%
8	DT	S2	Cross validation	SMOTE	83.33%

Table 6. DMMs with the best sensitivity for each DMT

DMM	DMT	S	SM	DA	Sensitivity
1	RF	S2	Split validation	SMOTE	93.52%
9	ANN	S1	Split validation	SMOTE	92.38%
10	LR	S1	Split validation	SMOTE	91.43%
11	NB	S1	Split validation	SMOTE	92.24%
5	DT	S2	Split validation	SMOTE	88.89%

Table 7. DMMs with the best specificity for each DMT

DMM	DMT	S	SM	DA	Specificity
12	RF	S2	Split validation	Without oversampling	96.30%
6	ANN	S2	Split validation	SMOTE	93.52%
13	LR	S1	Cross validation	Without oversampling	92.88%
14	NB	S2	Split validation	SMOTE	90.53%
15	DT	S1	Cross validation	Without oversampling	92.87%

Analyzing Tables 4, 5, 6 and 7 it can be observed that, overall the best results were obtained using the RF classifier, the S2 scenario, the Split Validation method and Oversampling (SMOTE), having achieved the best accuracy, sensitivity and specificity values, which were 93.06%, 93.52% and 96.30%, respectively. In what regards the precision metric, the best results were also achieved when using the S2 scenario, the Split Validation method and Oversampling (SMOTE), but this time using the ANN classifier.

For this context, the metrics applied don't have the same impact. A correct diagnose of PCOS (precision) and how many people with PCOS were correctly predicted (sensitivity) is more important than knowing, out of all healthy people how many were predicted as being healthy (specificity) and of all the people how many were correctly labeled (accuracy). In order to choose the most suitable model, a threshold was established, and the models were ranked according to their sensitivity results. In this case, sensitivity was selected as the most valuable since it decreases with the increasing of FN. These FN values correspond to a wrong diagnose of PCOS, in other words, it is when a patient with PCOS is diagnosed as a healthy individual. Therefore, high sensitivity reduces the chances of not correctly diagnosing a patient with PCOS, which is extremely important because early detection has a heavy impact in the treatment of this syndrome. Hence, this metric was selected because of the harmful consequences that can arise from high FN values, which refers to patients that have the disease, but the model is incapable of classifying them as having the disease, which is a matter of crucial importance when it comes to diagnosing PCOS. It is preferable to diagnose a person with PCOS when that is not true (FP) than to predict that a person does not have PCOS when, in fact, it has (FN). Hence, the defined threshold was every metric >88% and sensitivity >90%. Table 8 presents the four best models that achieved the threshold by their ranking order, according to sensitivity.

Table 8. DMMs with the best results within the threshold defined

DMM	DMT	S	SM	DA	Accuracy	Precision	Sensitivity	Specificity
1	RF	S2	Split validation	SMOTE	93.06%	92.66%	93.52%	92.59%
16	RF	S2	Cross validation	SMOTE	90.39%	90.43%	90.51%	90.25%
6	ANN	S2	Split validation	SMOTE	90.18%	92.86%	90.50%	93.52%
17	RF	S1	Split validation	SMOTE	90.95%	91.35%	90.48%	91.43%

For better visualization and easier comparison between the results obtained in each DMM and for each evaluation metric, it was decided to plot the results of Table 8 in the bar chart shown in Figure 8.

Figure 8. Comparison of the results obtained for the DMMs that fall within the defined threshold

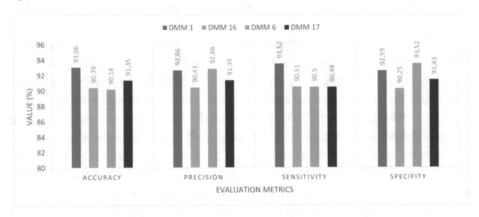

With the information collected in Table 8, it is easy to point out that the 4 best models (100%) used the data with oversampling, particularly the SMOTE Upsampling technique. Additionally, 3 out of the 4 models (75%) selected used the RF classifier. In what concerns the scenarios, it is possible to conclude that 3 out of the 4 models (75%) used the S2 scenario. On the other hand, for the sampling methods, Split Validation seem to perform better, as only 1 out of the 4 best models (25%) used Cross Validation. Lastly, the first model presents better values for every metric when compared to the other models. Thus, it is possible to claim that the most suitable model, from all the 60 induced models, is DMM = {Classification, S2, RF, Split Validation, With Oversampling, PCOS}.

As observed, generally, models with Cross Validation as the sampling method achieved worse results when compared to those with Split Validation, which is confirmed by the results in Table 8.

In the S3 scenario, there was a significant impact on the results because *Insulin levels*, *Follicle No (L)* and *Follicle No (R)* attributes, that are directly related with the target, were removed. In this scenario, the results for the great majority of the techniques were lower than the other scenarios, as it can be observed by the nonexistence of S3 in Table 8, the one that contains the best results. The scenario that obtained the best results overall was the S2 scenario. When comparing scenario S2 with scenario S3, the only difference found is the lack of *Follicle No (L)* and *Follicle No (R)* in the third scenario. By observing the values of these two, the S2 obtains better results, which means that *Follicle No (L)* and *Follicle No (R)* are relevant attributes for the classification of PCOS. In turn, when comparing S1 and S2, the difference is that S2 removes the attributes with a correlation weight lower than 0.1, which means that the removal of attributes with lower correlation weights seems to be beneficial for the forecasting of PCOS.

By analyzing the results obtained it is noticeable that the algorithms that had the best results were achieved with the RF classifier, which means that out of the five classifiers used in this study, this technique is the most suitable for the used dataset and the problem at hand. In contrast, the technique with the worst results was the DT classifier. Although being the one that achieved the lowest values, these are still acceptable, having achieved values around 80%.

Contrary to what has been found in (Bindha et al., 2019) where DT was the best performing classifier with an accuracy of 96.6%, in this study the DT classifier had the worst performance with an accuracy of 85.19%. These differences could be explained from the use of an unbalanced dataset in (Bindha et al., 2019) in which accuracy can be an unreliable measure of model's performance since the models created are unable to distinguish between the two classes and can only classify cases of the majority class.

Most of the studies mentioned in the Related Work section, (Satish et al., 2020), (Denny et al., 2019), and (Neto et al., 2021), concluded that RF was the best classifier for predicting cases of PCOS. The present work validates these findings, where RF was the best performing algorithm with an accuracy value of 93.06%.

Figure 9 shows the comparison of the Accuracy values obtained in this work and the ones obtained in the works mentioned in the Related Work Section.

Figure 9. Comparison between the accuracy results obtained and the Related Work

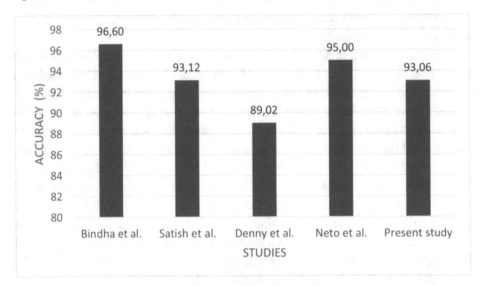

Although it has been obtained a greater accuracy value than the one obtained in (Denny et al., 2019), the results obtained in the present study were slightly lower than those obtained in (Satish et al., 2020) and (Neto et al., 2021). The lower results achieved in (Denny et al., 2019) are probably due to the reduced number of features selected for the study. In what concerns the study conducted in (Satish et al., 2020), although the difference is relatively small, it is probably caused by the use of all attributes, which includes the *Insulin Levels* attribute, the one that has an extremely high correlation with the target.

The work that stands out the most was the one previously carried out by the authors of the present paper (Neto et al., 2021), in which an accuracy of 95% was achieved. Furthermore, precision (96%), sensitivity (94%) and specificity (96%) values were also greater than the ones achieved in the present paper, as it can be seen in Figure 10.

Figure 10. Comparison between the results of the present study results and the ones obtained in a previous work

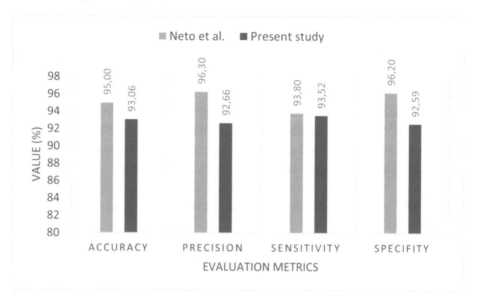

Hence, a more detailed comparison will be made. The meaningful differences found between the two papers are based on the use of the normalization technique, the use of different criteria to detect outliers, the use of distinct sampling techniques and the use of different feature selection techniques. The factors that stand out the most when explaining the difference in the results obtained are, respectively, the use of normalization and the use of a combination of different selection techniques; with both using, the correlation and the *f_classif* criteria (Scikit-learn, 2021). Since there were several attributes related to perimeters and measurements of substances found in the human body at varying scales, where higher scales could lead to an unrealistic influence, the use of a minmax normalization technique in (Neto et al., 2021) has been shown to result in a more accurate use of the data. Regarding the criteria used for feature selection, it can then be concluded that using only correlation-based criteria did not prove to be more efficient than using a combination of criteria.

CONCLUSION AND FUTURE WORK

The project developed focused on solving the binary classification of patients with PCOS based on scenarios defined according to correlation weight criteria. The application of such a model would be extremely efficient since many patients with PCOS can remain undiagnosed for a considerable amount of time. Thus, a DM model applied to a hospital database could warn doctors and nurses to further investigate and confirm the cases of PCOS identified by the model. In fact, it proves that the application of DM in the prediction of PCOS is viable. Some DMMs, were able to achieve levels of accuracy, precision, sensitivity and specificity as high as 93,06%, 92.66%, 93.52% and 96.30%, respectively. Additionally, the best model induced combined all the metrics above 92%, more specifically, 93.06% accuracy, 92.66% precision, 93.52% sensitivity and 92.59% specificity.

Although, these percentages seem to confidently support the viability of creating a model that correctly diagnoses PCOS in a clinical scenario, the approach taken in this research, by selecting the features based only on the correlation weight, was not the best when compared with the previous study conducted in this field by the authors. More specifically, the feature selection based only on the correlation weight decreased the values of accuracy by 1.9%, precision by 3.7%, sensitivity by 0.3%, and specificity by 3.6%.

In future work, it would be interesting to analyse and combine different techniques of feature selection in order to improve the results obtained. Furthermore, it would be interesting to study the implementation of intelligent feature engineering. As concluded in this study and also in a previous one, a balanced dataset is able to achieve better results. Hence, it would be valuable in the future to not replicate nor synthetically create new instances, but to collect more data of the minority class, or even more instances as long as a balanced distribution is guaranteed. Lastly, more DMTs could be tested, such as Gradient Boost, as well as optimizing the parameters for each of the techniques selected.

ACKNOWLEDGMENT

This work is funded by "FCT—Fundação para a Ciência e Tecnologia" within the R&D Units Project Scope: UIDB/00319/2020. D.F. and C. N. thank the Fundação para a Ciência e Tecnologia (FCT), Portugal for the grants 2021.06308.BD and 2021.06507.BD, respectively.

REFERENCES

Alqahtani, M., Gumaei, A., Mathkour, H., & Maher Ben Ismail, M. (2019). A genetic-based extreme gradient boosting model for detecting intrusions in wireless sensor networks. *Sensors (Basel)*, *19*(20), 4383. doi:10.339019204383 PMID:31658774

Azziz, R., Carmina, E., Dewailly, D., Diamanti-Kandarakis, E., Escobar-Morreale, H. F., Futterweit, W., Janssen, O. E., Legro, R. S., Norman, R. J., Taylor, A. E., & Witchel, S. F. (2009). The Androgen Excess and PCOS Society criteria for the polycystic ovary syndrome: The complete task force report. *Fertility and Sterility*, *91*(2), 456–488. doi:10.1016/j.fertnstert.2008.06.035 PMID:18950759

Balen, A., & Rajkowha, M. (2003). Polycystic ovary syndrome—A systemic disorder? *Best Practice & Research. Clinical Obstetrics & Gynaecology*, *17*(2), 263–274. doi:10.1016/S1521-6934(02)00119-0 PMID:12758099

Bhatt, H., Mehta, S., & D'mello, L. R. (2015). Use of ID3 decision tree algorithm for placement prediction. *International Journal of Computer Science and Information Technologies*, *6*(5), 4785–4789.

Bindha, P. G., Rajalaxmi, R. R., & Poorani, S. (2019). *Predicting the Presence of Poly Cystic Ovarian Syndrome using Classification Techniques*. Academic Press.

Chawla, N. V., Bowyer, K. W., Hall, L. O., & Kegelmeyer, W. P. (2002). SMOTE: Synthetic minority over-sampling technique. *Journal of Artificial Intelligence Research*, *16*, 321–357. doi:10.1613/jair.953

Chui, K. T., Liu, R. W., Zhao, M., & De Pablos, P. O. (2020). Predicting students' performance with school and family tutoring using generative adversarial network-based deep support vector machine. *IEEE Access: Practical Innovations, Open Solutions*, 8, 86745–86752. doi:10.1109/ACCESS.2020.2992869

Cutler, A., Cutler, D. R., & Stevens, J. R. (2012). Random forests. In *Ensemble machine learning* (pp. 157–175). Springer. doi:10.1007/978-1-4419-9326-7_5

Denny, A., Raj, A., Ashok, A., Ram, C. M., & George, R. (2019, October). i-HOPE: Detection And Prediction System For Polycystic Ovary Syndrome (PCOS) Using Machine Learning Techniques. In TENCON 2019-2019 IEEE Region 10 Conference (TENCON) (pp. 673-678). IEEE.

Dhiraj, K. (2019). *Top 5 advantages and disadvantages of Decision Tree Algorithm*. Available in: https://dhirajkumarblog.medium.com/top-5-advantages-and-disadvantages-of-decision-tree-algorithm-428ebd199d9a

El Hayek, S., Bitar, L., Hamdar, L. H., Mirza, F. G., & Daoud, G. (2016). Poly cystic ovarian syndrome: An updated overview. *Frontiers in Physiology*, *7*, 124. doi:10.3389/fphys.2016.00124 PMID:27092084

ESHRE. (2004). Revised 2003 consensus on diagnostic criteria and long-term health risks related to polycystic ovary syndrome. *Fertility and Sterility*, *81*(1), 19–25. doi:10.1016/j.fertnstert.2003.10.004 PMID:14711538

Ferreira, D., Silva, S., Abelha, A., & Machado, J. (2020). Recommendation system using autoencoders. *Applied Sciences (Basel, Switzerland)*, *10*(16), 5510. doi:10.3390/app10165510

Ghosh, D., & Vogt, A. (2012, July). Outliers: An evaluation of methodologies. In Joint statistical meetings (Vol. 2012). Academic Press.

Gibson-Helm, M., Teede, H., Dunaif, A., & Dokras, A. (2017). Delayed diagnosis and a lack of information associated with dissatisfaction in women with polycystic ovary syndrome. *The Journal of Clinical Endocrinology and Metabolism*, *102*(2), 604–612. PMID:27906550

Gmb, H. R. 2021. *Deep Learning - RapidMiner Documentation*. Available at: https://docs.rapidminer.com/latest/studio/operators/modeling/predictive/neural_nets/deep_learning.html

Graupe, D. (2013). *Principles of artificial neural networks* (Vol. 7). World Scientific. doi:10.1142/8868

Hand, D. J., & Adams, N. M. (2014). Data mining. *Wiley StatsRef: Statistics Reference Online*, 1-7.

Hofmann, M., & Klinkenberg, R. (Eds.). (2016). *RapidMiner: Data mining use cases and business analytics applications*. CRC Press. doi:10.1201/b16023

Kaggle.com. (2021). *Kaggle: Your Machine Learning and Data Science Community*. Available at: https://www.kaggle.com

Kottarathil, P. (2021). *Polycystic ovary syndrome (PCOS)*. Available at: https://www.kaggle.com/prasoonkottarathil/polycystic-ovary-syndrome-pcos

Leon, L. I. R., & Mayrin, J. V. (2020). *Polycystic Ovarian Disease*. StatPearls.

Martins, B., Ferreira, D., Neto, C., Abelha, A., & Machado, J. (2021). Data Mining for Cardiovascular Disease Prediction. *Journal of Medical Systems*, *45*(1), 1–8. doi:10.100710916-020-01682-8 PMID:33404894

Mijwel, M. M. (2018). *Artificial neural networks advantages and disadvantages*. Retrieved from LinkedIn https//www. linkedin. com/pulse/artificial-neuralnet Work

Myles, A. J., Feudale, R. N., Liu, Y., Woody, N. A., & Brown, S. D. (2004). An introduction to decision tree modeling. *Journal of Chemometrics: A Journal of the Chemometrics Society, 18*(6), 275-285.

Neto, C., Brito, M., Lopes, V., Peixoto, H., Abelha, A., & Machado, J. (2019). Application of data mining for the prediction of mortality and occurrence of complications for gastric cancer patients. *Entropy (Basel, Switzerland), 21*(12), 1163. doi:10.3390/e21121163

Neto, C., Peixoto, H., Abelha, V., Abelha, A., & Machado, J. (2017). Knowledge discovery from surgical waiting lists. *Procedia Computer Science, 121*, 1104–1111. doi:10.1016/j.procs.2017.11.141

Peng, C. Y. J., Lee, K. L., & Ingersoll, G. M. (2002). An introduction to logistic regression analysis and reporting. *The Journal of Educational Research, 96*(1), 3–14. doi:10.1080/00220670209598786

Pranckevičius, T., & Marcinkevičius, V. (2017). Comparison of naive bayes, random forest, decision tree, support vector machines, and logistic regression classifiers for text reviews classification. *Baltic Journal of Modern Computing, 5*(2), 221. doi:10.22364/bjmc.2017.5.2.05

Rish, I. (2001, August). An empirical study of the naive Bayes classifier. In IJCAI 2001 workshop on empirical methods in artificial intelligence (Vol. 3, No. 22, pp. 41-46). Academic Press.

Satish, C. N., Chew, X., & Khaw, K. W. (2020). *Polycystic Ovarian Syndrome (PCOS) classification and feature selection by machine learning techniques.* Academic Press.

Scikit-learn. (2021). *feature_selection: f_classif.* Available at: https://scikit-learn.org/stable/modules/generated/sklearn.feature_selection.f_classif.html

Silva, C., Oliveira, D., Peixoto, H., Machado, J., & Abelha, A. (2018, May). Data mining for prediction of length of stay of cardiovascular accident inpatients. In *International Conference on Digital Transformation and Global Society* (pp. 516-527). Springer. 10.1007/978-3-030-02843-5_43

Visa, S., Ramsay, B., Ralescu, A. L., & Van Der Knaap, E. (2011). Confusion matrix-based feature selection. *MAICS, 710*, 120–127.

Wang, Q., Cao, W., Guo, J., Ren, J., Cheng, Y., & Davis, D. N. (2019). DMP_MI: An effective diabetes mellitus classification algorithm on imbalanced data with missing values. *IEEE Access: Practical Innovations, Open Solutions, 7*, 102232–102238. doi:10.1109/ACCESS.2019.2929866

Witchel, S. F., Oberfield, S. E., & Peña, A. S. (2019). Polycystic ovary syndrome: Pathophysiology, presentation, and treatment with emphasis on adolescent girls. *Journal of the Endocrine Society*, *3*(8), 1545–1573. doi:10.1210/js.2019-00078 PMID:31384717

Witten, I. H., Frank, E., Hall, M. A., & Pal, C. J. (2005). Practical machine learning tools and techniques. Morgan Kaufmann.

Zhang, X. D. (2020). *A Matrix Algebra Approach to Artificial Intelligence*. Springer.

Chapter 7
A Psychometrics Approach to Entropy

Joana Machado
Centro ALGORITMI, Universidade do Minho, Portugal

Isabel Araújo
Cooperativa de Ensino Superior Politécnico e Universitário, Portugal

António Almeida-Dias
Cooperativa de Ensino Superior Politécnico e Universitário, Portugal

Jorge Ribeiro
https://orcid.org/0000-0003-1874-7340
Instituto Politécnico de Viana do Castelo, Portugal

Henrique Vicente
https://orcid.org/0000-0001-8456-7773
Universidade de Évora, Portugal

José Neves
Centro ALGORITMI, Universidade do Minho, Portugal

ABSTRACT

Today's metrics for women housework work (WHW) operate at a quantitative level, specifically measuring time expended on a task and the totality of tasks women perform, not considering that it is a process that is eminently qualitative in nature. To fill this gap, an innovative framework for representing and thinking about big data or knowledge is presented, borrowing from the field of artificial intelligence the methods and methodologies for problem solving, from logic programming the artifacts to improve practice through theory, and from the laws of thermodynamics the construct of entropy, interpreted as the degree of disorder or unpredictability in a system, a principle that may be used to understand system evolution. Last but not least, it also considers the relationship among the disciplines of psychometrics and psychology or sociology (i.e., how certain psychological and sociological concepts such as cognition, knowledge and personality affect WHW satisfaction).

DOI: 10.4018/978-1-7998-9172-7.ch007

INTRODUCTION

Social Norms

Social Norms are a widely intervention strategy for promoting positive health-related behaviors, specifically within a family. It operates on the premise that individuals misperceive their peers' behaviors and attitudes, with evidence of under and over-estimations of deeds and peer approval for a range of positive and negative conducts (Araújo, 2005; Bartz, 2010; Janzen & Hellsten, 2018). It is branded by assurance, joint judgements, and shared aims. Understanding the structure, function, and the course of action of a family are of the utmost importance to contribute to the individual and group well-being. Indeed, countless changes come about in ongoing families, but the most significant one is that of their structure, understood as *an orderly relationship between parts of the family and between the family and other social systems*, promoting its uniqueness (Hanson, 2005). Indeed, in the field of *Sociology*, people as Talcott Parsons that uttered the role of personally and function of devised individuals, both at the level of family structure and at the level of socialization, suggesting that women are expressions of the role of others, a fact that weigh in the well-being of the social unity (Black, 1961). On the other hand, the work of Burr (1998) on gender studies was fundamental to questioning family-related roles that produce, reproduce, and manifest the positions of the genre. In fact, the roles of behavior, duties and expectations correspond to a position of the individual in the social hierarchy. A role is consistent with one's own behavior, a kind of interaction that creates a specific situation between individuals and different norms, beliefs, and values. Indeed, in this work, four implicit roles in housework were acknowledged, namely physical, emotional, mental, and spiritual, that integrating housework with care work, includes all those who contribute to such kind of occupation. Under this setting, one has new questions on this issue, as well as a re-understanding of specific recognized roles in the situation of women, viz.

- *Housewife, i.e., do you do all kinds of household chores, including housekeeping and gardening?;*
- *Childminder, i.e., does it include taking care of children to meet their needs, namely basic safety and fun?;*
- *Socialization, i.e., does its aggregate interaction with other family members and external elements?; and*
- *Therapeutic, these include sharing concerns, being willing to listen to others, actively participating in problem-solving, namely promoting health and preventing disease, and seeking emotional support.*

just to name a few. Indisputably, a new tool with evidence for the representation, validity, and reliability of such constructs is needed to measure the *WHW* and to better describe their final outcomes, i.e., the level of satisfaction that they may or may not enjoy. Indeed, this article reports on the results of a study evaluating the psychometric evidence of *WHW*, including factor structure, internal consistency, reliability test and validity design. One's assessment of the validity of the *WHW* construct emphasizes the extent to which a measure of entropy provides a theoretically meaningful standard of performance, anticipating that there is a major connection among the *WHW's* scales and the answers to questionnaires such as *ChildMinder*, *Housewife Care, Therapy* and *Socialization* (Araújo, 2005). In fact, other types of tasks or work might have been considered, but to our understand and purpose, these are the ones that, once affect the process, may have a major impact on the results; this is the rationale behind our option. For a systematic comparison with other approaches and techniques to problem solving see Araújo (2005).

Presentation Planning

Indeed, what lies behind and beyond the subject here presented develops throughout the lines, i.e., succeeding the *Introduction* the basics followed in this work are established, i.e., the use of *Logic Programming* (*LP*) for *Knowledge Representation and Reasoning* (*KRR*) and its relation either to *Entropy* or to the discipline of *Psychometrics,* which is concerned with the question of how psychological constructs (e.g. *Intelligence*, *Neuroticism*, or *Depression*) can be optimally related to observables outcomes of psychological and sociological nature. It leads to an assessment of its entropic facets, the landscapes of which are understood as a process of energy depreciation (Wenterodt & Herwig, 2014). It then presents a case study on behavioral analysis of women's satisfaction with household chores, their translation into logical programs or logical theories and how evidence of *WHW* satisfaction is produced. Finally, conclusions are drawn, and future developments are outlined.

Preliminaries

A cohort of 50 (fifty) portuguese women born between 1970 and 2019 were observed during some phases of adulthood (ages 25 to 49 years old). On the other hand, to ensure that the problem-solving methodology is intelligible, it is given in pictorial mode. Therefore, and in terms of the *ChildMinder Questionnaire-Four-Item* (*CMQ-4*), one may have (Neves et al., 2019; Neves et al., 2021), viz.

- *Q1 – Do you usually bathe your children/grandchildren?;*
- *Q2 – Do you usually feed your children/grandchildren?;*

- *Q3 – Do you have help in the basic care of your children/grandchildren? and*
- *Q4 – Can you reconcile your profession with childcare?.*

The purpose of this questionnaire is to capture women's general feelings about their behavioral relationships, provided that the high scores on the ChildMinder scale led to positive outcomes and benefits. The scale used is an expanded version of a Likert type one, the expansion of which allows us to trace the evolution of the entropic state of a system's discourse universe, viz.

strongly agree (4), agree (3), disagree (2), strongly disagree (1), disagree (2), agree (3), strongly agree (4)

Moreover, it is included a neutral term, *neither agree* nor *disagree*, which stands for *uncertain* or *vague*. The reason for the individual's answers is in relation to the query depicted below, showing the way to Table 1.

As a family member, how much would you agree with each one of the CMQ – 4 referred to above?

Instead, to avoid biasing consent, the emphasis was on writing questions that would not lead the answerer to conclude that there was a correct or positive answer, i.e., preventing asking questions based on whether the interviewee agrees with a particular statement or not.

Table 1. One woman's answers to CMQ - 4 lead to the creation of the Best and Worst-case scenarios

Questions	Scale							
	(4)	(3)	(2)	(1)	(2)	(3)	(4)	Vagueness
Q1	×	×						
Q2					×	×		
Q3					×		×	
Q4								×
Leading to … Figure 1								

Figure 1. Graphic representation of a female perception of her entropic states in relation to the Best and Worst-case Scenarios

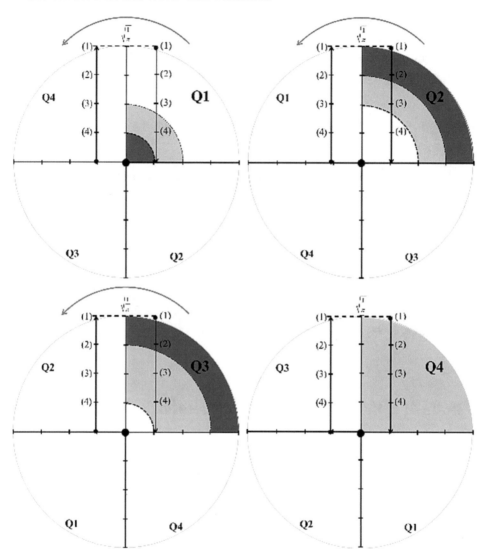

The dark areas denote exergy (i.e., the energy already used, a measure of the entropic state of the employed woman), the gray areas symbolize vagueness or blurring (i.e., the energy values that may have been shifted and consumed), and the white areas embody anergy (i.e., the energy potential that has not yet been reassigned and consumed). Indeed, once the input for *Q1* matches *(4) → (3)*, it states that the woman's entropic state tends to deteriorate. The inputs can be read from *(4) → (1)* (with increasing entropy of the woman entropic state) or from *(1)*

$\rightarrow$ *(4)* (with decreasing entropy of woman entropic state). The markers on the axis correspond to any of the possible scale options, which may be used from *bottom* $\rightarrow$ *top (from (4)* $\rightarrow$ *(1))*, indicating that the woman entropic state decreases as the entropy increases, or used from *top* $\rightarrow$ *bottom (from (1)* $\rightarrow$ *(4))*, indicating that the woman entropic state increases as entropy decreases. Table 2 gives an evaluation of the woman entropic states for the *Best* and *Worst-case* scenarios.

Table 2. The extent of cmq – 4's predicate obtained from a woman's perception of CMQ – 4 statements

Best-case Scenario					Worst-case Scenario				
E	*V*	*A*	*PE*	*QoI*	*E*	*V*	*A*	*PE*	*QoI*
0.24	0	0.76	0.97	0.76	0.24	0.49	0.27	0.68	0.27
Leading to ... Program 1									

where *PE* stands for *Psychometric Evidence*, i.e., a *Reliable Proof of WHW Satisfaction*, and *QoI* denotes the *Measure of the Validity of PE Sensitivity* (Robinson, 1965; Neves, 1994; Kakas, Kowalski & Toni, 1998).

{

$$\neg cmq - 4\big(E, V, A, PE, QoI\big) \leftarrow not \ cmq - 4\big(E, V, A, PE, QoI\big),$$

$$not \ abducible_{cmq-4}\big(E, V, A, PE, QoI\big).$$

cmq – 4(0.24, 0, 0.76, 0.97, 0.76)

}

Program 1. The extent of *cmq – 4's* predicate for the *Best-case scenario*.

The extent of cmq – 4's predicate for the *Worst-case Scenario* follows the same construction pattern.

The assessment of *PE* and *QoI* for the *CMQ – 4's* scope is now carried out in the form, viz.

- *PE* is figured out using $PE = \sqrt{1 - ES^2}$ (Fig. 2), where *ES* stands for the exergy's that may have been consumed, a value that ranges in the interval *0…1*. In the *Best-case Scenario (BcS)*, *ES=exergy*, while in the *Worst-case Scenario (WcS)*, *ES=exergy+vagueness*).

$$PE_{BcS} = \sqrt{1 - (0.24)^2} = 0.97;\ PE_{WcS} = \sqrt{1 - (0.24 + 0.49)^2} = 0.68$$

Figure 2. PE evaluation

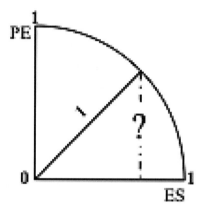

- *QoI* is evaluated in the form, *QoI=1 – ES/Interval length(=1)*, viz.

$$QoI_{BcS} = 1 - 0.24 = 0.76;\ QoI_{WcS} = 1 - (0.24 + 0.49) = 0.27$$

A Case Study on A Behavioral Analysis of Women's Satisfaction with Household Work

A family stands for a social system that consists of one or more persons living together with some expectations of mutual affection, responsibility, and temporary duration. It is characterized by commitment, joint decision-making, and goal achievement. Looking at the family in this way, one may consider different attitudes and arrangements that exist in today's society. Indeed, understanding its structure, function, and procedure is of utmost importance for its characterization and how it may contribute to the well-being of the individual or the group, and in particular of the *WHW*. This understanding will be addressed here in terms of questionnaires to assess *Women Household Caring*, *Therapeutic*, and *Socialization* practices.

Women Household Caring

In the circumstances mentioned above, one can cross gender boundaries and participate in household tasks; one must not rule, one must share. To decide in which extension this is the case, answer questions such as, viz.

Q1– Do you usually help with housework?;
Q2 – Do you usually participate in cooking?;
Q3 – Do you iron your clothes?; and
Q4 – Do you usually bring the trash on the street?.

once it is of the utmost importance to obtain as much information on the subject as possible. They represent the *Women Household Caring Questionnaire Four-Item* (*CQ – 4*), whose answers in terms of qualitative and quantitative values of consumed energy are shown in Tables 4 and 5, respectively.

Women Household Therapeutics

In order to be aware if someone feel happier, more relaxed or to be more healthy, answer questions such as, viz.

Q1 – Do you usually suggest to your family members to do health surveillance?;
Q2 – When someone complains of some symptoms gives advice to go to the doctor?;
Q3 – Do you care about the health of other family members?;
Q4 – Do you usually do routine appointments and screening tests?;
Q5 – When a family member goes to the doctor, do they usually accompany them?; and
Q6 – Discuss family problems?.

once it is of the utmost importance to obtain as much information on the subject as possible. They stand for the *Women Household Therapeutics Questionnaire-Six-Item* (*TQ – 6*), whose answers in terms of qualitative and quantitative values are shown in Tables 3 and 4, respectively.

Women Household Socialization

Socialization is a process that introduces people to social norms and customs, i.e., a person learns to become a member of a group, community, or society. Answer questions such as, viz.

- *Socialization prepares people to participate in a social group by teaching them its norms and expectations;*
- *Socialization has some primary goals, namely teaching impulse control and developing a conscience, preparing people to perform certain social roles or cultivating shared sources of meaning and value; and*
- *Socialization is culturally specific, but this does not mean certain cultures are better or worse than others.*

that stand for the *Women Household Socialization Questionnaire-Four-Item* (*SQ – 4*), viz.

Table 3. A woman's answers to questionnaires CQ–4, TQ–6 and SQ–4 in qualitative terms at time t(ime)=0

Questionnaires	Questions	Scale							
		(4)	**(3)**	**(2)**	**(1)**	**(2)**	**(3)**	**(4)**	*Vagueness*
CQ–4	Q1				×		×		
	Q2		×						
	Q3								×
	Q4						×		
TQ–6	Q1						×	×	
	Q2					×			
	Q3		×	×					
	Q4						×		
	Q5								×
	Q6		×	×					
SQ–4	Q1		×	×					
	Q2								×
	Q3	×	×						
	Q4					×		×	
Leading to … Table 4									

Table 4. The assessment of a woman answers in terns of her entropic state with regard to the questionnaires CMQ – 4, CQ – 4, SQ – 6 and TQ – 4 at time t(ime)=0

Questionnaires	Best-case Scenario						Worst-case Scenario				
	E	V	A	PE	Qol		E	V	A	PE	Qol
CMQ – 4	0.24	0	0.76	0.97	0.76		0.24	0.49	0.27	0.68	0.27
CQ – 4	0.28	0	0.72	0.96	0.72		0.28	0.42	0.30	0.71	0.30
TQ – 6	0.34	0	0.66	0.94	0.66		0.34	0.45	0.21	0.61	0.21
SQ – 4	0.14	0	0.86	0.98	0.86		0.14	0.40	0.46	0.84	0.46
catch-all clause	**0.25**	**0**	0.75	0.96	0.75		**0.25**	**0.44**	0.34	0.71	0.34
Leading to ... Program 2											

Q1 – Do you maintain close relationships with neighbors?;
Q2 – Do the different family members relate to the neighbors?;
Q3 – Do neighbors often come to your house?; and
Q4 – Do you attend church/religion regularly?.

whose answers in terms of qualitative and quantitative values are shown in Tables 3 and 4, respectively.

where catch-all-clause denotes a term that cover all possibilities not covered by individual terms. On the other hand, $0.25 = (0.24 + 0.28 + 0.34 + 0.14)/4$. It stands for the entropic state of the employed woman at time *t(ime)=0* in the *Best-case Scenario*. The remaining values were computed in a similar way.

The Computational Framework

One's work that went step-by-step to understand the problem and come up with a solution was possible due to the power of *Logic Programming* (*LP*), a set of problem-solving methods that involve expressing problems and their solutions in ways that a computer may execute, i.e., it describes the decision-making process used in programming to turn up one's decisions into algorithms. Here it is used deduction, i.e., starting from a conjecture and considering a fixed set of relations (axioms and inference rules), try to construct a proof of the conjecture. It is a creative process. *LP* works with a proof search for a defined strategy (Neves, 1994; Neves et al., 2021). Therefore, and for the *Best-case Scenario*, one may have, viz.

Best-Sase Scenario

{

$$\neg cmq - 4\left(E, V, \text{A}, PE, QoI\right) \leftarrow not\ cmq - 4\left(E, V, \text{A}, PE, QoI\right),$$

$$not\ abducible_{cmq-4}\left(E, V, \text{A}, PE, QoI\right).$$

cmq – 4(0.24, 0, 0.76, 0.97, 0.76)

$$\neg cq - 4\left(E, V, \text{A}, PE, QoI\right) \leftarrow not\ cq - 4\left(E, V, \text{A}, PE, QoI\right),$$

$$not\ abducible_{cq-4}\left(E, V, \text{A}, PE, QoI\right).$$

cq – 4(0.28, 0, 0.30, 0.96, 0.72)

$$\neg tq - 6\left(E, V, \text{A}, PE, QoI\right) \leftarrow not\ tq - 6\left(E, V, \text{A}, PE, QoI\right),$$

$$not\ abducible_{tq-6}\left(E, V, \text{A}, PE, QoI\right).$$

tq – 6(0.34, 0, 0.21, 0.94, 0.66)

$$\neg sq - 4\left(E, V, A, PE, QoI\right) \leftarrow not\ sq - 4\left(E, V, A, PE, QoI\right),$$

$$not\ abducible_{sq-4}\left(E, V, A, PE, QoI\right).$$

sq – 4(0.14, 0, 0.46, 0.98, 0.86)

}

Program 2. The extent of *cmq – 4, cq – 4, tq – 6 and sq – 4's* predicates for the *Best-case Scenario*

In fact, woman's behavior (Fig. 3) is obtained as a side effect when the proposition below is proven, being in harmony with the *Timeline* and *Program 2* (i.e., enforced a number of times that match the number of weeks (months) under study (Robinson, 1965), viz.

$$\forall\left(E_1,V_1,A_1,PE_1,QoI_1,\cdots,E_4,V_4,A_4,PE_4,QoI_4\right),\ \left(cmq-4(E_1,V_1,A_1,PE_1,QoI_1),\right.$$
$$\left.cq-4\left(E_2,V_2,A_2,PE_2,QoI_2\right),\ tp-6\left(E_3,V_3,A_3,PE_3,QoI_3\right),\ sq-4\left(E_4,V_4,A_4,PE_4,QoI_4\right)\right)$$

leading to Fig.3. A similar framework is created for the Worst-case Scenario.

Figure 3. Evolution of the ES of a women worker in terms of a Best and Worst-case Scenarios

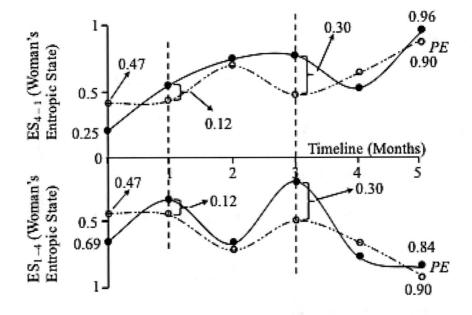

To explain it more clearly, at time *t(ime) = 0*, her *ES* has a value of *0.25* (Table 4), expressed in the *Best-case Scenario*, which means that she can be satisfied with her housework or, in other words, their degree of uncertainty or randomness about satisfaction with housework is low; however, over time, her *ES* tend to a value close to *1 (one)* at the end of the 5th month, creating a situation of distress, i.e., not having clearly distanced at the right time from various forms of unsatisfaction with housework, she is completely dysfunctional. Similar conclusions can be drawn for the *Worst-case Scenario*, that presents an *ES* with a value of 0.69 at time *t(ime) = 0*. Indeed, despite technological developments in several areas of work, few developments have been made in research to meet the expectations of working women with housework. Therefore, new methods and methodologies for problem solving that stem from the scientific areas referred to above were used to assess the womens' sentiments and feelings in order to provide a window to support their insertion in the system of corporate work; a way to help managers and politicians in support of actions that can lead to women's expectations being met.

CONCLUSION

Women's adaptive performance becomes a key factor in maintaining persistence throughout the *PE (Psychometrics Evidence of WHW Satisfaction)* and the measure of its sustainability (*QoI*). This was the main objective of this work, delivered as a computational agency that integrates the phases of data gathering, anticipating a logic representation of uncertainty and vagueness, plus the stages of data processing and results' analysis. A vision was also presented of how the outcome or desired outcomes can be assessed in terms of a multi-valued logic, a subject that in the past has only been addressed generally, i.e., a narrative about the *WHW* they enjoy doing and to the level of satisfaction with which they do it, a value that ranges in the interval *0 (undeniably satisfied) … 1 (undeniably unsatisfied)* (Fig. 3). Future work will examine the issues that may arise in this context in relation to *Justice*, *Power* and *Leadership* forces that develop in a family setting, and their impact on a woman satisfaction with household work. Last but not least, it will be also study why satisfaction with housework declined in women and increased in men. These diverging trends contrast with concurrent shifts in time spent on housework. We will be looking and compare changes in individual gender role attitudes *vs.* changes in couple evaluations of fairness.

ACKNOWLEDGMENT

This work has been supported by FCT – Fundação para a Ciência e Tecnologia within the R&D Units Project Scope: UIDB/00319/2020 and UIDB/50006/2020.

REFERENCES

Araújo, I. (2005). Family Roles Assessment Scale: Assessment of Psychometric Properties. *Journal of Nursing Reference*, *IV*(4), 51–59.

Bartz, C. (2010). International Council of Nurses and person-centered care. *International Journal of Integrated Care*, *10*(5), 24–26. doi:10.5334/ijic.480 PMID:20228907

Black, M. (1961). *The Social Theories of Talcott Parsons: A Critical Examination*. Prentice Hall.

Burr, V. (1998). *Gender and Social Psychology*. Routledge.

Hanson, S. M. (2005). *Family Health Nursing: Theory, Practice and Research*. Lusodidacta.

Janzen, B., & Hellsten, L. (2018). Does the psychosocial quality of unpaid family work contribute to educational disparities in mental health among employed partnered mothers? *International Archives of Occupational and Environmental Health*, *91*(5), 633–641. doi:10.100700420-018-1310-y PMID:29691657

Kakas, A., Kowalski, R., & Toni, F. (1998). The role of abduction in logic programming. In D. Gabbay, C. Hogger, & I. Robinson (Eds.), *Handbook of Logic in Artificial Intelligence and Logic Programming* (Vol. 5, pp. 235–324). Oxford University Press. doi:10.1093/oso/9780198537922.003.0007

Neves, J. (1984). A logic interpreter to handle time and negation in logic databases. In R. Muller, & J. Pottmyer (Eds.), *Proceedings of the 1984 annual conference of the ACM on the 5th Generation Challenge* (pp. 50–54). Association for Computing Machinery. 10.1145/800171.809603

Neves, J., Maia, N., Marreiros, G., Neves, M., Fernandes, A., Ribeiro, J., Araújo, I., Araújo, N., Ávidos, L., Ferraz, F., Capita, A., Lori, N., Alves, V., & Vicente, H. (2019). Entropy and Organizational Performance. In H. Pérez García, L. Sánchez González, M. Castejón Limas, H. Quintián Pardo, & E. Corchado Rodríguez (Eds.), Lecture Notes in Computer Science: Vol. 11734. *Hybrid Artificial Intelligent Systems* (pp. 206–217). Springer. doi:10.1007/978-3-030-29859-3_18

Neves, J., Maia, N., Marreiros, G., Neves, M., Fernandes, A., Ribeiro, J., Araújo, I., Araújo, N., Ávidos, L., Ferraz, F., Capita, A., Lori, N., Alves, V., & Vicente, H. (2021). Employees Balance and Stability as Key Points in Organizational Performance. *Logic Journal of the IGPL*, jzab010. Advance online publication. doi:10.1093/jigpal/jzab010

Robinson, J. A. (1965). A Machine-Oriented Logic Based on the Resolution Principle. *Journal of the Association for Computing Machinery*, *12*(1), 23–41. doi:10.1145/321250.321253

Wenterodt, T., & Herwig, H. (2014). The Entropic Potential Concept: A New Way to Look at Energy Transfer Operations. *Entropy (Basel, Switzerland)*, *16*(4), 2071–2084. doi:10.3390/e16042071

Chapter 8
Electronic Health Records Structuring Based on the OpenEHR Standard

Daniela Oliveira
Centro ALGORITMI, Universidade do Minho, Portugal

Francini Hak
Centro ALGORITMI, Universidade do Minho, Portugal

Helia Guerra
University of the Azores, Portugal

António Abelha
Centro ALGORITMI, Universidade do Minho, Portugal

ABSTRACT

The growth of electronic health records (EHR) produced by health facilities has been exponential, leading to massive and heterogeneous data storage. This raises the need for secure, continuous, and interoperable data structuring between different legacy systems. The OpenEHR standard provides open data specifications that aim to overcome recognized gaps in the collection, storage, and management of clinical records. In this sense, this chapter describes a case study applied in an emergency context, where 14-year clinical records were restructured to an interoperable and standardized environment, according to the OpenEHR specifications.

DOI: 10.4018/978-1-7998-9172-7.ch008

INTRODUCTION

Aside from the significant evolution of the Electronic Health Records (EHR), the digitalization of clinical records has resulted in the creation of extravagant amounts of data every day, stored in dedicated repositories and afterwards used or not. In this context, multidisciplinary teams in the fields of Information Systems (IS) and Medical Informatics (MI) have arisen in healthcare institutions, particularly the biomedical engineer specializing in MI, which has proven to be crucial in data control, developing tools to use them and managing healthcare institution's Health Information Systems (HIS), to provide a complete symbiosis and interoperability between all systems (Bernstam et al., 2010). Therefore, research in this area has opened new horizons in recent years, through innovative techniques and solutions to reach more and more in terms of HIS efficient use, adopting new methodologies and worldwide recognized clinical standards for its ergonomic use.

The continuous marathon of data structuring contributes to the knowledge extraction following a specific purpose. In the healthcare field, a lot of information present in diaries and clinical reports are written in an unstructured way and may not be possible to acquire the necessary knowledge about a specific clinical case. Furthermore, nowadays, many clinical encounters and procedures still occur in an isolated way, making it difficult to access more patient information in real time, which can negatively influence decision-making (Murdoch & Detsky, 2013).

This massive and heterogeneous creation of clinical records raises concerns regarding the processing and storage of these data. The use of unstructured data generated some problems in the use of HIS, such as failure in communication between systems, lack of data standardization, difficulty in acquiring clinical knowledge, and others.

In a particular Portuguese Healthcare Institution, the described problem scenario also exists. Millions of 20-year Electronic Health Records were stored in an unused Legacy System (LS). This uselessness and non-use of data generated data loss due to the lack of a standard and data structuring, leading to the inability to interoperate with each other. In addition, data held in the LS could have been leveraged for data analysis and to support decision making.

In order to respond to the identified problem, a preventive and collaborative approach to developing the widely used HIS by healthcare professionals is proposed. Thus, this book chapter will describe a case study in a Portuguese Healthcare Institution where millions clinical records were recovered from a discontinued and offline system that was used in emergency context, being mapped to an intelligent and standardized way. To maintain standardization and data interoperation, an open data model strategy was adopted resorting the specifications of the OpenEHR standard.

This chapter is structured in five sections. First, the research background is presented. Secondly, it is described the methods used to develop the present study. The third section presents the results obtained. In section four, a discussion of the findings is held and the direction of future work is pointed out. Finally, some conclusions are drawn.

BACKGROUND

Healthcare Information Systems

Nowadays, large amounts of data are produced and consumed daily in the healthcare industry. With the exponential growth of clinical data in recent years, there has been an emerging need for its better organization to automate, collect, and analyze it whenever necessary. As a result, in the mid-1990s, hospitals began allowing Information Technologies (IT) to intervene in the clinical process at multiple levels. These IT systems enabled more effective and efficient hospital management, from the development of clinical reports to the registration of clinical exams, among other functionalities. All these advancements and advantages are facilitated and coordinated by Information Systems (IS). To make a precise clinical decision, it's necessary to have access to patient information, including retrospective and prospective data. It is critical that all this information is readily available, not only during health care delivery but also to support clinical research or any other activity that may contribute scientifically to continuous improvement in the healthcare field.

The not-for-profit Healthcare Information and Management Systems Society (HIMSS) has emerged in the mid-1960s promoting the adoption of Healthcare Information Systems (HIS), having a significant impact on healthcare and clinical practices from the administrative data management to the clinical data management and communication (Laudon & Laudon, 2011). Thereby, hospital information management depends on the use of specialized information systems applied to the medical domain. The IT professionals, insurance and pharmaceutical companies, and governments use a variety of IS in the healthcare area, such as Data Entry Systems (DES) and Decision Support Systems (DSS). A HIS has a complex integration of several solutions inside a healthcare facility. The collecting, processing, and reporting of data are critical aspects that place the interoperability at forefront in a hospital environment, according to this:

A HIS is a collection of data, procedures, people, and information technology that work together to collect, store, process, and provide the information needed for health care.

Every day, because of technological progress new and modern systems arise with unique approaches to provide decision makers with enhanced healthcare data. So, the term *e-Health* is now used as a natural mode and represents not only the electronic concept, but also a set of words that are also important, such as efficacy, enhancing quality, evidence-based, empowerment, and encouragement, as well as education, enabling, extending, ethical, and equity. The expression also means easy-to-use, entertaining, and even exciting (Eysenbach, 2001). However, the main concern is how to establish communication between HIS and the already existing Legacy Systems. Without this mindset, the separated mounts of information will continue to exist and grow inside healthcare organizations and countries (Miranda et al., 2012; Whitten et al., 1989).

Within a healthcare institution, several units and departments collect pertinent and necessary information that will assist the professionals in the decision process. The Electronic Health Record (EHR) system collects, organizes, analyzes, and processes this data to present essential information in a simple, intelligible, and accessible way to the users. Thus, the EHR is the basis for the effective management of a wide variety of information types, including the patient's medical history, demographics and personal metrics, clinical diaries and hospitalizations, as well as problem lists, prescribed and administered medication, allergies, clinical analyses and exams, and vital signs measurements (McDonald, 1997; A. Pereira et al., 2015; R. Pereira et al., 2012).

Although the continuous evolution of digital clinical records and patient data access improvement, the way that information is entered and stored in the EHR differs significantly, causing confusion among users due to data heterogeneity (Dick et al., 1997). Many platforms for physicians to interact with EHRs have been developed, but the underlying information model of how clinical, demographic, and administrative data should be recorded and stored has been the responsibility of IT professionals. As a result, depending on the systems structure of each institution, different methodologies and technologies were adopted. One of the most challenging aspects of dealing with the many LS is that most of them do not employ clinical information standards. The software providers generate their own data models, and it is expected that this data be exchanged properly between different systems in other institutions, which rarely happens (Grandia, 2017). To ensure the viability and functionality of the entire ecosystem, it is vital to promote interoperability between all LS and to implement globally recognized standards. Thus, all patient information will be centered in only one place, with all updated data from other systems, and will be accessed and retrieved easily and quickly. Additionally, all existing data can be analyzed to construct alert or recommendation systems. Furthermore, implementing an EHR-oriented system enables the creation of a big database for doing research on several human health-related topics (Dick et al., 1997; Duarte et al., 2010). The

EHR features such as Availability, Readability, Completeness and Consistency, Flexibility, and Reuse, are based on the following principles: "it's important to have clear and structured information and exchanging health information between different LS" (ISO, 2011).

Hodach et al. (2014) recognized the lack of standards and interoperability for dealing with large data scenarios, compromising data storage and, therefore, knowledge discovery. Consequently, there is a need for innovative approaches to define new clinical information workflows, that is, how the information will be recorded, exchanged, and retrieved in the EHR. For these approaches to be viable, HIS must share information in a symbiotic and interoperable way.

Interoperability

It is critical to emphasize the importance of openness and shared features in *e-Health* solutions. A medical operating protocol technology can only address a limited number of needs. A solution is frequently part of a collection of supporting resources for other protocols, and this is the crux of the problem. The environment has been populated with hastily generated new technical inputs with no consideration for mutual interaction. As a result, the time to market for each solution is limited. However, in response to the claim, the protocol's implementation must be viable and straightforward. In medical terms, the enormous number of solutions makes it difficult for healthcare providers to integrate a patient's situation immediately. Interoperability is desirable because of its ability to interact harmoniously with a wide range of technologies, ensuring that all modules operate at optimal efficiency and communicate with one another effortlessly and consistently (Lamine et al., 2017).

Some organizations, such as HIMSS, International Organization for Standardization (ISO), Institute of Electrical and Electronics Engineers (IEEE), and European Committee for Standardization (CEN), define *e-Health* interoperability as a technological contribution that operates primarily at the software and data layers of the overall system architecture, hence benefiting actors during some of their collaborative acts. However, its definition must go beyond this, considering organizational, cultural, ethical, economic, financial, and legal aspects. Each of these aspects is a key source of information that might be critical in the creation of collaborations among different HIS (Lamine et al., 2017; Miranda et al., 2009).

From Mari Greenberger's point of view, as a senior director of informatics at HIMSS, the organization is trying to achieve global interoperability by adding an additional "organizational" level to address the need for a robust interoperability infrastructure, considering non-technical aspects that contribute to the success of interoperability. According to the most recent HIMSS interoperability definition, interoperability can be classified into four distinct levels:

- Foundational level: Establishes the inter-connectivity requirements for a system or application to securely communicate with and receive data from each other.

- Structural level: It defines the syntax for data exchange, i.e., the format, syntax, and organization, including at the data field level interpretation.

- Semantic level: Provides the ability for two or more systems to understand the meaning in same way of the models and data encoding exchanged, including the use of data elements derived from publicly available value sets and encoding vocabularies.

- Organizational level: Includes governmental, political, social, legal, and organizational aspects to facilitate communication and safe use of the systems. These components enable shared consent, trust, and integrated end-user processes and workflows.

While current solutions and technologies can solve most basic and structural interoperability issues, semantic interoperability is still the main concern, with a special research development focus. The necessity to make health information understandable and automatically computerizable by external IS increases the challenge of establishing the semantic interoperability level. According to the European Commission (EC), semantic interoperability is a critical factor in realizing the benefits of EHR, as it allows us to improve the quality and safety of health care delivery, public health, and its management (Stroetman et al., 2009). A knowledge-oriented HIS development, including ontologies and clinical terminologies, is emerging to represent and share complex medical meaning. This development must ensure a viable, maintainable, and adaptable patient-centric EHR system.

Healthcare Data Standards

International coordinated efforts have resulted in the ongoing development of standards and guidelines for defining an EHR as one or more open access information repositories by different HIS. The CEN, HL7, ISO, and the OpenEHR Foundation are non-profit organizations dedicated to international frameworks and standards development, including terminologies, EHR specifications, and information models, to support the exchange, integration, and retrieval of electronic health information (Stroetman et al., 2009).

As already mentioned, the most difficult level to achieve and guarantee is the semantic interoperability level. According to Stroetman et al., (2009), semantic interoperability will only be feasible if there are agreements on standards, information models, terminologies, and semantic definitions used for data sharing. In addition, social, cultural, and legal aspects within each organization, region, or country will influence the implementation of semantically interoperable systems. It is recommended that such a high level of semantic interoperability be initially implemented and practiced only in specific, priority clinical areas of high relevance to patient safety. Current efforts to standardize clinical data gathering, representation, and communication consider three artefact layers: the Reference Model (RM), Clinical Data Structure, and Clinical Terminologies (Stroetman et al., 2009).

On the one hand, the RM can guarantee data in a complete, homogeneous, and secure way. On the other hand, a clinical data structure definition allows to build precise clinical information models with a unique meaning and use. To complement this, clinical terminologies are precious, ensuring unified meanings through specific vocabulary. So, the main question that arises here is:

"What is the importance of standards in the clinical environment?"

To answer this question, we have to take into account that, for a long time, HIS were designed to satisfy certain functional requirements defined by specific users. Therefore, over time, many of these existing systems became limited in different contexts of use or even obsolete in the face of new user requirements. Besides that, many of these older systems tended to record only the minimum information required for each clinical act. Consequently, additional valuable information for diagnosis and clinical decision support was continuously lost.

Clinical standards should give flexibility to data structures so that new relevant information can be added. Thus, EHR standards define generic data models that can be linked to specific clinical concepts and information structures. In addition, standards should ensure the complete representation of clinical act context information, such as the participants and location of the clinical act, which may influence the clinical data interpretation contained in the EHR. Also, clinical data is complemented by information necessary to support audit or control tasks (Moreno-Conde et al., 2015).

Costa et al. (2011) recommend using standards with duo architecture to ensure semantic interoperability using a basic unit called *Archetypes* based on their extensive literature review and international guidelines. These are the minimum units of information that HIS can transmit to each other. An archetype combination gives rise to complex *Templates* capable of demonstrating sequential clinical workflows. ISO 13606, OpenEHR, and HL7 are examples of dual-architecture standards that are used globally (Costa et al., 2011).

Also, the Garde et al. (2007) work research classifies the EHR as patient-centered, longitudinal, extensive, and prospective, and must retain all the care provided to the patient, not just an isolated episode. Its longitudinal and comprehensive character means it encompasses not only past events but also future perspectives and preventive planning. Therefore, the sharing of clinical data between different healthcare professionals and institutions, through different HIS, must be efficient and fast. For this, clinical data will have to be of high quality, reliable, and flexible. Thus, highly standardized structures will have to be developed, as well as each institution's governance rules for managing them. As a viable solution, the researchers propose the use of the OpenEHR standard. They argue that various levels of interoperability can be achieved using it (Garde et al., 2007).

Figure 1. OpenEHR dual-model approach

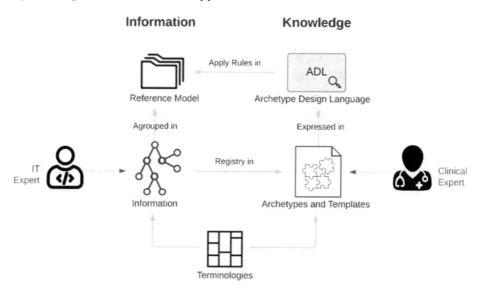

Figure 1 shows the two-level architecture proposed by OpenEHR, where information and knowledge are in two different layers. All clinical data needs context information, i.e., each clinical act must be accompanied by additional information such as how and by whom the data was recorded, and where it was recorded. This additional data is very useful for improving the interpretation of clinical data, supporting the organization of tasks, supporting audits, and legislative issues.

Currently, one of the major concerns in the healthcare IT area is information modeling, which describes how information should be organized and structured. Previously, most IT solutions and their underlying information models for storing clinical information have been left exclusively to the developers. Thus, over the years, issues of linking different types of information from different systems or, e.g., the difficulty of interoperating multiple devices into a single database have arisen (Huff et al., 1995). It was then increasingly important to develop standards that provide functional and consistent information models across different situations.

Nowadays, the most advanced EHR architectures and standards are based on a dual model approach architecture such as ISO EN 13606 and OpenEHR, defined by a Reference Model (RM) and an Archetype Model (AM). Thus, important and generic concepts should be defined (Martínez-Costa et al., 2010):

- Reference Model (RM): A collection of entities that serve as the generic building blocks of an EHR and include non-volatile EHR features such as clinical information and contextual data.
- Archetype Model (AM): It presents the clinical concepts in a combined structured way, restricted to the entities contained in the RM.
- Archetypes: A unit base used for consistently building clinical compliance in dual model approaches, and they are regarded as critical for providing fully interoperable EHRs. These structures define clinical concepts through the combinations of entities presented in RM, defining clinical knowledge.
- Templates: Combination of two or more archetypes, representing a full clinical act.

Compared to OpenEHR, the ISO EN 13606 specification is simpler, consisting of four main packages: context, clinical and demographic information, and data types. ISO EN 13606 also represents the information in an EHR. However, it does not provide support for other relevant modules such as the representation of local information models and a query language for the EHR. This component is very important and has a specific purpose: to extract information from EHRs between HISs.

Due to its wide coverage, support, and flexibility, the OpenEHR standard was chosen to develop this research work. Its open and continuously evolving nature has led to the development over the last few years of a large international community with the same main goal: to create comprehensive and interoperable clinical EHRs.

METHODS

In this section, it will be described the methods used to develop this case study. It comprises data gathering, data selection, data mapping and data structure. OpenEHR dual-model approach

Data Gathering

This case study addresses an offline Legacy System (LS) used in an emergency context in a Portuguese Healthcare Facility. The data stored in this system covered millions of clinical records over 20 years old and, which were not being used. In this sense, the need arose to recover the data kept in the LS, to transform and migrate them to a standardized and interoperable structure.

The millions of records kept in the LS were stored in a relational database. In order to proceed with the extraction and collection of clinical records, an algorithm was developed capable of executing the queries of the intended data, obtaining their extraction to a staging area.

Data Selection

In a first phase, it was necessary to define the interval of years for the selection of the clinical records. In order to respond to the needs of the Portuguese Healthcare Facility, 14-year data were selected, covering the period from 2004 to 2018. Second, an analysis was performed on the data stored in the Legacy System, where clinical records were selected guided by its context. As shown in Table 1, selected clinical contexts include emergency admissions, triage, diagnosis, history, prescriptions, requested MCDT's (exams), procedures, administrations, and measured vital signs.

Table 1. Selected Legacy System data

Data Context	Count of Records	Selection
Emergency Admissions and Discharge	1356193	
Triage	1817819	
Complaints	1962131	
Diagnosis	1693894	
Requested Exams	1139600	
Vital Signs	2307358	
History	4016822	
Prescription	1184171	
Problem List	13391	
Procedures	1619204	
Administrations	2149006	

In summary, more than 1300000 emergency room admissions were collected, making an average of 265 admissions per day. Regarding the patient's admission in the emergency context, it involves triage, and discharge. Furthermore, in order to identify the emergency room diagnosis, it is usually necessary to collect information through the measurement of vital signs, analysis of procedures, tests, or analyses required by health professionals. The emergency system under study also relates to the patient's problem list. The patient's complaints and problem history data were not selected for this case study.

Process Design

After extracting and selecting the data, the process of mapping the records extracted from the Legacy System to the standardized data structure was planned. To this end, the specifications of the OpenEHR open data standard were used in order to support the structuring and standardization process, as shown in Figure 2.

Figure 2. Modeling process for OpenEHR structures

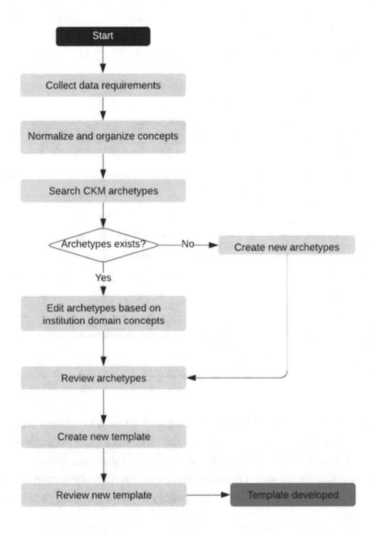

Throughout the data collection process, requirements were raised to determine which concepts should be stored and how they should be represented. These datasets were organized and context oriented. In order to relate the retrieved data to the new data structure, the Clinical Knowledge Management (CKM) data repository was used, where in-depth research was carried out using archetypes and templates, with the purpose of reusing structures already developed by the community. If there were no archetypes available in CKM, new archetypes were created according to the desired purpose.

The modeling phase was carried out with the collaboration of health professionals, where, through an appropriate tool, they managed to modulate data structures based on data extracted from the Legacy System. After the creation of archetypes and templates, the new data structure was modeled. The next phase regards to map the new structure with the retrieved data. With this development, it is possible to extract clinical knowledge to support the health process and store all relevant patient information.

OpenEHR Data Structure and Data Mapping

To make the retrieval process as realistic as possible, the clinical domain experts collaborated with the IT experts to analyze the relevant information for this case study. This symbiotic collaborative environment is essential for information retrieval as well as the continuous evolution of OpenEHR systems. Table 3 represents the result of mapping data from the Legacy System to the new standardized structure based on OpenEHR.

Table 3. Templates modeled in OpenEHR and the archetypes reused

Original Data	Template	Archetypes
Emergency Admissions, and Triage, Complaints	urg_admission.opt	OpenEHR-EHR-COMPOSITION.encounter OpenEHR-EHR-SECTION.adhoc OpenEHR-EHR-OBSERVATION.story OpenEHR-EHR-CLUSTER.symptom_sign OpenEHR-EHR-ADMIN_ENTRY.admission OpenEHR-EHR-EVALUATION.reason_for_encounter OpenEHR-EHR-ADMIN_ENTRY.triage OpenEHR-EHR-CLUSTER.demographic
Discharge	urg_discharge.opt	OpenEHR-EHR-COMPOSITION.administrative OpenEHR-EHR-ADMIN_ENTRY.episode_institution
Diagnosis	diagnosis.opt	OpenEHR-EHR-COMPOSITION.encounter OpenEHR-EHR-EVALUATION.problem_diagnosis
Procedures	procedures.opt	OpenEHR-EHR-COMPOSITION.encounter OpenEHR-EHR-ACTION.service

Continued on following page

Table 3. Continued

Original Data	Template	Archetypes
History	disease_history.opt	OpenEHR-EHR-COMPOSITION.progress_note OpenEHR-EHR-OBSERVATION.progress_note
Vital Signs	vital_signs.opt	OpenEHR-EHR-COMPOSITION.encounter OpenEHR-EHR-OBSERVATION.laboratory_test_result OpenEHR-EHR-CLUSTER.laboratory_test_analyte OpenEHR-EHR-CLUSTER.demografico_sonho OpenEHR-EHR-OBSERVATION.blood_pressure OpenEHR-EHR-OBSERVATION.pulse OpenEHR-EHR-OBSERVATION.glasgow_coma_scale OpenEHR-EHR-OBSERVATION.respiration OpenEHR-EHR-OBSERVATION.pulse_oximetry OpenEHR-EHR-OBSERVATION.body_temperature
Requested Exams	requests.opt	OpenEHR-EHR-COMPOSITION.request OpenEHR-EHR-SECTION.adhoc OpenEHR-EHR-INSTRUCTION.service_request

Based on the analysis of the extracted metadata, domain experts modeled the new structure from archetypes and templates, available in the CKM. Templates resulted from the joining of one or more archetypes and, when these did not exist in CKM, they were created.

In this sense, data mapping consists of the representation of existing data to the new modeled structure. First, all the metadata corresponding to each context, and the chain between them, were surveyed. Then, the information to be considered went through a validation of its permanence, based on the relevance of each attribute and its sufficiency of data. After defining the dataset for each context, the data were modeled using selected archetypes and templates. It is possible to notice that each data context previously selected from the Legacy System originated a template built from a set of archetypes.

It should be mentioned that the most difficult aspect of this initial phase was the existence of unstructured data with no standardization. This information can be found, for example, in the patient's disease history or in the patient's complaints during the emergency episode. The clinicians in these situations recorded their observations without any uniformity. These same observations were inconsistent, as the same term was frequently recorded in different ways in different records. In these circumstances, modulation was restricted to open text type.

RESULTS

Converting data from the current systems of a healthcare institution is one of the most critical parts of developing a Healthcare Information System (HIS) based on the OpenEHR standard. Legacy Systems (LS) on the one hand, may be in operation and constantly updated, while others may no longer be in clinical practice but may still include valuable clinical knowledge acquired from years of data accumulation. The distinction between online and offline LS is related to changes in how they are translated for usage in the newly developed OpenEHR system.

Data Migration from Legacy Systems

One of the most important aspects of building a HIS based on the OpenEHR standard is converting data from a healthcare institution's current systems. LS, on the other hand, could be in use and in continuous updating, and others may no more be in the field of clinical practice, but may still include useful clinical information from years of data collection.

A mapping system for offline LS migration was created and afterwards included in the new OpenEHR structure. Furthermore, the mapping system developed consists in a Multi-Agent System (MAS) composed by autonomous and intelligent agents that retrieve relevant information from the already existing offline LS database, and then bind that information to the new respective OpenEHR structure. This new structure is always saved in the form of a *Composition* that corresponds to a determined template that has been specifically designed for the purpose of storing it. At the same time as filling out the composition, the Reference Model (RM) of the template that will be used in each context is filled out and saved as well. Since the data from the offline systems is already immutable, the conversion to the new structure can be done in bulk as a big data batch process, and the meaning and value of the data remains intact and saved.

There were multiple data sources that supplied the offline system under study, requiring connections to different old versions of databases and, as a result, the use and installation of different database clients. To handle the different versions of the existing databases and the multiple templates generated by modeling, a control structure was created to ensure that all of the essential requirements were connected. A retrievalData algorithm had to be created in order for the data conversion to actually occur. The main function of this method is to process each record of the control structure before proceeding with the data conversion. Each control record includes the SQL query created by IT experts, its respective template id, and the binding structure of its items, as well as the source database to be queried. The algorithm runs in the background for a set amount of time, depending on the number of records to be processed, until the last record is retrieved. The records are then transformed into their target composition, coupled with their respective RM, and stored in the staging area. Consequently, a MAS system is triggered after the creation of a new record in this staging repository. All the processes described are shown in the schema presented in figure 3 below. Online and offline LS are distinguished in this project due to the differences in the ways in which they are transformed and used in the newly built OpenEHR system.

Figure 3. A novel data retrieval process for the OpenEHR approach

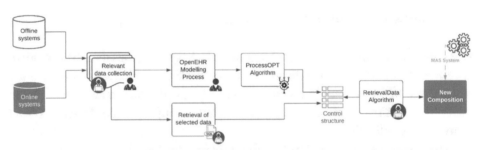

MAS Versioning and Managing Developed

To increase the flexibility of the EHR structure, OpenEHR provides the option of adopting a set of folders and their respective root directories. This feature allows for more flexibility in clinical record structure as well as the linking of profiles with the physician who is consulting or modifying a specific EHR at the time. A dynamic folder system was implemented in this case study to configure not only how users wanted to view the displayed data, but also how they wanted to view the organized information of a particular patient in a specific context.

It was required to create a consistent versioning and organizing system in order to create a long-lasting EHR that is easy to access and manage. The versioning system created was based on OpenEHR principles, and it was organized using a Folders and Directories system. The number of folders produced, as well as their content, can be volatile or persistent over time, giving the OpenEHR a high degree of flexibility. Persistent folders are built up of persistent compositions that contain information that is transversal throughout the patient's life and can readily summarize his health state. Persistent folders also can be divided into categories such as problem lists, vaccines, and allergies, among other clinical topics. Otherwise, folders based on episodic or event data, with their corresponding types of compositions as content, can also be generated. The MAS shown in Figure 4 was developed in a flexible way for any data source and OpenEHR target structures.

Figure 4. MAS proposed to versioning and organizing OpenEHR data

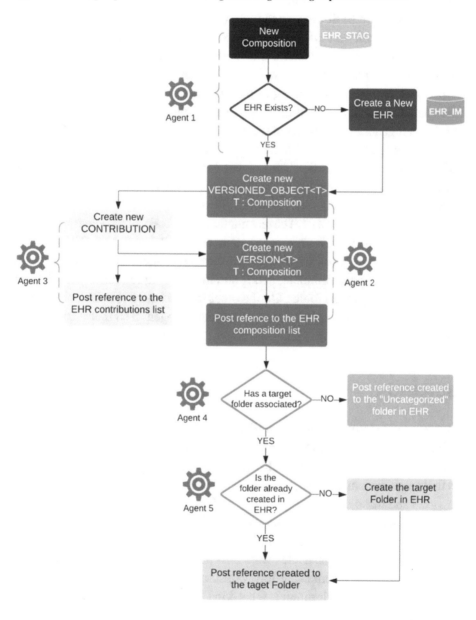

As the figure above demonstrates, new records and records that are not yet "completed" are kept in a staging area. Agent 1 is constantly looking for complete records in the staging area for the system to proceed. This agent takes care of querying the staging area to discover new *Compositions* to integrate into a given EHR. Once it finds a new record, it will check if the UID of the patient associated with the record has a specific EHR associated with it. If it does, it sends a message to agent 2 telling it that it can process the new record for that EHR. If agent 1 doesn't find an EHR associated with the patient, it will create one and then send the message to agent 2. The occurrence of new data leads to the creation of a new *VERSIONED_COMPOSITION* for the versioning of the information to be possible. This task is in the charge of agent 2, which only initializes it after the message is received by agent 1. After generating the UID of the new *VERSIONED_COMPOSITION*, agent 2 sends a message to agent 3 with the respective *OBJECT_REF* of the new version so that it can perform its tasks. Thus, agent 3 can create a new *CONTRIBUTION* and save its reference in the list of contributions of the respective EHR, and agent 2 finishes its task by saving the versioning reference of the new record in the list of compositions of the same EHR. The termination of the tasks of the versioning agents happens when agent 3 sends a message to agent 4 with its respective *OBJECT_REF* created and the record's source. With that information, agent 4 can check if there is any target folder for that template, and if not, the received reference will be stored in a default uncategorized folder. On the other hand, if there is a folder associated with the template in use, agent 4 sends a message to agent 5 so that it can save the reference to the new information in the target folder within the EHR.

DISCUSSION

This case study aimed to retrieve millions of records from a Legacy System to a standardized and interoperable approach based on the OpenEHR standard. The choice of this open data standard fulfilled the expected objectives. By mapping the data to the new structure, it was possible to retrieve clinical data that were no longer being used and make them interoperate with other active systems in the Portuguese Healthcare Facility. Therefore, it allowed the discovery of new clinical knowledge through the big amount of transformed data.

Some challenges and obstacles were also part of this process. Firstly, the data extraction phase was a somewhat time-consuming process as it was necessary to understand the work environment, what kind of records were stored, and other concerns. The connection to old version databases was also a challenge. Furthermore, resistance from health professionals and lack of resources made it difficult to model and create a faster collaborative environment in the modeling phase.

Based on the retrieved data, 474,645 EHR structures were created, organized by 5 distinct folders: Encounters, Medication, Problems List, Procedures, and MCDTs (exams). Each of these folders is composed of a list of references, of type *<OBJECT_REF>*, for each assigned composition. In terms of compositions, all structures created were classified as episodic for their temporal character limited to the emergency episode.

The retrieved data was converted to 1,356,072 emergency department admissions, resulting in an equal number of compositions created based on the *urg_admission. opt* template, as well as their consequent discharge, through the *urg_discharge.opt* structure. At the level of diagnoses, new 1,193,560 compositions were generated based on the *diagnosis.opt* template. Note that not every hospital discharge is associated with a particular diagnosis. On the other hand, the procedures performed in the context of emergency care gave rise to 1,201,315 compositions through the template *procedures.opt*.

Regarding the exams and clinical analysis requested during the clinical episodes, 576,648 compositions were created through the template *requests.opt* modeled. This template contains an *INSTRUCTION* archetype, which led to the grouping of requests through the *history<INSTRUCTION>* attribute in form of the list.

At the clinical observation level, two templates were developed for this purpose and are named *disease_history.opt* and *vital_signs.opt*. Each of them has at least one archetype of the *OBSERVATION* type associated with it, thus allowing, through the *history<OBSERVATION>* attribute type in form of the list, to group its records on a time scale. Were also generated 576,648 compositions through the *disease_history. opt* template and 673,117 compositions with vital signs measurement information through the *vital_signs.opt* template.

CONCLUSION

This chapter describes a case study applied in a Portuguese Healthcare Facility, where clinical records of 14 years of an emergency context were extracted and mapped to a standardized structure. This structure was based on the OpenEHR standard that promotes interoperability between Health Information Systems through the modeling of knowledge and clinical information. In this way, millions of records were restored from an offline system. This strategy allowed to create a structured and open clinical repository, interoperable with other systems.

We conclude that sharing and modeling data in OpenEHR structures is challenging and rewarding. Some obstacles were encountered during the process, but they were overcome and compensated for by the result. Furthermore, this case study allowed opening doors to new challenges in the sense of implementing the proposed solution in other similar cases, and even solving other problems still identified in the healthcare institution worked. Thus, it was essential to determine the most viable approach of establishing interoperability between existing systems and the newly developed OpenEHR system. At security level of working with already immutable records, this process could be cyclical and evolutionary.

This encourages further research work on open data approaches and globally recognized standards. The existence of a high number of free-text records made the conversion from an outdated offline system challenging. Furthermore, one of the main conclusions extracted from this case study, was the future necessity for the development of a Nature Language Processing (NLP) module using Named Entity Recognition (NER) methods, which would result in improved clinical modulation and knowledge discovery. This NLP module would overcome both the existence of non-standard text, and the improvement of collection of reliable and shareable clinical information in a future central open repository. We therefore encourage the continued adoption of internationally recognized open data standards for the Health Information Systems research community.

ACKNOWLEDGMENT

F.H. thanks the Fundação para a Ciência e Tecnologia (FCT), Portugal for the Ph.D. Grant 2021.06230.BD.

REFERENCES

Bernstam, E. V., Hersh, W. R., Sim, I., Eichmann, D., Silverstein, J. C., Smith, J. W., & Becich, M. J. (2010). Unintended consequences of health information technology: A need for biomedical informatics. *Journal of Biomedical Informatics*, *43*(5), 828–830. doi:10.1016/j.jbi.2009.05.009 PMID:19508898

Costa, C. M., Menárguez-Tortosa, M., & Fernández-Breis, J. T. (2011). Clinical data interoperability based on archetype transformation. *Journal of Biomedical Informatics*, *44*(5), 869–880. doi:10.1016/j.jbi.2011.05.006 PMID:21645637

Dick, R. S., Steen, E. B., & Detmer, D. E. (1997). *The computer-based patient record: an essential technology for health care*. National Academies Press.

Duarte, J., Salazar, M., Quintas, C., Santos, M., Neves, J., Abelha, A., & Machado, J. (2010). Data Quality Evaluation of Electronic Health Records in the Hospital Admission Process. *2010 IEEE/ACIS 9th International Conference on Computer and Information Science*, 201–206. 10.1109/ICIS.2010.97

Eysenbach, G. (2001). What is e-health? *Journal of Medical Internet Research*, *3*(2), e20. doi:10.2196/jmir.3.2.e20 PMID:11720962

Garde, S., Knaup, P., Hovenga, E. J. S., & Heard, S. (2007). Towards semantic interoperability for electronic health records. *Methods of Information in Medicine*, *46*(03), 332–343. doi:10.1160/ME5001 PMID:17492120

Grandia, L. (2017). Healthcare information systems: a look at the past, present, and future. *Health Catalyst*, 1–4.

Hodach, R., Chase, A., Fortini, R., Delaney, C., & Hodach, R. (2014). *Population health management: A roadmap for provider-based automation in a new era of healthcare*. Institute for Health Technology Transformation. Http://Ihealthtran. Com/Pdf/PHMReport. Pdf

Huff, S. M., Rocha, R. A., Bray, B. E., Warner, H. R., & Haug, P. J. (1995). An event model of medical information representation. *Journal of the American Medical Informatics Association: JAMIA*, *2*(2), 116–134. doi:10.1136/jamia.1995.95261905 PMID:7743315

Lamine, E., Guédria, W., Rius Soler, A., Ayza Graells, J., Fontanili, F., Janer-García, L., & Pingaud, H. (2017). An Inventory of Interoperability in Healthcare Ecosystems: Characterization and Challenges. *Enterprise Interoperability: INTEROP-PGSO Vision*, *1*, 167–198. doi:10.1002/9781119407928.ch9

Laudon, K. C., & Laudon, J. P. (2011). *Essentials of management information systems*. Academic Press.

Martínez-Costa, C., Menárguez-Tortosa, M., & Fernández-Breis, J. T. (2010). An approach for the semantic interoperability of ISO EN 13606 and OpenEHR archetypes. *Journal of Biomedical Informatics*, *43*(5), 736–746. doi:10.1016/j. jbi.2010.05.013 PMID:20561912

McDonald, C. J. (1997). The barriers to electronic medical record systems and how to overcome them. *Journal of the American Medical Informatics Association: JAMIA*, *4*(3), 213–221. doi:10.1136/jamia.1997.0040213 PMID:9147340

Miranda, M., Duarte, J., Abelha, A., Machado, J. M., & Neves, J. (2009). *Interoperability and healthcare*. Academic Press.

Miranda, M., Salazar, M., Portela, F., Santos, M., Abelha, A., Neves, J., & Machado, J. (2012). Multi-agent systems for hl7 interoperability services. *Procedia Technology*, *5*, 725–733. doi:10.1016/j.protcy.2012.09.080

Moreno-Conde, A., Moner, D., da Cruz, W. D., Santos, M. R., Maldonado, J. A., Robles, M., & Kalra, D. (2015). Clinical information modeling processes for semantic interoperability of electronic health records: Systematic review and inductive analysis. *Journal of the American Medical Informatics Association: JAMIA*, *22*(4), 925–934. doi:10.1093/jamia/ocv008 PMID:25796595

Murdoch, T. B., & Detsky, A. S. (2013). The Inevitable Application of Big Data to Health Care. *Journal of the American Medical Association*, *309*(13), 1351. doi:10.1001/jama.2013.393 PMID:23549579

Pereira, A., Marins, F., Rodrigues, B., Portela, F., Santos, M. F., Machado, J., Rua, F., Silva, Á., & Abelha, A. (2015). Improving quality of medical service with mobile health software. *Procedia Computer Science*, *63*, 292–299. doi:10.1016/j.procs.2015.08.346

Pereira, R., Duarte, J., Salazar, M., Santos, M., Abelha, A., & Machado, J. (2012). Usability of an electronic health record. *2012 IEEE International Conference on Industrial Engineering and Engineering Management*, 1568–1572. 10.1109/IEEM.2012.6838010

Standardization, I. O. (2011). *Health informatics-Requirements for an electronic health record architecture*. Author.

Stroetman, V., Kalra, D., Lewalle, P., Rector, A., Rodrigues, J., Stroetman, K., Surjan, G., Ustun, B., Virtanen, M., & Zanstra, P. (2009). *Semantic interoperability for better health and safer healthcare*. Academic Press.

Whitten, J. L., Bentley, L. D., & Dittman, K. C. (1989). *Systems analysis and design methods*. Irwin Homewood.

Chapter 9

A New Approach to E–Health Application Development Using Blockchain

Vedant Singh Bhanote
VIT University, India

Ayush Kumar Pandey
VIT University, India

Achyut Agrawal
VIT University, India

Sujatha Manohar
VIT University, India

ABSTRACT

Drugs are a marvel of modern medicine. With the huge drug market present in the world today, there is also a huge bane to the existence of drugs which is the presence of counterfeit drugs in the market that may cause irreversible damage to us. This chapter proposes a solution to counter this menace and save lives. After exploring the existing solutions in the global market and reviewing academic literature, it was found that such a comprehensive solution has not yet been implemented in India or the world. A comprehensive, affordable, easily accessible mobile application and website is proposed as the outcome of this research work. The application can provide the consumer with necessary details like the constituent salts, side effects, age barrier, safe consumption limit, and the purpose of the drug. To achieve this, a database of all known drugs and their images will be created and will be continuously updated with the help of machine learning and artificial intelligence. The chapter also discusses the business model to make it commercially viable.

DOI: 10.4018/978-1-7998-9172-7.ch009

INTRODUCTION

Regulating drugs to keep them authentic and safe is a huge task for any organization. The governments of different countries are working together to provide their citizens with safe drugs enclosed within authentic packaging and proper transportation. The growing counterfeit drugs menace is very difficult to handle, especially at lower levels of the supply chain, because many factory workers branch out and use their knowledge of "how the drug looks" to produce counterfeit drugs that may be chalk or powder or other harmful substances that may be used to give it a touch of authenticity. The problem with this is that these combinations sometimes prove to be fatal or inert and can cause severe problems to the patient's/consumer's health. Consumers have a right to know what they are buying and whether it is safe and clinically approved before it hits the market. Usage of counterfeit drugs has caused the unsuspecting consumer huge problems (WHO factsheet, 2018).

This book chapter aims to provide a solution to the above-mentioned problem by proposing the application "Checked-It," a feasible, cheap, easily accessible, and comprehensive solution. It aims to wipe out the use of counterfeit drugs through the chemist store or online, with the use of a simple mobile application that scans and tells the consumer if the medicine they have brought is authentic or not. It will be available on Android and IOS devices as well.

The proposed solution is based on a framework that utilizes the two incredible advancements - blockchain and AI for the protected stock of clinical medications all through the production network. Every item inside the blockchain can be moved between verified elements of the chain utilizing an "occasion demand reaction component." All exchanges between elements are recorded into the blockchain, thereby utilizing "brilliant agreements" with the assistance of which an item can be followed to its source.

This chapter includes the literature review regarding various health care applications and throws light upon the menace of counterfeit drugs, and emphasizes the need for a solution. The results of a qualitative study to understand customer requirements from such a solution are also included. The proposed solution and the technical specifications are discussed. It also provides a viable business model which will achieve the target of providing safety to the consumers and regulating the drug market.

MOTIVATION

It's hard enough to detect errors in the entire process of manufacturing and distributing one's pharmaceutical products, but pharmaceutical companies must also address the challenge of counterfeit medications that, at best, are ineffective and, at worst, are deadly. Drugs have been a marvel of modern medicine. Nowadays, drugs are present for every aspect of our lives, be it viral infections, bacterial infections, pain suppressors, or dopamine rushers. With the huge drug market present in the world today, there is also a huge bane to the existence of drugs which is the presence of counterfeit drugs in the market. The problem with these counterfeits is that they are random mixtures of unapproved chemicals that may cause irreversible damage to consumers. A study by Interpol indicates that about one hundred thousand to one million people die due to fake drugs every year. Last year about two hundred and fifty thousand children lost their lives to fake drugs, and that's just in the United States. The number shoots up exponentially when it comes to developing countries like India and Brazil. To counter this menace and save lives, the authors have come up with a comprehensive, cheap, and easily accessible application/website. The authors plan to reach out to the governments of different countries to help them in spreading awareness among people through different advertisement processes as it will also help them in eradicating fake drugs from the market. A big part of their motivation was them watching people lose their close ones just because of the greed of some people. People get into the counterfeit business for huge profits and greed. The most sophisticated counterfeiters may add an insignificant layer of active ingredients to avoid detection. The results can be deadly, particularly to children. Counterfeiters count on the fact that these patients are already ill to quell suspicions about the integrity of their fake drugs. Hence, the author's felt like it was their moral and ethical duty as citizens of the world to provide a means for people to have knowledge about what they are purchasing and to save as many lives as possible from the greed of people who pursue illegal activities like counterfeiting life-saving drugs. The authors strive for a better tomorrow and a counterfeit, free world where the safety of every person is paramount.

LITERATURE REVIEW

In this section, we first look at the Global and Indian scenario of the market for mobile healthcare applications, the market gap, and the need for a comprehensive solution.

Health Care Applications and their Adoption

The availability of fast internet speeds at lower costs, an ever-increasing number of smartphone users, advancements in the healthcare sector and, demand for the best healthcare privileges have resulted in the launch of various healthcare apps.

Health care apps are software applications on your smartphones that act as a tool for improving healthcare by providing valuable insights regarding the health information of consumers. Healthcare apps are gaining huge popularity due to the ease of access, low maintenance cost, better satisfaction to the users due to fair competition in the market, freedom from clinical paper records, and the ability to communicate vital treatment details. (Mosa, Yoo, and Sheets, 2012).

The unwillingness of the healthcare sector to consider new software or new technology is because of the involvement of sensitive patient information in the apps. This has been a hurdle in the development and adoption of healthcare applications. However, according to data by FDA (Food and Drugs Administration), there has been tremendous growth in the launch of new healthcare apps. It is expected that this growth will escalate at a faster pace as the internet disruptions will deplete. The trendy adoption of personalized medical solutions in people's homes for self-monitoring purposes is another major thing increasing the growth of the health care app market.

The healthcare application markets are extremely competitive as the tech market witnesses new players that are capable of investing in the market. Also, the go-to-market strategies of freshers aim to release sustainable and trustworthy mobile apps as quickly as every couple of weeks or so.

Europe and North America retain as major market holders with high growth potential due to investment capacity, prevalent technological adoption, and increasing population. The ASEAN region, especially India and China, is estimated to grow at robust CAGR during the forecast period of 2020-2027 due to the availability of high-speed internet, rising patient population, and government aid for the digitization of healthcare (Rivers and Glover, 2008)

Customer Requirements in Health Care Applications

"Simply having a mobile app is not enough," said Brian Kalis, managing director in Accenture's Health practice. "Apps are failing to engage patients by not aligning their functionality and user experience with what consumers expect and need. Consumers want ubiquitous access to products and services as part of their customer experience, and those who become disillusioned with a provider's mobile services – or a lack thereof – could look elsewhere for services." (Fajardo, 2021)

People are more intended to download applications that meet the following requirements:

a) **Functionality- Easy To Use**
   People want user-friendly applications, which don't take much time, are easy to use and are ready to serve the way customers want. This requires

comprehensive research on customer reviews and feedback and keeps improving to make their usage easier and more efficient.

b) **Accessibility**

"The healthcare app needs to provide clear and actionable information for all users." (Fajardo, 2021)

It needs to provide to-the-point information with additional data, to make it an application of purpose not the application of greed.

c) **Access to Online Community**

"According to the Journal of Medical Internet Research, social features in healthcare apps enhanced patients' ability to commit to treatment plans and healthier habits. Online communities provide a space to interact with others going through similar situations. Fostering a positive and helpful community for end-users will yield a great return on investment for all." (Fajardo, 2021)

Market Players

There already are good players in the market who dominate the healthcare sector. Some of them are OpenXcell, Swenson He, Consagous Technologies, Algoworks, Hidden Brains InfoTech, Abbott India Ltd., Lybrate India Pvt. Ltd., Zoctr Health Pvt. Ltd., MediIT Health Solutions India Pvt. Ltd, Portea Medical, HealthifyMe Wellness Pvt. Ltd.

According to research by statista.com, there are around 54,300 health care applications on Google Play, out of which 50% of them are based on booking appointments getting trends about a disease, or knowing about a particular type of symptoms, simply by adding details about the stuff you want to know.

Another Half of the applications majorly cover applications about fitness, wellness, or exercise. It majorly involves how a person could prevent a major disease how he/she could keep themselves fit and fine to never step on any harmful boat of dangerous diseases.

Coming to the point of medicines, many applications work for ordering and distribution of pharmaceutical drugs. Many applications are working to tell the usage or prescription of the medicines, but no application works for the authentication of any medicine. It simply works based on trust, we trust, and we buy. It's a huge market out there; we never know what is being offered to us or what's authentic. There is an urgent need to tackle this case by introducing an application which we can break the barriers of doubt over any pharmaceutical drug we buy (Gan, Koshy, Nguyen, and Haw, 2016)

According to the www.pharmacytimes.com website, the following Healthcare Apps have been listed as among the most convenient for users:

Epocrates:
- Reviews prescription drug and safety information
- Runs drug-drug interactions
- Scans health care insurance formularies for medication coverage
- Calculates body mass index
- Identifies medications by physical characteristics or imprint
- Available for Android and iOS devices

iPharmacy:
- Analyses drug tablet or capsule based on colour, shape, and/or imprint
- Provides detailed medication profiles
- Available for Android and iOS devices

Pharmacy Lab Values:
- Includes more than 150 different lab values that are organized and divided into categories
- Works offline
- Available for Android devices only

MPR:
- Provides detailed drug information
- Checks drug-drug interactions
- Offers up-to-date, concise prescription and OTC drug monographs
- Distributes daily drug news and warnings
- Contains personalized bookmarks for frequently accessed contents
- Accommodates more than 120 different clinical tools, such as calculators
- Available for Android and iOS devices

Pharmacist's Letter:
- Delivers concise recommendations for patient care
- Contains subscription options for continuing education found in the letter
- Available for Android and iOS devices

Pocket Pharmacists:
- Provides complete drug profile
- Runs drug-drug interactions, precautions, and adverse effects between 2 or more drugs
- Incorporates online resources for medications
- Available for Android and iOS devices

Shots Immunizations:
- Encompasses vaccine schedules and footnotes from the US Centers for Disease Control and Prevention
- Supplies graphics, images, and commentary for vaccines
- Maintains important up-to-date information for each vaccine

　　　◦　　Available for Android and iOS devices
PharmEasy:
　　　◦　　Home-delivered access to prescriptions.
　　　◦　　OTC pharmaceutical
　　　◦　　Other consumer healthcare products
　　　◦　　Comprehensive diagnostic test services
　　　◦　　Teleconsultations
　　　◦　　Available for Android and iOS devices

III Effects of Counterfeit Drugs

The progress that humankind has made in terms of medicine, health, and safety is nothing short of marvelous. However, due to the avarice of organizations and individuals, innocent people are being taken advantage of without them having any knowledge about it. The problem is huge and, if not addressed immediately, may result in unnecessary loss of life. Studies and statistics indicate that every year there are about five to seven million people affected by counterfeit drugs. A small percentage of those who have used these get away unscathed. However, a large majority is not so lucky. Counterfeit drugs have been known to cause severe mutations in the human DNA, which might cause other significant issues in the body. Sometimes it causes malfunctioning of the kidney or other vital organs. In other mild cases, it can cause rashes and discomfort all over the body, and the patient might just think that it is the side-effect of the medicine.

In the US alone, over 251,000 patients died in 2016 due to medical errors making it the 3rd largest cause of death in the country. A large portion of the mortalities resulted from the consumption of incorrect medications. Worldwide sales of counterfeit drugs crossed over $75 billion in 2010, with more than 75 percent of the counterfeit drugs connected to the Indian export of generic drugs.

The pandemic era has exacerbated this counterfeit drug crisis with Interpol's global pharmaceutical crime-fighting unit - Operation Pangea - capturing COVID-19 related counterfeit drugs worth over $14 million in April alone (Interpol Study, 2020).

Studies have shown that about one million die each year due to counterfeit drugs alone. The problem is also that these drugs are made out of cheap knockoff substances like chalk and potassium compounds that, when taken orally, can cause chemical imbalances in the body. The other side of this coin is that some substances used to make these drugs are inert, like flour or powder. Thus, those who need specific drugs for their health and life do not receive them. Since these drugs have no active chemical composition, the patients often die. These deaths are unnecessary and can be completely avoided if there is a system to detect counterfeits at the ground level.

GAP ANALYSIS – NEED FOR A COMPREHENSIVE SOLUTION

The authors acknowledge the existence of healthcare solutions in India and the rest of the world but highlight the need for an affordable, innovative, and easy-to-use solution to combat the problem of counterfeit drugs discussed in the previous section.

A qualitative study was conducted to understand the perception and requirements of the potential stakeholders in our app. Mr. Uchit Aggarwal, the COO of HBR chemicals, was interviewed in-depth, and the excerpts from his interview have been discussed below.

"There are several layers through which a manufactured medicine is passed before launching it in the market, like the approvals from various concerned authorities and medical experts," explains Mr. Uchit Aggarwal, director of Operations and Research in HBR chemicals and an investor, who is keenly interested in bringing about a change in the healthcare sector.

For example, "Atorvastatin," a drug used for lowering blood cholesterol and preventing heart attack and strokes, had to go through a 4-phase process defined by the FDA (taking the example of the US's Drug Administration). After the development and research of cholesterol-lowering medication, the drug is ready to further encourage the processes. Atorvastatin is tested on dogs, pigs, hamsters, etc., to study cholesterol behaviour. Then FDA inputs all the data and processes it for accurate mixture and components identification, including texture and quantity.

After a thorough examination by FDA, like what is mentioned above, a drug is launched.

"Launching a drug is a tedious process and on top of it, having an application that looks upon the drug's authenticity might just be a baby thing in front of FDA's approval status, hence stressing on the target audience and improving the trust exponentially on our AI application-based software must be a concern," explains Mr. Uchit Aggarwal.

If anyone comes from a family working in pharmaceutical knows how medicines are processed from the root level. Identifying the roots, the basic functionalities involved in making a drug has to be mandatory knowledge for someone trying to bring about a change in healthcare, Mr. Aggarwal further added, who, along with his family, has seen huge strides in healthcare.

PROPOSED SOLUTION

An application/website (checked-it) has been developed that is easily accessible and free to download on all platforms. This application is simple to use and user-friendly. It has been made in such a way that everyone with an internet connection and a smartphone can use the app with ease.

The app can be downloaded from the android play store or the IOS Appstore, and after entering the user's age, it will be ready to use. A database will be created for all the drugs that are available on the market. This will be achieved by signing contracts with pharmaceutical companies and by contacting the governments of various countries. The database can later also be updated regularly by the consumers who have been verified. Thus, it becomes an open-end operation rather than a back-end application. However, the data uploaded by users will be scrutinized to verify its authenticity.

The application/website employs smart image engines, artificial intelligence, and machine learning to detect counterfeits. The working of the app is very simple. A step-by-step tutorial is also given to the new user. The first step is to take a snapshot of the barcode and upload the sealed strip of medicine that has been bought from the pharmacy. This will verify the batch number, manufacturing date, and expiry date of the strip. Next, the user will take a snapshot of the drug capsule/tablet. What happens now is that a rigorous database check takes place with the help of our machine learning technology. The image processing AI module compares the original images of the capsule/tablet to the picture that the consumer has taken. The reason for this is that more than 95% of the available counterfeits have a different texture/colour/imprint/size than the original ones. Once this process is complete, a display message will tell the customer if the drug is safe for them to use or not. After this, the consumer will be shown all the details about that drug ranging from the manufacturing date of the drug to the constituent salts used. They will also be displayed with the safe age range to consume the drug, the proper dosage, and side effects, if any.

Blockchain technique tracks the route of the drug strip to the origination point to help eradicate counterfeit drugs from the market. If the image that has been processed by the platform suggests any trace of a counterfeit, a warning message will be displayed, and the relevant authorities will be intimated. The pharmacy where the drug was bought from will also be notified, and if there is another lapse, the pharmacy will automatically be registered on a black list. This list will be regularly updated and sent to the relevant authorities for appropriate action.

In the later stages of the app, once there is a strong user base, implementation of a review system will be done where advice can be given by fellow members in terms of the side effects of the drug or the efficiency of the medicine. There will be a forum where patients can address their doubts and speak to each other freely. It will provide a sense of community to the patients that are undergoing similar treatments/drug therapy.

With fast and responsive software, ***Checked-it*** offers a wide variety of features and privileges to the customers. While all other players in the health care application industry are into delivery and consultations mostly, checked, it stands out to be a different and quite a unique experience for the customers.

User Interface

Checked-It is focused on providing an easy-to-use application. It facilitates 3 step medicine verification without much trouble. It will be accurately designed to make its use simple and efficient. The application should feel the same for any platform they use it in, be it android or IOS.

Figure 1 shows the application in use on a smartphone.

Figure 1.

Problem	Solution	Unique Value Proposition	Unfair Advantage	Customer Segments
Worldwide sales of counterfeit drugs crossed over $75 billion in 2010 with more than 75 percent of the counterfeit drugs are connected to Indian export of generic drugs. Combat false claims and improper medicine usage by empowering users with increased information accessibility and convenience.	When the consumer scans the medicine or upload the image of medicine or its package, our database will run tests which include, image comparison, since the counterfeit ones tend to have some difference in the structure, logo, colour, packaging and whether it is approved by the drugs association or not. Blockchain technique will keep track of the route of the medicine as to from where they originate in order to help eradicate counterfeit drugs from the market.	The project not only helps consumers in making informed choices, but also educates them about the ups and downs of the condition they will impede upon themselves by doing so. Ensuring the understandability and approaching in such a way that domain for non-medical users are also befitted. While using technologies like blockchain, will help us locate the fraudsters at the source level and will help government to ensure authentic products in the market.	• Community • Team with industry experience • First of its kind **Channels** • Paid advertising • Sales People • Medical stores	• Young(18-24 years old) 20% • Adults(24-44 years old) 50% • Old aged(44- years old)30%

Cost Structure:

At first our team will, generate funding through crowd funding or personal funding. But after a ray of profit , we will be more inclined towards angel investors for the first round of capital improvement. Our angel investors will be mostly targeted for the companies in pharmaceuticals. But we will obviously be look for an angel inventor from another MNC.

Revenue Streams: Name of the medicine.
Company manufactured in.
And expected manufacturing month
Authenticity of the medicine.
But only these 4 will be displayed on the device while scanning for authenticity.
The greater part of the feature will be unlocked for premium user only who has to pay a 150 rupees/month membership with *checked-it*, to access more features. Like-
Name of the nearest chemist where this medicines are available in real time.
The symptoms under which the medicine will work and all the information about the cure for every symptoms.
The authenticity in a more elaborative manner.
Expected expiry month

Figure 2 shows the website in use on a personal computer.

222

Figure 2.

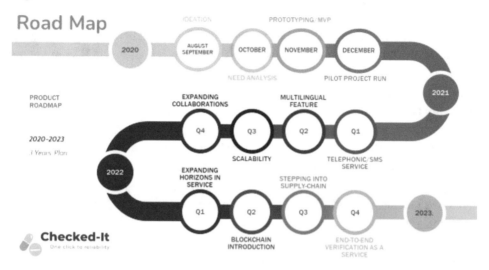

Checked-it has various information in addition to the scanning and getting medicinal information, which will make it much more attractive and smooth.

TECHNICAL SPECIFICATIONS

This section deals with the technical specifications and the various technologies that the authors have used in the creation of this application.

Blockchain

Blockchain is another innovation that is, bit by bit, arising with the expanding ubiquity of advanced monetary forms like Bitcoin. It is a 'disseminated record information base.' Blockchain records exchanges that have happened by setting up an information base of all organization hubs, and the whole process is open, straightforward, and irreversible. (Pandey, and Litoriyaf, 2020). It can be separated into public Blockchain, consortium blockchain, and private Blockchain. The consortium blockchain and private blockchain are considered permission blockchains. The public blockchain is decentralized in the genuine sense whenever any hub joins or passes on the choice to fabricate another square. However, in the permissioned blockchain, the choice to fabricate another square is made by a specific block confided in hubs. It has been applied to copyright the executives, personality validation, and information stockpiling administrations.

Ethereum and Smart Contracts

Smart Contracts need to be deployed on the blockchain, and here Ethereum is used for the same. Bitcoin's comprehensiveness is low since it is fabricated distinctly for virtual cash situations and isn't Turing-finished. Subsequently, a few other blockchain-based advancements have been developed, and different sorts of programming will currently be addressed on the blockchain as smart contracts. Ethereum previously understood the total attack of blockchain and smart contracts. (Bocek, Rodrigues, Strasser, and Stiller, 2017). Assuming a brilliant agreement is conveyed on the blockchain, it would be carried out as per predefined rules, and nobody will want to adjust it. The smart contract in Ethereum is written in a stack-based low-level bytecode language called EVM code, which is executed by the Ethereum Virtual Machine. (geeksforgeeks.org)

System Overview

This subsection deals with the various terminologies used in the implementation of RASA. The function and workflow of these terminologies have been explained.

1. Proprietor
   a. Make another client be added to the chain.
   b. Peruse the data of any client.
   c. Update the jobs of a client.
   d. Erase a client from the chain.
2. Carrier
   a. Check the bundle (Raw Material or Medicine).
   b. Pick the bundle from a substance (given carrier type).
   c. Convey the item to a substance.
3. Provider
   a. Make a Raw Material.
   b. GET the addresses of the Raw Materials made.
4. Producer
   a. Get the Raw Material from the Supplier through the Transporter.
   b. Check the wellspring of the item got.
   c. Make another Medicine utilizing got unrefined components.
5. Distributer
   a. Get the medication from the maker through the Transporter.
   b. Check the wellspring of the medication.
   c. Move the responsibility for medication.
6. Merchant

       a.   Get the medication from the Wholesaler through the Transporter.

       b.   Check the wellspring of the medication.

       c.   Move the responsibility for medication.

7.   Client

       a.   Get the medication from the Distributor through the Transporter.

       b.   Check the wellspring of the medication.

       c.   Place orders utilizing the Rasa chatbot.

       d.   Get clinical medication data.

Blockchain Implementation

The following steps take place during the implementation of the blockchain:

1.   The proprietor sends the shrewd agreements to the Ethereum Blockchain.

2.   The Owner verifies and registers the substances (drugs) of the chain.

3.   The Provider enrolls another Raw Material.

4.   Unrefined substance Contract is conveyed for the recently made unrefined substance.

5.   Comparing Transaction Contract is likewise sent for the recently made unrefined substance.

6.   Unrefined substance enrolled effectively.

7.   Provider moves the unrefined substance to the Transporter.

8.   Provider refreshes the item status and makes a Transaction in the Transaction Contract.

9.   Carrier moves the unrefined substance to the maker.

10.   Producer checks the wellspring of the natural substance.

11.   Producer refreshes the item status and makes a Transaction in the Transaction Contract.

12.   Producer enrolls another medication.

13.   Medication Contract is conveyed for the recently made medication.

14.   Related Transaction Contract is additionally sent for the recently made medication.

15.   Medication enlisted effectively.

16.   Producer moves the natural substance to the Transporter.

17.   Producer refreshes the item status and makes a Transaction in the Transaction Contract.

18.   Carrier moves the unrefined substance to the Wholesaler.

19.   Distributer confirms the wellspring of the natural substance.

20.   Distributer refreshes the item status and makes a Transaction in the Transaction Contract.

21. Distributer moves the natural substance to the Transporter.
22. Distributer refreshes the item status and makes a Transaction in the Transaction Contract.
23. Carrier moves the natural substance to the Distributor.
24. Merchant confirms the wellspring of the unrefined substance.
25. Wholesaler updates the item status and makes a Transaction in the Transaction Contract.
26. Merchant moves the unrefined substance to the Transporter.
27. Merchant refreshes the item status and makes a Transaction in the Transaction Contract.
28. Merchant moves the unrefined substance to the customer.
29. Client confirms the wellspring of the medication through an impermanent hub.
30. Client refreshes the situation with the item through an impermanent hub.

The truffle system helps to better the aggregation and organization of brilliant agreements. Truffle is an improved device for the Ethereum Solidity language and gives a test structure, making DApp advancement more straightforward. The test climate for the proposed arrangement is recorded. Visual Studio Code is an incredible, free, and open-source word processor that can assemble a strong IDE by downloading some modules. Web3.js is a JavaScript library given by Ethereum. It offers a total arrangement of JavaScript items and capacities that assist the customer side associated with the blockchain. The authors order and move their agreements, which gives them a form variant of their agreements that incorporates the agreement reflection into the content to utilize the agreement deliberation given by the truffle straightforwardly in the JavaScript code. The way to DApp advancement is to compose the smart contracts and collaborate with them through the front-end website pages. The code for the front-end, alongside the association foundation and communication rationale, is written in JavaScript with the ReactJS structure's assistance. Clients can communicate with contracts through the UI to utilize the unique functionalities given by the DApp.

RASA

A chatbot is required to enable ordering, tracing back medicines, and enhancing blockchain-based credit evaluation. Rasa is an open-source AI structure for mechanized text and voice-based discussions. Rasa can be utilized to get messages, hold discussions, and associate with informing channels and APIs. (D'souza, Nazareth, Vaz, and Shetty, 2021). Following are the means of how a collaborator worked with Rasa reacts to a message:

1. The "got message" is directed into the translator, which interprets it into a word reference of the first message, purpose, and substances found. This is taken care of by NLU.
2. The tracker object records the present status of the discussion. It gets the data that another message has come in.
3. The approach gets the tracker's present status.
4. The arrangement figures out the activity to do straightaway.
5. The tracker logs the picked activity.
6. A reaction is shipped off to the client.

RASA Implementation

The Rasa Open-Source engineering NLU Pipeline processes client expressions, utilizing an NLU model that is produced by the prepared pipeline. Given the specific circumstance, the exchange of the board perspective characterizes the following activity in a discussion. This is portrayed in the outline as the Discourse Policies. The pipeline utilized comprises of the accompanying parts:

1. Spacy center model: This is a pre-prepared model to foresee named elements, allocate grammatical feature labels (POS) and parse syntactic conditions.
2. Whitespace Tokenizer: Creates a token for each whitespace-isolated person arrangement utilized for aims and reactions
3. Regex Featurizer: An element will be set to check whether a regex in the preparation dataset was found in the client's message or not.
4. Lexical Syntactic Featurizer: This takes a contribution of tokens and makes highlights for substance extraction.
5. Count Vector Featurizer: Converts assortment of text reports to an inadequate network of token counts. It makes highlights for message goal grouping and reaction determination.
6. DIET Classifier: DIET (Dual Intent and Entity Transformer) is a perform various tasks engineering that can deal with both plan arrangement and substance acknowledgment together anticipated through a Conditional Random Field (CRF) labeling layer. It produces a result of elements, aim, and goal positioning.
7. Substance Synonym Mapper: This part will guarantee that the identified preparing element will be planned to similar equivalent word esteem.
8. Reaction selector: Used to anticipate bot's reaction from a bunch of applicant reactions. It implants client information sources and reaction names into something very similar space.
9. Spacy Entity Extractor: This part predicts the elements of a message.

The model is prepared on more than 12k web scratched and pre-processed drug names. This web-scratching script is composed utilizing Selenium and Beautiful Soup. At the point when a client demands a medication name like the ones in this dataset, the model concentrates the right medication name, a substance with the assistance of DIET Classifier, alongside Regex Featurizer and questions a rundown of comparative medications and subtleties like its producer name, parts, and so on. The portable application is assembled utilizing Flutter, which is a half and half application advancement system that can make applications for both android and iOS simultaneously.

This is associated with our rasa bot utilizing attachments, and messages are spilled to and from the application to the server. Each message is then shipped off to the server, and the rasa bot decides the goal from the text. An important message is then received back to the client dependent on the goal.

Rasa Chatbot fundamental Features Carried out are:

1. Structure for Ordering Medicines: Customers can choose the medication and determine the amount required. In light of the clients' bits of feedback and legitimacy check, the request is put, and a bill is produced. These request subtleties and a timestamp are then put away on the firebase cloud firestore while the client's discussion history and trackers are put away in MongoDB.
2. Setting clients' close-by area: Customers can set their close-by area by text. This creates a question to bring and store their area arranged in the information base.
3. Follow orders: Customers can check the ID (address) of the bought medication to know whether it is a confirmed medication and view its production network exchange history, following it back to the wellspring of its part unrefined components utilized in the creation of that medication. Along these lines, it permits drug stores/clients to know the genuine worth of the medication.

To check the performance of the system deployed on Ethereum and accessed through Ganache, capacity is calculated using TPS (Transaction per second).

$Throughput = capacity = TPS = (block\ size) * (block\ time)(Note: considered\ average\ values)\ (1)\ TPS = (transactions\ per\ block) * (block\ per\ second)$

Smart Contract Design

Supply Chain Contract: This agreement is sent by the Owner of the chain. It comprises numerous elements related to the inventory network, i.e., Owner, Provider, Transporter,

Manufacturer, Wholesaler, Distributor, Customer. It additionally comprises of different Solidity occasions used to speak with the front end continuously. Each capacity in the agreement must be arrived at by its separate job given to it. This is finished with the assistance of "modifiers" in Solidity. In this way, no element without a specific job can get to a particular capacity. This assists with expanding the security and openness of information put away or questioned from the blockchain.

Raw Material Contract: A separate Supplier sends the Raw Material Contract. When an unrefined substance is made genuinely, it is then added to the chain by the provider that made the unrefined substance. While making an unrefined substance to be added to the chain, information like EA (Ethereum Address) of the Supplier, Date-Time, EA of Transporter, Transaction Contract Address, and so on are mentioned from the provider. It additionally contains occasions that can register the whereabouts of the bundle progressively. The EA of Receiver (Manufacturer) is subsequently refreshed depending on the occasion demand reaction instrument. It likewise stores the current status of the medication, i.e., which substance at present has the unrefined substance.

Medicine Contract: The separate maker conveys the Medicine Contract. When a medication is made genuinely, it is then added to the chain by the producer that made the medication. While making medication to be added to the chain, information, for example, EA (Ethereum Address) of Raw Material used to make medication, Date-Time, EA of Transporter, Transaction Contract Address, and so on, is mentioned from the maker. It additionally contains occasions that can register the whereabouts of the bundle progressively. The EA of Wholesaler, EA of Distributor, and EA of Customer are refreshed later dependent on the occasion demand reaction component. It additionally stores the current status of the medication, i.e., which substance right now has the bundle.

Transaction Contract: The Transaction Contract is sent naturally by the Raw Material and Medicine smart contracts at whatever point made. The contract takes information like Date Time, sender EA, recipient EA, area, exchange hash, and the hash of the past exchange. The exchange hash is 32 bytes. The past exchange hash is put away for elements to confirm the wellspring of items in the chain.

Traceability and Source Verification

1. To start with, the purchaser starts a buy demand. The buyEvent() occasion in the Supply Chain contract is then set off. The occasion incorporates the purchaser's, furthermore, dealer's Ethereum address (Buyer EA and Seller EA), the location of the unrefined substance/medication to be bought, alongside the mark which is endorsed with the private key of the requester(buyer) and timestamp of the solicitation. The mark is sent along on the occasions to affirm

the character of the two players and the credibility of the solicitation. The Seller addresses are ordered so every dealer can inquiry their records dependent on their Ethereum Address.

2. Then, at that point, the Seller questions the log records identified with himself as per his Ethereum address and checks the legitimacy of the mark contained in the occasions. Assuming the confirmation is passed, an occasion respondent() is set off by the dealer to react to the purchaser's solicitation alongside a mark that is endorsed with the private key of the dealer.

3. Then, the Seller sends the item to the purchaser through the Transporter. An occasion sendEvent() is set off to demonstrate that the unrefined components/meds have been transported, including the Seller's and purchaser's Ethereum address (Seller EA and Buyer EA), the item address, alongside the mark which is endorsed with the private key of the Seller and timestamp of the exchange of the item.

4. At last, an occasion received event() is set off by the purchaser upon receipt of the merchandise to confirm that the products have been gotten. For instance, assume the producer requires a natural substance to make new medication. All things considered, the producer goes about as the purchaser, and the provider, which requires the unrefined substance, goes about as the vendor. When the above cycle is finished, the Supplier will refresh the exchange data as per the item address in the comparing Transaction contract, and the new collector of the natural substance is refreshed in the Raw Material agreement. The framework accepts that solely after the two players of the exchange have honestly enacted the above occasions, and the exchange subtleties will be changed. The item's source will be viewed as dependable.

BUSINESS MODEL

In this section, the authors propose a viable business model for the commercialization of the solution discussed above.

Business Model Canvas

Figure 3 represents the Business model canvas.

Figure 3.

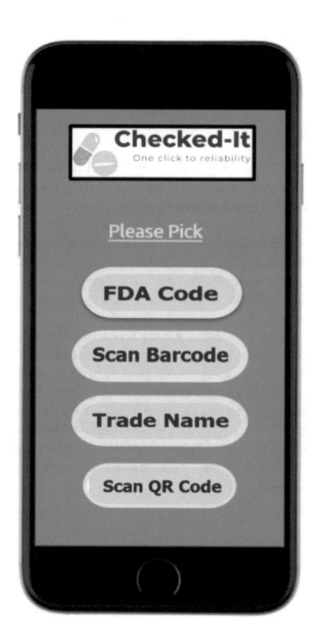

Marketing Strategy

The company plans to reach out to governments and pharmaceutical companies for creating awareness through advertisements on television, radio, newspapers, etc. To save a company's reputation, one will surely promote the application. Conducting drives or online campaigns against fake drugs and medicines would be mass publicity for this new application.

Encouraging drug retail stores to advertise the application to anyone who comes by their shop and the application will return the favour by promoting their pharmacies to the users.

Revenue Model

With flawless availability on Play Store and App store, Checked-it targets a freeware strategy among the users. Information will be limited and will only include authenticity, manufacturer, date, and month of manufacturing.

For unlocking a more detailed version of the application, the user has to purchase a premium version of the application, which includes the name of the nearest pharmacy where the medicine is available, the symptoms under which the medicine will work, and all the information about the cure for every symptom, the authenticity of the drug in a more elaborate manner and expected expiry month, and all the regular customer features as well.

Another revenue plan involves the introduction of the "SAVIOUR BADGE" scheme targeted to have maximum screen time from the customers. The badge will have ten levels in which each level unlocks a new feature and a discount voucher for the next medicine the consumer purchases from any pharmacy registered with the application. To ensure profit, sales, and advertising for the pharmaceutical company that has contracts with us, there will be a universal discount feature that will only be available for premium customers. This will entitle the premium customer to greater discounts and deals. These schemes will also give a push to more customers opting for the premium service.

Road Map

Figure 4 shows the Road map to be followed for the Business model.

Figure 4.

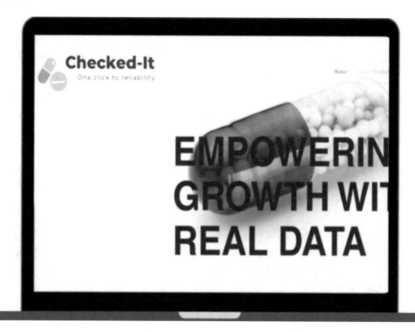

CONCLUSION

In conclusion, this book chapter emphasizes the need for techniques like blockchain ML/AI to tackle the counterfeit drug market menace. It is of imminent importance for people to come together and say NO to fake drugs that cause so many deaths every year. The plan is to provide a unique platform to every consumer to flag their grievances and for people to form a community of safe spaces for individuals in need. The app aims to provide concerned authorities with relevant information about the procurement and distribution of counterfeit manufacturers so that necessary action can be taken. The main aim is to provide a better and healthier future and to tackle the current obstacles that are faced by the everyday consumer in terms of information, dosage, safety usage, and efficiency. Checked-it strives for excellence, and this platform shall be available to everyone with a smartphone so that we can curb this problem once and for all.

REFERENCES

Ahad, M. A., Paiva, S., & Zafar, S. (Eds.). (2021). Sustainable and Energy Efficient Computing Paradigms for Society. EAI/*Springer Innovations in Communication and Computing*. *doi:10.1007/978-3-030-51070-1*

Best Free Mobile Apps for Pharmacists. (2021, March 5). Pharmacy Times. Retrieved 2021, from https://www.pharmacytimes.com/*view/best-free*-mobile-apps-for-pharmacists

Blackstone, E. A., Fuhr, J. P. Jr, & Pociask, S. (2014). The health and economic effects of counterfeit drugs. American Health & Drug Benefits, 7(4), 216–224. PMID:25126373

Bocek, T., Rodrigues, B. B., Strasser, T., & Stiller, B. (2017). Blockchains everywhere - a use-case of blockchains in the pharma supply-chain. 2017 IFIP/IEEE Symposium on Integrated Network and Service Ma*nagement (IM). https://doi:10.23919/ inm.2017.7987376*

Bose, S. (2018). A comparative study: Java vs Kotlin programming in Android application development. International Journal of Advanced Research in Computer Scie*nce, 9(3), 41–45. https://doi.org/10.26483/ijarcs.v9i3.5978*

*D'*souza, S., Nazareth, D., Vaz, C., & Shetty, M. (2021). Blockchain and AI in Pharmaceutical Supply Chain. SSRN Electronic Journal. doi:10.2139/ssrn.3852034

Fa*jardo, A. (2021, Decemb*er 8). 8 Best Healthcare Apps for Patients | Top Mobile Apps in 2021 - Rootstrap. Rootstrap - Call Rootstrap Today. Retrieved 2021, fr*om https://www.rootstrap.com/blog*/healthcare-apps/

Gan, S. K. E., Koshy, C., Nguyen, P. V., & Haw, Y. X. (2016). An overview of clinically and healthcare-related apps in Google and Apple app stores: Connecting patients, drugs, and clinicians. Scientific Phone Apps and Mobile Devices, 2(1), 8. *Advance online publication. doi:10.1186/1070-016-0012-7*

GeeksforGeeks. (2020, November 13). Creating dApps using the Truffle Framework. ht*tps://www.geeksforgeeks.org/creating-dapps*-using-the-truffle-framework/

Jayatilleke, B. G., Ranawaka, G. R., Wijesekera, C., & Kumarasinha, M. C. (2018). Development of mobile application through design-based research. Asian Association of Open Universities Jour*nal, 13(2), 145–168. doi:10.1108/aaouj-02-2018-0013*

Kern, C. (2012). Hospitals Need To Renew Their Digital St*rategies To Reclaim Patient Engagement. Retrieved 2021, from https://www.health*itoutcomes.com/doc/hospitals-need-renew-digital-strategies-patient-engagement-0001

Kostecka-Jurczyk, D. (2019). Tying on the mobile apps market and competition rules. Ekonomia, 25(3), 43–54. doi:10.19195*/2084-4093.25.3.4*

Mosa, A. S. M., Yoo, I., & Sheets, L. (2012). A Systematic Review of Healthcare Applications for Smartphones. BMC Medical Informatics and Decis*ion Making, 12(1). https://doi.org/10.1186/1472*-6947-12-67

Pandey, P., & Litoriya, R. (2020). Securing E-health Networks from Counterfeit Medicine Penetration Using Blockchain. Wireless Personal Communication*s, 117(1), 7–25. https://doi.org*/10.*1*007/s11277-020-07041-7

Parsazadeh, N., Ali, R., & Rezaei, M. (2018). A framework for cooperative and interactive mobile learning to improve online information evaluation skills. Computers & Education, 120, *75–89. doi:10.1016/j.*compedu.2018.01.010

Pharmaceuticals in the environment: a growing problem. (2015). The Pharmaceutical Journa*l. doi:10.1211/PJ.2015.20*067898

Rivers, P. A., & Glover, S. H. (2008b). Health care competition, strategic mission, and patient satisfaction: Research model and propositions. Journal of Health Organ*ization and Management, 22(6), 627–641. doi:*10.*1*108/14777260810916597 PMID:19579575

Samsudin, M. R., Sulaiman, R., Guan, T. T., Yusof, A. M., & Yaacob, M. F. C. (2021). Mobile Application Development Trough ADDIE Model. International Journa*l of Academic Research in Progressive Education and Development, 10(2), 1017–1027.*

Sylim, P., Liu, F., Marcelo, A., & Fontelo, P. (2018). Blockchain Technology for Detecting Falsified and Substandard Drugs in Distribution: Pharmaceutical Supply Chain Intervention. JMIR Research P*rotocols, 7(9), e10163. ht*tps://doi.org/10.2196/10163

West, J. H., Belvedere, L. M., Andreasen, R., Frandsen, C., Hall, P. C., & Crookston, B. T. (2017). Controlling Your "App" site: How Diet and Nutrition-Related Mobile Apps Lead to Behavior Change. JMIR mHealth *and uHealth, 5(7), e95*. doi:10.2196/mhealth.7410 PMID:28694241

WHO Factsheet. (2018, January 31). Substandar*d and falsified medical products. Retrieve*d December 16, 2021, from https://www.who.int/news-room/fact-sheets/detail/substandard-and-falsified-medical-products

Chapter 10

Generation of Synthetic Data:
A Generative Adversarial Networks Approach

André Ferreira
(iD) https://orcid.org/0000-0002-9332-0091
Centro ALGORITMI, Universidade do Minho, Portugal

Ricardo Magalhães
NeuroSpin, CEA, CNRS, Paris-Saclay University, France

Victor Alves
(iD) https://orcid.org/0000-0003-1819-7051
Centro ALGORITMI, Universidade do Minho, Portugal

ABSTRACT

Artificial intelligence is growing, but techniques like deep learning require more data than is usually available, especially in the medical context. Usually, the available data sets are not representative of reality, meaning that more samples have to be acquired, which is very costly. The demand for tools that can generate as much data as needed has increased. Traditional data augmentation tools are used to expand the available data, but they are not able to generate new data. The use of generative adversarial networks to generate synthetic data has proven revolutionary for big data as it increases the amount of available data without much cost. To this end, an adaptation of alpha-GAN for 3D MRI scans was developed to create a pipeline for generating as many synthetic scans of rat brains as needed. The applicability of the synthetic data was tested in a segmentation test and the realism by visual assessment.

DOI: 10.4018/978-1-7998-9172-7.ch010

INTRODUCTION

Every day, various medical imaging techniques are used to assess the health condition of many patients, e.g. Computed Tomography (CT), X-rays and Magnetic Resonance Imaging (MRI). The latter has a great advantage over other methods: it has no known side effects; it can produce multiplanar and three-dimensional images of in vivo structures with high spatial resolution; it does not expose the user to high levels of radiation (Cleary & Guimarães, 2014). Normally, these images, called scans, are evaluated by specialists who can detect anomalies, but this process can be very time-consuming. To solve this problem, several artificial intelligence-based decision support systems are currently being developed. A specific branch of artificial intelligence called Deep Learning (DL) has already been used for many applications such as decision support systems (Kose et al., 2021). However, DL usually requires a large amount of data to achieve high performance.

Collecting large amounts of medical imaging data can be very expensive, time-consuming or even impossible due to restrictive laws such as the ethical 3Rs rule (Russell & Burch, 1959), and often these data cannot be freely shared due to data protection laws (Foroozandeh & Eklund, 2020; Shin et al., 2018). The UK Biobank (Collins, 2020) in the United Kingdom is a successful attempt to overcome the problem of data scarcity by building huge long-term data repositories. This data can be used by the public or private sector without restriction. This initiative was very successful as it would support many researchers with a wide range of data.

Traditional data augmentation (Nalepa et al., 2019) and generative models have also been used to address the problem of lack of data. These techniques have shown some improvements in DL models, but only to a very limited extent (Foroozandeh & Eklund, 2020; Kodali et al., 2017). Conventional data augmentation does not fill all existing gaps in the data set distribution and some generative models are not sufficiently realistic and representative. Therefore, there is a need to develop better tools that can generate big data to better fill the gaps in the data set distribution. This tool can be created using Generative Adversarial Networks (GANs) (I. J. Goodfellow et al., 2014). With a well-trained generator, it is possible to create as many realistic scans as necessary.

In this paper, the use of GANs, in particular, α-GAN (Kwon et al., 2019; Rosca et al., 2017), to generate synthetic MRI scans was investigated, reviewing the literature on the subject, analysing successful experiments and examining the authors' experiments. The advantages and disadvantages of this method for generating large amounts of data were also analysed. Since the lack of information is not unique to human MRI scans, a study was conducted using rat brain MRI scans. The contributions of this work are:

- a new architecture that can be used to train a generator to produce realistic synthetic MRI scans of the rat brain;
- a pipeline that generates as many synthetic MRI scans of rats brains as needed;
- proof that synthetic data can be successfully applied and is realistic.

LITERATURE REVIEW

DL belongs to a subfield of machine learning called representation learning based on artificial neural networks, which is inspired by the structure and functions of neurons in the brain. DL can extract the most important features of a data set without human intervention, e.g. without labels (I. Goodfellow et al., 2016; Hao et al., 2016). DL has achieved good results when the available data is abundant, but this is not always the case. Sometimes it is very difficult to obtain data and medical data cannot usually be shared freely (Foroozandeh & Eklund, 2020). If the data set is small and it is not possible to collect more samples, there are two possible solutions: Generative Models or Few-Shot Learning. The approach in this paper is based exclusively on generative models to enable the generation of Big Data.

Few-Shot Learning

One approach to overcome the lack of data is to use few-shot learning, although this is not applied in this work. Few-shot learning aims to improve DL networks rather than increase the amount of data available. This method attempts to mimic human learning, as humans can learn with few samples and rare cases can be more easily learned by the models and not treated as outliers. These networks can handle imbalanced data sets better than other DL architectures and generalise more quickly to new classes that contain few samples. The goal is to train a function that can predict similarity, i.e., learn a deep distance metric, instead of detecting the images in the training set and then generalising to the test set (Sung et al., 2018; Wang et al., 2020).

Some works have been developed using these techniques. (Feng et al., 2021) have designed an Interactive Few-shot Learning (IFSL) approach to improve segmentation tasks when only small data sets are available. (Prabhu et al., 2019) proposed a scalable few-shot learning method to improve the classification of dermatological images.

Generative Networks

Generative networks are artificial neural networks that learn efficient coding of unlabelled data, also known as unsupervised learning (Kramer, 1991). The network attempts to capture the data distribution from the data set and produce data that should be very similar to that of the data set. Ideally, the model should be able to produce the same data without artefacts, blurring and other unwanted changes. These networks are typically used to reduce the dimensionality of data, e.g. data compression (Hinton & Salakhutdinov, 2006) and generate more data that is different from the original (Tanaka & Aranha, 2019).

Figure 1 shows three of the main types of deep generative networks that have been used, namely AutoEncoder (AE), Variational AutoEncoder (VAE) and Generative Adversarial Networks. The AE is characterised by having an input layer, one or more hidden layers and an output. The hidden layers are bottlenecks to reduce the size of the latent vector required to represent the data distribution. The latent vector is characterised by the fact that it has a lower dimensionality and is usually located in the middle of the network. Since the latent vector stores all relevant information, i.e., main features, the size of the latent vector affects the level of compression and the output quality so that an optimal balance must be achieved (Hinton & Salakhutdinov, 2006).

The VAE is an evolution relative to the AE, where the latent vector is a probability distribution rather than a fixed vector. Assuming that x denotes the input data, z denotes the latent encoding vector ($z{\sim}N(0,I)$), $\varnothing$ denotes the parameters, $q_{\varnothing}$ and $p_{\varnothing}$ denotes the encoder and decoder distribution, respectively, $q_{\varnothing}(z\,|\,x)$ and $p_{\varnothing}(x\,|\,z)$ are the probabilistic encoder and decoder (X. Chen et al., 2017; Kingma & Welling, 2014b).

Similar to VAE and AE, GANs consist of two networks trained simultaneously, but instead of being called Encoder and Decoder, they are called Discriminator and Generator respectively. They are characterised by the simultaneous training of two networks that compete to outperform the other, also called Generator vs. Discriminator Game where one generates an image and the other detects whether the generated image is real or synthetic. The generator produces synthetic data and attempts to fool the discriminator (D). The discriminator classifies the realism of each image generated by the generator, i.e. it gives a probability value for truth each time it receives an image, with higher values corresponding to higher realism. When the discriminator is unable to distinguish real images from synthetic ones, the maximum potential of the GAN is reached, i.e. optimal solution (Alqahtani et al., 2019; Gui et al., 2020). These networks have attracted much attention in the computer vision community due to their realistic data generation capacity compared to other generative networks.

(Costa et al., 2018) recognized the same problem as the researchers in this paper: "the availability of the large amounts of annotated data is becoming increasingly critical" adding that "annotated medical data is often scarce and costly to obtain".

For this reason, they explored adversarial learning to synthesize retinal coloured images. The problem was divided into two parts: An adversarial autoencoder was implemented to generate images of retinal vessels, and these images were then used to generate retinal coloured images. An end-to-end system was created, capable of synthesizing as many labelled retinal images as the user desires. To verify the quality of their system, they used visual and quantitative methods, proving that the images generated were different from the original but anatomically correct, i.e. with high visual quality and realism).

(Han et al., 2018) highlights one of the most important applications of the generated data, namely "improve diagnostic reliability". They focused on generating multi-sequence magnetic resonance images of the brain using GANs. The main difficulties were intra-sequence variability and consistency of brain anatomy due to the low-contrast images used. The data set used was BraTS 2016, resized from 240x155 to 64x64 and 128x128 to avoid artefacts and speed up training. The capabilities of DCGAN (Radford et al., 2016) and WGAN (Arjovsky et al., 2017) to generate synthetic images were tested. To assess the quality of the generated images, a visual Turing test was performed, which proved that the generated images looked realistic, as the experts were unable to distinguish the real images from the synthetic ones.

Figure 1. Representation of an AutoEncoder, a Variational Auto Encoder and a basic GAN architecture

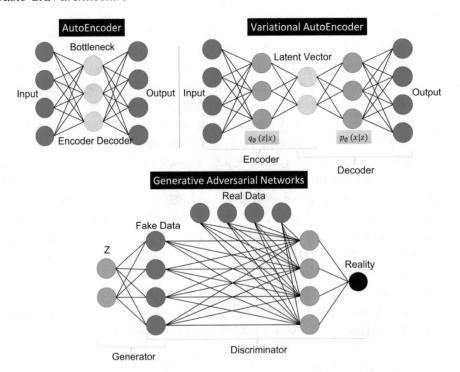

(Sun et al., 2020) has done one of the most recent works with 3D scans of the liver and brain, using a conditional GAN model, a Multi-Modal GAN, MM-GAN more specifically, to scale up the training data set. The problem of pathology morphology violation was solved with this architecture, leading to the possibility of translating the label maps into 3D MRI scans. This was probably the first GAN-based method to use MRI scans of the liver for data augmentation. The data set of brain tumors used was BraTS17 to perform data augmentation, but also to test the data anonymization capacity of the GAN models. Understanding the main application of these techniques, they tested the segmentation capacity of two different segmentation networks, 3D U-Net and Triple-Cascaded-Net, using different proportions of real and synthetic scans. This approach improved the Dice score for the whole tumor and tumor core by 0.17 and 0.16, respectively. The LIVER100 data set was also used to test the capacity of the MM-GAN model, with an equivalent improvement as when tested with the BraTS17 data set. The generator was based on the 3D U-net architecture with some optimizations, such as replacing ReLU with LeakyReLU, using instance normalization instead of batch normalization layers, and adding spectral normalization after each convolutional layer. The discriminator was inspired by the SimGAN discriminator (Shrivastava et al., 2017) but adapted to 3D cases. An image pool was also introduced to improve the stability of the discriminator. This consisted of a buffer of 4 tuples judged by the discriminator in each iteration, instead of only one tuple per iteration.

Unbalanced data sets are another problem that leads to the poor performance of DL models. (Shaker et al., 2020) solves this problem by using GANs to generate synthetic data of electrocardiograms. Their approach was able to improve accuracy, precision, specificity and sensitivity, and outperform several other electrocardiogram classification methods. The data set used, the MIT-BIH arrhythmia data set (Moody & Mark, 2001), has 15 imbalanced classes. The network is trained with each class independently to allow balancing. The lack of data may occur due to protection laws (Foroozandeh & Eklund, 2020) that prevent the possibility of free data sharing between researchers. This situation can be solved by relying on GANs, as shown in Shin et al. (Shin et al., 2018), since the synthetic images generated do not correspond to anyone, i.e., it is completely new information.

The main problems with the generality of GANs are that they require high computational power, are time-consuming and their training is characterised by high instability leading to mode collapse. Some stabilization techniques such as Spectral Normalization (Miyato et al., 2018), Gradient Penalty (Gulrajani et al., 2017), Batch Normalization and Instance Normalization have been developed to overcome the problem of instability, but they do not completely solve the problem and may increase the processing time required. Another problem is the introduction of blurriness and artefacts, although this is not exclusive to this generative method (Alqahtani et al., 2019; Karras et al., 2018; Kodali et al., 2017).

Alpha-GAN Generative Networks

The architectures used in this work are based on the Alpha-GAN architecture adapted to 3D MRI scans. Alpha-GAN also referred to as α-GAN (Rosca et al., 2017), is a generative model that combines a Deep Convolutional Generative Adversarial Network (DCGAN) (Radford et al., 2016) with a VAE (Kingma & Welling, 2014a; Rezende et al., 2014). The DCGAN is similar to the basic GAN architecture (I. J. Goodfellow et al., 2014), but consists of convolutional layers without fully connected hidden layers.

The introduction of this architecture aims to prevent both blurring and mode collapse. Mode collapse is characterized by the inability of the generator or discriminator to learn, resulting in a steady state of the generator, i.e. always producing similar images. This can be observed when the discriminator is unable to distinguish between real and synthetic images or when the discriminator is too good, and the generator cannot learn from the discriminator's feedback. This problem is solved when a VAE is used, but this architecture is known to produce blurred images, which is solved by the GvsD-GAN game.

Figure 2 shows the main differences between a DCGAN and a α-GAN, where a VAE is added and instead of only one discriminator, there are two ($D_\varnothing$ and C_ω). The Encoder encodes a real image ($xr_{eal)}$, and this vector ($\hat{Z}$) is discriminated by the Code Discriminator (C_ω) considering a random vector (Z) as real and $\hat{Z}$ as synthetic. Then $\hat{Z}$ and Z are used to generate two synthetic images (x_{rec} and $x_{gen,}$ respectively). Those images are discriminated by the discriminator and the feedback is passed to the *Encoder* and to the *Generator* (Kwon et al., 2019; Rosca et al., 2017).

(Kwon et al., 2019) was probably the first work able to generate new 3D brain MRI scans from a random distribution. Since this work was conducted to produce 3D MRI scans, the complexity of the problem increased exponentially. The computational power required, the problem of mode collapse and instability all increase when the whole scan is used instead of just a slice. The model created takes advantage of the α-GAN architecture (Rosca et al., 2017), and solved the mode collapse and blurring problem. Three different data sets were used, one with only healthy MRI data and the other two with different diseases (tumor and stroke). In the healthy MRI data set, qualitative (Principal Component Analysis, PCA) and quantitative (Mean Discrepancy, MMD and Multi-Scale Structural SIMilarity, MS-SSIM) measurements were performed to ensure the quality of the images generated. For the other two data

242

sets, only qualitative measurements were performed. Compared to other state-of-art architectures, this new approach achieved significantly better results.

Figure 2. Representation of two architectures, without VAE (DCGAN) and with VAE (α-GAN) (Rosca et al., 2017)

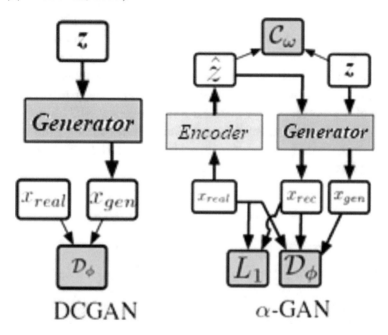

NETWORK ARCHITECTURE FOR 3D MRI DATA GENERATION

An adaptation of the α-GAN architecture for 3D MRI scans was developed to create a pipeline for generating synthetic scans of rat brains. The workflow of the training process and the corresponding evaluation is illustrated in Figure 3. The Image Resources block (Figure 3 A)) represents the creation of the data set, i.e. acquisition of the scans with an 11.7T Bruker scanner from NeuroSpin, CEA. The pre-processing block (Figure 3 B)) is the pre-processing of the data set, such as resizing by constant padding with zero value (from 64x64x40 to 64x64x64), conventional data augmentation and intensity normalization between -1 and 1. The deep learning application block (Figure 3 C)), where the models are trained and evaluated. The best model was selected based on quantitative, namely MS-SSIM, MMD, Peak Signal-to-Noise Ratio (PSNR), Root Mean Squared Error (RMSE), Mean Absolute Error (MAE), Normalized Cross-Correlation (NCC) and Dice Score, and qualitative metrics, i.e. visualization by the authors. These metrics were based on the works of (Baumgartner et al., 2018; Y. Chen et al., 2018; Kwon et al., 2019; Li et al., 2017; Sánchez & Vilaplana, 2018; Yi & Babyn, 2018; Zhao et al., 2018).

Several models were trained, of which only the two bests will be described here. Each model took about 6 days (approximately 150 hours) to train. This time varied because a shared machine was used.

To be able to share the generated scans when needed, some post-processing was necessary, namely cropping the constant paddings (from 64x64x64 to 64x64x40), flipping if necessary, and normalization between -1 and 1, as illustrated in Figure 4. Then, the metadata of an original file was copied into the generated file, resulting in a realistic NIfTI file. In the end, all that is needed is a trained model, a noise vector, e.g., a noise vector from a Gaussian distribution, and an original file to take advantage of the metadata and generate a completely new NIfTI file.

The input vector was sampled from a Gaussian distribution with mean 0 and variance 1 since the data set was normalized between -1 and 1. The size of the input vector was 500 or 1000 for each architecture.

Figure 3. Overall training and evaluation process workflow

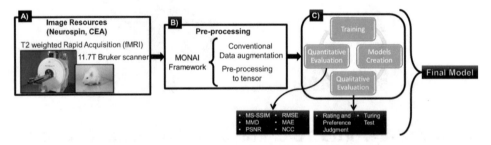

Figure 4. Generation workflow

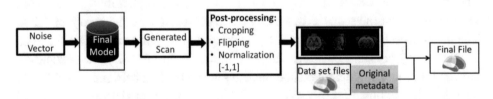

Data Representation and Pre-Processing

MRI is a non-invasive medical imaging technique used in radiology as it allows visualization of physiological functions, anatomical structures and molecular composition of tissues (Chan et al., 2019; Natarajan et al., 2012). The human body is composed of multiple tissues with different molecular constitutions, which means that the density and composition (e.g., water content) of each tissue is different. MRI uses these properties to create contrasts (Chou & Carrino, 2007; Duran et al., 2013).

Equally important as the method of acquisition is the evaluation of the data obtained. An MRI scan file essentially consists of three blocks of information: Header, affine transformation, and the actual image data. The header contains the meta-information of the file such as data type, name of the subject and much more important information that needs to be preserved. The affine transformation is a matrix that allows linear coordinate changes such as rotation, scaling, translation, etc. (Jenkinson, 2009). The real image data is a three-dimensional array consisting of two-dimensional arrays (each array is called a slice). A scan is a stack of slices, as shown in Figure 5. The scan shape is organized by the x-plane, the y-plane, the number of slices and the number of channels, e.g. [64,32,40,1] denotes a greyscale scan consisting of 40 slices of resolution 64x32. Usually, the fourth dimension is ignored as it does not provide any relevant information outside of functional studies.

There are many visualizers and software packages that help data analysis, such as Statistical Parametric Mapping (SPM), FMRIB Software Library (Jenkinson et al., 2012) and Python libraries (e.g., NiBabel and NumPy). Python is often used in this context because it has several libraries and frameworks for training DL models, handling and processing imaging data.

Figure 5. Slices of an MRI scan with shape [x-Plane, Y-Plane, nº Slices]

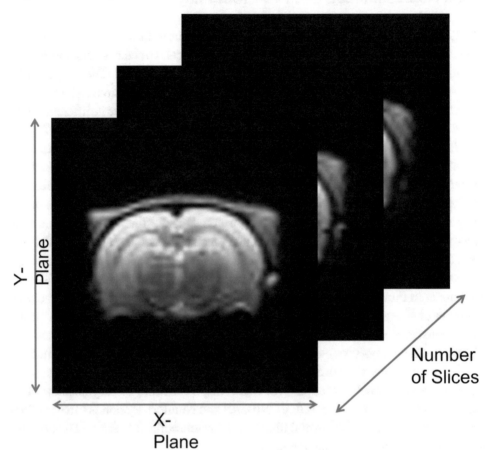

In this work, a Wistar rat brain MRI data set from the Sigma project was used to test whether GANs can be used for data augmentation. A total of 210 scanning sessions were performed using an ultra-high field 11.7 Tesla Bruker scanner and a 4 x 4 surface coil. A T2 weighted Echo Planar Imaging (EPI) sequence was used with a resolution of 0.375_{mm}x0.375_{mm}x0.5_{mm} over a matrix of 64x64x40, a TR of 2000ms and a TE of 17.5ms and 9 averages. Figure 6 shows slices from three different planes of a sample MRI rat brain. This data set is already pre-processed and ready to be used. For more information see (Barrière et al., 2019; Magalhães et al., 2018).

Figure 6. Sample scan from SigmaRat data set in all three planes (coronal, sagittal and axial slices, respectively)

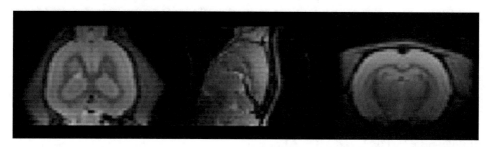

However, additional pre-processing was required. All scans had to be resized from 64x64x40 to 64x64x64, using constant padding so that the size could be resized back to 64x64x40 in a post-processing step, and the intensity of all scans was normalised to a value between -1 and 1. The data was augmented in a conventional way, i.e. by zooming, inserting Gaussian noise, flipping, scaling the intensity and shifting.

Methods

In this work, two architectures were developed, SigmaRatGAN1 and SigmaRatGAN2. Both are based on the architecture of (Kwon et al., 2019) applied to the SigmaRat data set. For the first architecture, some improvements were made based on (Miyato et al., 2018; Sun et al., 2020). Spectral Normalization was added after each convolutional layer to stabilize the training. Here, this normalization was applied in each network, although spectral normalization was created to stabilize the discriminator training (Miyato et al., 2018). The resulting architecture is illustrated in Figure 7 (left).

In the second architecture, spectral normalisation was removed from the generator and encoder, as this normalisation was created specifically to normalise discriminator training (Miyato et al., 2018). The batch normalization was removed from the code discriminator and the instance normalization was dropped from the discriminator to reduce the computational effort. The resulting architecture is illustrated in Figure 7 (right).

Training Procedure

The architecture of (Kwon et al., 2019) was used as the baseline for this work without any modifications for comparison. Then, it was trained SigmaRatGAN1 and SigmaRatGAN2. As mentioned in (Kwon et al., 2019), the size of the input vector was an important decision. The larger the vector, the more learning parameters the network had. It was very important that the network had enough learning parameters to be able to learn, but it could not have too many learning parameters to avoid overfitting when the model does not generalise. Therefore, the sizes 500 and 1000 were chosen.

The specifications of the workstation used are an ubuntu operating system (18.04.3 LTS (64 bits)) with CPU Intel Xeon E5-1650, 64 Gb of RAM, and secondary memory of: 2 Disks of 2TB; 1 Disk of 512Gb. The graphic card was: GPU – NVIDIA P6000; Cuda Parallel-Processing Colors 3840; GPU 24 GB GDDR5X; FP32 Performance 12 TFLOPS. It was used the programming language Python with the machine learning frameworks PyTorch and MONAI.

Figure 7. SigmaRatGAN1 architecture (left) and SigmaRatGAN2 (right) architecture

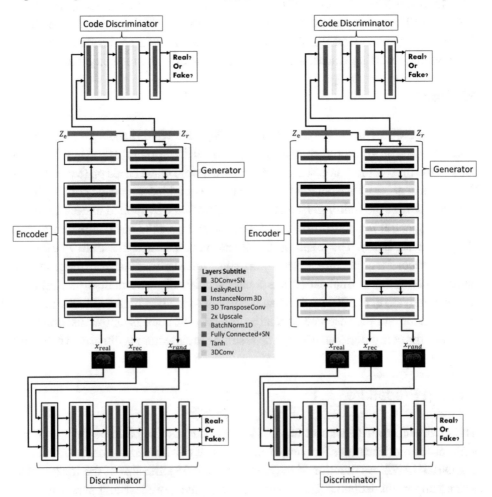

Loss Functions

For the baseline, the loss functions used for the discriminator, code discriminator, encoder/generator were Equation 1, Equation 3 and Equation 4, respectively, as explained in (Kwon et al., 2019). Equation 2 is the adversarial loss, with $\lambda 1 = \lambda 2 = 0$.

For the remaining architectures, all loss functions remained the same except for the encoder/generator. In the SigmaRatGAN1 training, the MSE loss was added in the encoder and the generator loss functions, Equation 5. For SigmaRatGAN2, the L1 loss was replaced by the gradient difference loss (GDL) (Mathieu et al., 2016) as used in recent super-resolution works, Equation 6 (Y. Chen et al., 2018; Miyato et al., 2018; Sánchez & Vilaplana, 2018). For this architecture the $\lambda 1 = \lambda 2 = 10$ and $\lambda 3 = 0.01$

$$L_D = \mathbb{E}_{z_e}\left[D\left(G\left(z_e\right)\right)\right] + \mathbb{E}_{z_r}\left[D\left(G\left(z_r\right)\right)\right] - 2\mathbb{E}_{x_{real}}\left[D\left(x_{real}\right)\right] + \lambda_1 L_{GP-D} \tag{1}$$

$$L_{GD} = -\mathbb{E}_{z_e}\left[D\left(G(z_e)\right)\right] - \mathbb{E}_{z_r}\left[D\left(G(z_r)\right)\right] \tag{2}$$

$$L_C = \mathbb{E}_{z_e}\left[C(z_e)\right] - \mathbb{E}_{z_r}\left[C(z_r)\right] + \lambda_1 L_{GP-C} \tag{3}$$

$$L_{G1} = L_{GD} - \mathbb{E}_{z_e}\left[C(z_e)\right] + \lambda_2 \left\| x_{real} - G\left(z_e\right) \right\|_{L1} \tag{4}$$

$$L_{G2} = L_{GD} - \mathbb{E}_{z_e}\left[C(z_e)\right] + \lambda_1 \left\| x_{real} - G\left(z_e\right) \right\|_{L1} + \lambda_1 \left\| x_{real} - G\left(z_e\right) \right\|_{MSE} \tag{5}$$

$$L_{G3} = L_{GD} - \mathbb{E}_{z_e}\left[C(z_e)\right] + \lambda_3 \left\| x_{real} - G\left(z_e\right) \right\|_{GDL} + \lambda_2 \left\| x_{real} - G\left(z_e\right) \right\|_{MSE} \tag{6}$$

D, G and C denote the Discriminator, Generator and Code Discriminator, respectively. z_e and z_r denote the latent vector of the encoder and the input random vector, respectively. x_{real} denotes a real scan. L_{GP-D} and L_{GP-C} denote the gradient penalty of Discriminator and Code Discriminator, respectively. L1, MSE and GDL denote the L1 loss, mean squared error and gradient difference loss, respectively. $\mathbb{E}$ denotes the total distribution.

Optimization

The SigmaRatGAN1 was trained with the Adam optimizer (Kingma & Ba, 2015) with default parameters. The learning rate was crucial and it was not easy to choose the best one (Ma et al., 2008; Smith, 2017). After surveying similar works (Baumgartner et al., 2018; Y. Chen et al., 2018; Han et al., 2018; Kwon et al., 2019; Li et al., 2017; Sánchez & Vilaplana, 2018; Yi & Babyn, 2018; Zhao et al., 2018) the value of $2*10^{-4}$ was chosen for all networks. The generator was always updated twice compared to the other networks, based on (Rosca et al., 2017). The optimiser for SigmaRatGAN2 was changed from Adam to AdamW (Loshchilov & Hutter, 2019) with the default parameters, as it can perform weight decay more stably. The other parameters were the same as the previous model. All models were trained for 200000 iterations.

RESULTS AND DISCUSSION

Table 1 summarizes the quantitative results. For the two new architectures, only the results with an input size of 500 are shown, as the results with an input size of 1000 did not achieve any relevant results. All metrics were calculated with 21000 comparisons, except for MS-SSIM, which has only 2100 comparisons for both real and synthetic data sets. First of all, it is possible to verify that the created models outperformed the base model. The SigmaRatGAN1 model had the best quantitative metrics, but this does not necessarily mean that the scans produced with this model are more realistic than those produced with the SigmaRatGAN2 model.

Specialists were asked to visually evaluate the scans generated. Figure 8 shows three different examples, the first being an original scan, the second a scan generated with the SigmaRatGAN1 model and the last one generated with the SigmaRatGAN2 model in three different planes, coronal, sagittal and axial. Figure 9 is composed of the same scans, but only shows the axial plane, which is the original plane, i.e. the scanning was performed in this plane. The first two rows are slices from the original scans, the next two rows were generated with the SigmaRatGAN1 model and the last two with the SigmaRatGAN2 model. The experts confirmed that the synthetic scans generated with the SigmaRatGAN2 model looked more realistic than the scans generated with the SigmaRatGAN1 model, considering only the axial plane. The SigmaRatGAN2 model also showed more potential since it could produce realistic scans more frequently and more detailed than the other models. That being said, these metrics may not be very reliable for comparing GAN models, at least there is no consensus on the best metrics and approaches for this comparison (Borji, 2019). However, it can be seen that SigmaRatGAN2 achieved better PSNR and RMSE values, which is consistent with the visual judgement. Although it is not possible to say with certainty, the assessment of the quality of the scans produced can pass through the use of this metric or a variant.

The MS-SSIM is a very interesting metric since it gives a value of similarity inside the data set. A value close to 1 corresponds to a data set made up of very identical scans, so to check whether the model fully represents the original data set this value should correspond to the real value (0.7490 in this case). The value 0.8118 is higher than the original one, which means that the model is not able to produce scans in the whole distribution. The value is still very far from 1, so this is not a big problem in this case.

Table 1. Quantitative results(mean and standard deviation). In bold are the best results for each metric. MS-SSIM values should be close to the real value (0.7490±0.0070), a higher value is better for NCC and PSNR, a lower value is better for RMSE, MAE and MMD

	Input Size	MS-SSIM	NCC	PSNR	RMSE	MAE	MMD
Base Line	1000	0.6860 ±0.0066	0.7241 ±0.0071	19.8245 ±0.1034	0.1029 ±0.0011	0.0316 ±0.0004	779.4653 ±27.2016
SigmaRatGAN1	500	**0.8118 ±0.0051**	**0.7887 ±0.0041**	20.2641 ±0.1158	0. 0979 ±0.0012	**0.0305 ±0.0004**	**753.1584 ±24.8816**
SigmaRatGAN2	500	0.8236 ±0.0056	0.7527 ±0.0037	**20.6033 ±0.0700**	**0.0955 ±0.0009**	0.0325 ±0.0003	819.3409 ±20.4437

Figure 8. Visualization of an original sample and a sample generated by each model (SigmaRatGAN1 and SigmaRatGAN2) in coronal, sagittal and axial planes

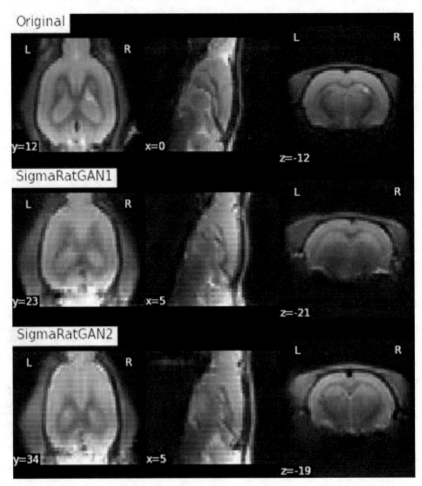

Looking at Figure 8 and Figure 9, it is very difficult to say which of the two models is better, but it can be said that overall, the generated scans are of good quality, i.e. they look realistic in both cases. When the specialists used a visualisation tool that allowed better visualisation of the slicing, they recommended using the SigmaRatGAN2 model for the next test. This model was then used to generate 348 synthetic scans. To test the ability of these scans to integrate the original data set, a DL based segmentation algorithm from (Rodrigues, 2018) was used that can create a segmentation mask for White Matter (WM), Grey Matter (GM) and CerebroSpinal Fluid (CSF). Table 2 summarizes the segmentation results. The test without synthetic data was performed by (Rodrigues, 2018) and the test with synthetic data by the authors. The combined use of 348 synthetic and 174 real scans improved substantially the global Dice score by 0.0172 and improved the GM, WM and CSF Dice scores by 0.0031, 0.0129 and 0.0712, respectively. This shows that GANs can generate large amounts of data and that the data is representative and realistic enough to improve DL models.

Table 2. Segmentation of the whole brain, Grey Matter (GM), White Matter (WM), and CerebroSpinal Fluid (CSF) Dice score. R denotes real and S denotes synthetic scans

	Without synthetic data	With synthetic data
Data set	174 Real; 0 Synthetic	174 Real; 348 Synthetic
Global Dice	0.8969	**0.9141**
GM Dice	0.9381	**0.9412**
WM Dice	0.8969	**0.9098**
CSF Dice	0.7468	**0.8180**

Figure 9. Coronal visualization of an original sample (first two rows), synthetic slices generated with the SigmaRatGAN1 model (next two rows), and slices of another sample generated with the SigmaRatGAN2 (last two rows)

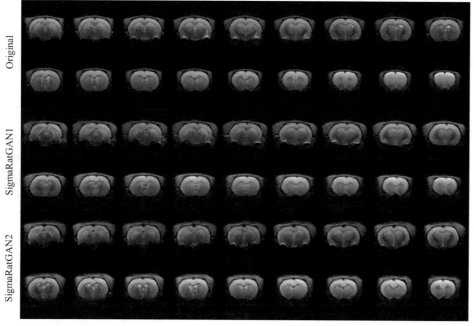

CONCLUSION

The problem identified here was the lack of available data, the difficulty of acquiring more and the urgency of having large amounts of it available, especially for DL training processes.

The use of traditional data augmentation can fill some gaps, but it is very limited compared to the possibilities offered by Generative Adversarial Networks. It was found that the α-GAN architecture has great potential when trained with MRI scans. This was confirmed when the generated scans were used to train a segmentation model and the Dice scores were improved compared to the baseline. The improvements of the segmentation of the CerebroSpinal Fluid were very impressive since this one is the most difficult structure to segment. The manual visualization of the scans also confirmed that GANs is able to produce very realistic scans. Only 348 synthetic scans were generated, but it is possible to generate many more and quickly if necessary, as the generator model is already trained and ready to be used.

Since the results in rats were so positive, it is expected that these models will have a great performance on the synthetic generation of MRI scans in humans, contributing to expanding the available data and improving healthcare. This approach enables the generation of multiple data sets that can be used in various artificial intelligence approaches in the healthcare industry.

For this work, it would be very interesting to test other GANs architectures or other approaches (e.g., changing the loss function of the networks) to confirm if the α-GAN architecture and the parameters used are best suited for use with MRI scans of rat's brains. To improve the world of GANs, exploring new metrics for evaluating models and new loss functions should be the main focus in improving GANs, as mentioned by (Borji, 2021). There are already many different GAN architectures focusing on different aspects, such as image, video and even sound, but they all have one serious problem: no metric comes close enough to human judgement.

ACKNOWLEDGMENT

This work of André Ferreira and Victor Alves has been supported by FCT- Fundação para a Ciência e a Tecnologia within the R&D Units Project Scope: UIDB/00319/2020.

REFERENCES

Alqahtani, H., Kavakli-Thorne, M., & Kumar, G. (2019). Applications of Generative Adversarial Networks (GANs): An Updated Review. *Archives of Computational Methods in Engineering*. Advance online publication. doi:10.100711831-019-09388-y

Arjovsky, M., Chintala, S., & Bottou, L. (2017). *Wasserstein GAN*. https://arxiv.org/abs/1701.07875

Barrière, D. A., Magalhães, R., Novais, A., Marques, P., Selingue, E., Geffroy, F., Marques, F., Cerqueira, J., Sousa, J. C., Boumezbeur, F., Bottlaender, M., Jay, T. M., Cachia, A., Sousa, N., & Mériaux, S. (2019). The SIGMA rat brain templates and atlases for multimodal MRI data analysis and visualization. *Nature Communications*, *2019*(1), 1–13. doi:10.103841467-019-13575-7 PMID:31836716

Baumgartner, C. F., Koch, L. M., Tezcan, K. C., Ang, J. X., & Konukoglu, E. (2018). Visual Feature Attribution Using Wasserstein GANs. *Proceedings of the IEEE Computer Society Conference on Computer Vision and Pattern Recognition*, 8309–8319. 10.1109/CVPR.2018.00867

Borji, A. (2019). Pros and cons of GAN evaluation measures. *Computer Vision and Image Understanding*, *179*, 41–65. doi:10.1016/j.cviu.2018.10.009

Borji, A. (2021). *Pros and Cons of GAN Evaluation Measures: New Developments*. https://arxiv.org/abs/2103.09396

Chan, R. W., Lau, J. Y. C., Lam, W. W., & Lau, A. Z. (2019). Magnetic Resonance Imaging. In R. Narayan (Ed.), *Encyclopedia of Biomedical Engineering* (pp. 574–587). Elsevier. doi:10.1016/B978-0-12-801238-3.99945-8

Chen, X., Kingma, D. P., Salimans, T., Duan, Y., Dhariwal, P., Schulman, J., Sutskever, I., & Abbeel, P. (2017). Variational lossy autoencoder. *5th International Conference on Learning Representations, ICLR 2017 - Conference Track Proceedings*, 1–17.

Chen, Y., Shi, F., Christodoulou, A. G., Xie, Y., Zhou, Z., & Li, D. (2018). Efficient and accurate MRI super-resolution using a generative adversarial network and 3D multi-level densely connected network. Lecture Notes in Computer Science (Including Subseries Lecture Notes in Artificial Intelligence and Lecture Notes in Bioinformatics), 11070 LNCS, 91–99. doi:10.1007/978-3-030-00928-1_11

Chou, E. T., & Carrino, J. A. (2007). Magnetic Resonance Imaging. In S. D. Waldman & J. I. Bloch (Eds.), *Pain Management* (pp. 106–117). W.B. Saunders. doi:10.1016/B978-0-7216-0334-6.50014-5

Cleary, J. O. S. H., & Guimarães, A. R. (2014). Magnetic Resonance Imaging. In L. M. McManus & R. N. Mitchell (Eds.), *Pathobiology of Human Disease* (pp. 3987–4004). Academic Press. doi:10.1016/B978-0-12-386456-7.07609-7

Collins, R. (2020). Accessing UK Biobank Data. *Scientia*, (October), 1–50.

Costa, P., Galdran, A., Meyer, M. I., Niemeijer, M., Abràmoff, M., Mendonça, A. M., & Campilho, A. (2018). End-to-End Adversarial Retinal Image Synthesis. *IEEE Transactions on Medical Imaging*, *37*(3), 781–791. doi:10.1109/TMI.2017.2759102 PMID:28981409

Duran, C., Sobieszczyk, P. S., & Rybicki, F. J. (2013). Chapter 13 - Magnetic Resonance Imaging. In M. A. Creager, J. A. Beckman, & J. Loscalzo (Eds.), *Vascular Medicine: A Companion to Braunwald's Heart Disease* (2nd ed., pp. 166–183). W.B. Saunders.

Feng, R., Zheng, X., Gao, T., Chen, J., Wang, W., Chen, D. Z., & Wu, J. (2021). Interactive Few-Shot Learning: Limited Supervision, Better Medical Image Segmentation. *IEEE Transactions on Medical Imaging*, *40*(10), 2575–2588. doi:10.1109/TMI.2021.3060551 PMID:33606628

Foroozandeh, M., & Eklund, A. (2020). *Synthesizing brain tumor images and annotations by combining progressive growing GAN and SPADE.* ArXiv Preprint ArXiv:2009.05946.

Goodfellow, I., Bengio, Y., & Courville, A. (2016). *Deep learning*. MIT Press.

Goodfellow, I. J., Pouget-Abadie, J., Mirza, M., Xu, B., Warde-Farley, D., Ozair, S., Courville, A., & Bengio, Y. (2014). Generative adversarial nets. *Advances in Neural Information Processing Systems*, *3*(January), 2672–2680.

Gui, J., Sun, Z., Wen, Y., Tao, D., & Ye, J. (2020). *A Review on Generative Adversarial Networks: Algorithms, Theory, and Applications.* https://arxiv.org/abs/2001.06937

Gulrajani, I., Ahmed, F., Arjovsky, M., Dumoulin, V., & Courville, A. (2017). *Improved training of wasserstein GANs.* Advances in Neural Information Processing Systems.

Han, C., Hayashi, H., Rundo, L., Araki, R., Shimoda, W., Muramatsu, S., Furukawa, Y., Mauri, G., & Nakayama, H. (2018). GAN-based synthetic brain MR image generation. *Proceedings - International Symposium on Biomedical Imaging*, 734–738. 10.1109/ISBI.2018.8363678

Hao, X., Zhang, G., & Ma, S. (2016). Deep learning. *International Journal of Semantic Computing*, *10*(03), 417–439. doi:10.1142/S1793351X16500045 PMID:28113886

Hinton, G. E., & Salakhutdinov, R. R. (2006). Reducing the dimensionality of data with neural networks. *Science*, *313*(5786), 504–507. doi:10.1126cience.1127647 PMID:16873662

Jenkinson, M. (2009). Image Registration and Motion Correction. *Image Processing*, *28*(3), 2009–2009.

Jenkinson, M., Beckmann, C. F., Behrens, T. E. J., Woolrich, M. W., & Smith, S. M. (2012). Fsl. *NeuroImage*, *62*(2), 782–790. doi:10.1016/j.neuroimage.2011.09.015 PMID:21979382

Karras, T., Aila, T., Laine, S., & Lehtinen, J. (2018). Progressive growing of GANs for improved quality, stability, and variation. *6th International Conference on Learning Representations, ICLR 2018 - Conference Track Proceedings*, 1–26.

Kingma, D. P., & Ba, J. L. (2015). Adam: A method for stochastic optimization. *3rd International Conference on Learning Representations, ICLR 2015 - Conference Track Proceedings*, 1–15.

Kingma, D. P., & Welling, M. (2014a). Auto-encoding variational bayes. *2nd International Conference on Learning Representations, ICLR 2014 - Conference Track Proceedings*, 1–14.

Kingma, D. P., & Welling, M. (2014b). Stochastic Gradient VB and the Variational Auto-Encoder. *2nd International Conference on Learning Representations, ICLR 2014 - Conference Track Proceedings*, 1–14.

Kodali, N., Abernethy, J., Hays, J., & Kira, Z. (2017). *On Convergence and Stability of GANs*. https://arxiv.org/abs/1705.07215

Kose, U., Deperlioglu, O., Alzubi, J., & Patrut, B. (2021). *Deep Learning for Medical Decision Support Systems*. Springer. https://link.springer.com/content/pdf/10.1007/978-981-15-6325-6.pdf

Kramer, M. A. (1991). Nonlinear principal component analysis using autoassociative neural networks. *AIChE Journal. American Institute of Chemical Engineers*, *37*(2), 233–243. doi:10.1002/aic.690370209

Kwon, G., Han, C., & Kim, D. (2019). Generation of 3D Brain MRI Using Auto-Encoding Generative Adversarial Networks. Lecture Notes in Computer Science (Including Subseries Lecture Notes in Artificial Intelligence and Lecture Notes in Bioinformatics), 11766 LNCS, 118–126. doi:10.1007/978-3-030-32248-9_14

Li, Z., Wang, Y., & Yu, J. (2017). Reconstruction of thin-slice medical images using generative adversarial network. *International Workshop on Machine Learning in Medical Imaging*, 325–333. 10.1007/978-3-319-67389-9_38

Loshchilov, I., & Hutter, F. (2019). Decoupled weight decay regularization. *7th International Conference on Learning Representations, ICLR 2019.*

Luo, J., & Huang, J. (2019). Generative adversarial network: An overview. *Yi Qi Yi Biao Xue Bao. Yiqi Yibiao Xuebao, 40*(3), 74–84. doi:10.19650/j.cnki.cjsi.J1804413

Ma, Y., Smith, D., Hof, P. R., Foerster, B., Hamilton, S., Blackband, S. J., Yu, M., & Benveniste, H. (2008). In vivo 3D digital atlas database of the adult C57BL/6J mouse brain by magnetic resonance microscopy. *Frontiers in Neuroanatomy, 2*(APR), 1–10. doi:10.3389/neuro.05.001.2008 PMID:18958199

Magalhães, R., Barrière, D. A., Novais, A., Marques, F., Marques, P., Cerqueira, J., Sousa, J. C., Cachia, A., Boumezbeur, F., Bottlaender, M., Jay, T. M., Mériaux, S., & Sousa, N. (2018). The dynamics of stress: A longitudinal MRI study of rat brain structure and connectome. *Molecular Psychiatry, 23*(10), 1998–2006. doi:10.1038/mp.2017.244 PMID:29203852

Mathieu, M., Couprie, C., & LeCun, Y. (2016). Deep multi-scale video prediction beyond mean square error. *4th International Conference on Learning Representations, ICLR 2016 - Conference Track Proceedings, 2015*, 1–14.

Miyato, T., Kataoka, T., Koyama, M., & Yoshida, Y. (2018). Spectral normalization for generative adversarial networks. *6th International Conference on Learning Representations, ICLR 2018 - Conference Track Proceedings.*

Moody, G. B., & Mark, R. G. (2001). The impact of the MIT-BIH arrhythmia database. *IEEE Engineering in Medicine and Biology Magazine, 20*(3), 45–50. doi:10.1109/51.932724 PMID:11446209

Nalepa, J., Marcinkiewicz, M., & Kawulok, M. (2019). Data Augmentation for Brain-Tumor Segmentation: A Review. *Frontiers in Computational Neuroscience, 13*(December), 1–18. doi:10.3389/fncom.2019.00083 PMID:31920608

Natarajan, P., Krishnan, N., Kenkre, N. S., Nancy, S., & Singh, B. P. (2012). Tumor detection using threshold operation in MRI brain images. *2012 IEEE International Conference on Computational Intelligence and Computing Research, ICCIC 2012.* 10.1109/ICCIC.2012.6510299

Niemeijer, M., Abràmoff, M. D., & van Ginneken, B. (2006). Image structure clustering for image quality verification of color retina images in diabetic retinopathy screening. *Medical Image Analysis*, *10*(6), 888–898. doi:10.1016/j.media.2006.09.006 PMID:17138215

Prabhu, V., Kannan, A., Ravuri, M., Chablani, M., Sontag, D., Amatriain, X., & Tech, G. (2019). Few-Shot Learning for Dermatological Disease Diagnosis. *Proceedings of Machine Learning Research, 106*(Icd), 1–15. http://www.dermnet.com/

Radford, A., Metz, L., & Chintala, S. (2016). Unsupervised representation learning with deep convolutional generative adversarial networks. *4th International Conference on Learning Representations, ICLR 2016 - Conference Track Proceedings*, 1–16.

Rezende, D. J., Mohamed, S., & Wierstra, D. (2014). Stochastic backpropagation and approximate inference in deep generative models. *31st International Conference on Machine Learning, ICML 2014*, *4*, 3057–3070.

Rodrigues, M. F. (2018). *Brain Semantic Segmentation: A DL approach in Human and Rat MRI studies.* http://hdl.handle.net/1822/64177

Rosca, M., Lakshminarayanan, B., Warde-Farley, D., & Mohamed, S. (2017). *Variational Approaches for Auto-Encoding Generative Adversarial Networks.* https://arxiv.org/abs/1706.04987

Russell, W. M. S., & Burch, R. L. (1959). *The principles of humane experimental technique.* Methuen.

Sánchez, I., & Vilaplana, V. (2018). Brain MRI super-resolution using 3D generative adversarial networks. *ArXiv, Midl*, 1–8.

Shaker, A. M., Tantawi, M., Shedeed, H. A., & Tolba, M. F. (2020). Generalization of Convolutional Neural Networks for ECG Classification Using Generative Adversarial Networks. *IEEE Access: Practical Innovations, Open Solutions*, 8, 35592–35605. doi:10.1109/ACCESS.2020.2974712

Shin, H.-C., Tenenholtz, N. A., Rogers, J. K., Schwarz, C. G., Senjem, M. L., Gunter, J. L., Andriole, K. P., & Michalski, M. (2018). Medical image synthesis for data augmentation and anonymization using generative adversarial networks. *International Workshop on Simulation and Synthesis in Medical Imaging*, 1–11. 10.1007/978-3-030-00536-8_1

Smith, L. N. (2017). Cyclical learning rates for training neural networks. *Proceedings - 2017 IEEE Winter Conference on Applications of Computer Vision*, 464–472. 10.1109/WACV.2017.58

Sun, Y., Yuan, P., & Sun, Y. (2020). MM-GAN: 3D MRI data augmentation for medical image segmentation via generative adversarial networks. *Proceedings - 11th IEEE International Conference on Knowledge Graph, ICKG 2020*, 227–234. 10.1109/ICBK50248.2020.00041

Sung, F., Yang, Y., & Zhang, L. (2018). Relation Network for Few-Shot Learning. *Cvpr*, 1199–1208.

Tanaka, F. H. K. dos S., & Aranha, C. (2019). *Data augmentation using GANs.* ArXiv Preprint ArXiv:1904.09135.

Wang, Y., Yao, Q., Kwok, J. T., & Ni, L. M. (2020). Generalizing from a Few Examples: A Survey on Few-shot Learning. *ACM Computing Surveys*, *53*(3), 1–34. doi:10.1145/3386252

Yi, X., & Babyn, P. (2018). Sharpness-Aware Low-Dose CT Denoising Using Conditional Generative Adversarial Network. *Journal of Digital Imaging*, *31*(5), 655–669. doi:10.100710278-018-0056-0 PMID:29464432

Zhao, M., Wang, L., Chen, J., Nie, D., Cong, Y., Ahmad, S., Ho, A., Yuan, P., Fung, S. H., Deng, H. H., & ... (2018). Craniomaxillofacial bony structures segmentation from MRI with deep-supervision adversarial learning. *International Conference on Medical Image Computing and Computer-Assisted Intervention*, 720–727. 10.1007/978-3-030-00937-3_82

ADDITIONAL READING

Brock, A., Donahue, J., & Simonyan, K. (2019). Large scale GaN training for high fidelity natural image synthesis. *7th International Conference on Learning Representations, ICLR 2019*, 1–35.

Chen, Y., Shi, F., Christodoulou, A. G., Xie, Y., Zhou, Z., & Li, D. (2018). Efficient and accurate MRI super-resolution using a generative adversarial network and 3D multi-level densely connected network. Lecture Notes in Computer Science (Including Subseries Lecture Notes in Artificial Intelligence and Lecture Notes in Bioinformatics), 11070 LNCS, 91–99. doi:10.1007/978-3-030-00928-1_11

Costa, P., Galdran, A., Meyer, M. I., Niemeijer, M., Abràmoff, M., Mendonça, A. M., & Campilho, A. (2018). End-to-End Adversarial Retinal Image Synthesis. *IEEE Transactions on Medical Imaging*, *37*(3), 781–791. doi:10.1109/TMI.2017.2759102 PMID:28981409

Goodfellow, I. J., Pouget-Abadie, J., Mirza, M., Xu, B., Warde-Farley, D., Ozair, S., Courville, A., & Bengio, Y. (2014). Generative adversarial nets. *Advances in Neural Information Processing Systems*, *3*(January), 2672–2680.

Karras, T., Laine, S., Aittala, M., Hellsten, J., Lehtinen, J., & Aila, T. (2020). Analyzing and improving the image quality of stylegan. *Proceedings of the IEEE Computer Society Conference on Computer Vision and Pattern Recognition*, 8107–8116. 10.1109/CVPR42600.2020.00813

Sun, Y., Yuan, P., & Sun, Y. (2020). MM-GAN: 3D MRI data augmentation for medical image segmentation via generative adversarial networks. *Proceedings - 11th IEEE International Conference on Knowledge Graph, ICKG 2020*, 227–234. 10.1109/ICBK50248.2020.00041

KEY TERMS AND DEFINITIONS

Adversarial Networks: Networks that compete with each other. In GANs, the generator tries to fool the discriminator by producing realistic data and the discriminator has to penalize the production of bad synthetic data.

Alpha-GANs: Junction of a VAE architecture with a GAN architecture to solve mode collapse and blurriness problems.

Big Data: Large amounts of information on a topic that are sometimes difficult to manage. It can be structured or unstructured. This term is often associated with Data Bases or Deep Learning.

GANs: Specific generative networks called Generative Adversarial Networks.

Generative Models: A set of operations that involve the distribution of the data set itself and can generate synthetic data. This can be divided into two approaches: generative (joint distribution) and discriminative (conditional distribution).

MRI Scans: Medical imaging modality to observe soft parts of the body. Very useful to study and observe the brain, breasts, joints, heart, and other organs.

Static Magnetic Field: Coil surrounding the in vivo object. This field must be constant and homogeneous in the entire object volume. The higher the field, the higher the spatial resolution.

Synthetic Data: Information generated in a non-natural way, i.e., not by measuring or performing the usual operations.

Chapter 11
Importance of E–Health in Human Life

B. Hemavathi
Sri Padmavati Mahila Visvavidyalayam, India

Depuru Bharathi
Sri Padmavati Mahila Visvavidyalayam, India

A. Suvarna Latha
Sri Padmavati Mahila Visvavidyalayam, India

ABSTRACT

E-health plays a significant role in giving valuable information to the people about human life. E-health is commercial and protected use of data about the health, information and communication technology (ICT), and its associates with the health-related directions and human health activities. ICT or e-health includes different interventions like telehealth, telemedicine, m-health (mobile health) e-health registers (EHR), big data, wearables, and uniform artificial intelligence. In life there is no time for paper and pen work in the countries, and they are change completely to the digitalization and sharing health information and patient health data through the online mode, which is more simple and successful healthcare improvements. Such healthcare apps are useful to us to lead better, well, and more fruitful lives. E-health can be one of the important hopeful aspects for providing community health benefits which incorporates a predictable medical system.

DOI: 10.4018/978-1-7998-9172-7.ch011

INTRODUCTION

With the help of internet and other related latest technologies E-health distributes the information about the medical health informatics, health of the public, business issues and important health services which are useful to the public. E-health means transfer of health information and health precautions through electronic media. The advanced electronic devices like telecommunications, electronics and informatics help E-health in health caring process (Sandesh, 2019).

E-health is a wide word and it discusses the use of health related data and advanced communication technologies that is used for the newest data and advanced communication technologies in health related areas, for example gathering information, keeping data, returning data, evaluating and super vision the information, merging the automated health registers, circulating and distributing health related therapeutic data, operations and isolated health care units, extra informative and useful E-health care cards. The main goal of E-health is to communicate with patients to know their health condition and to upgrade their health conditions (Yousef, 2012).

For development, evaluation and planning of E-health the different premediated methods are needed and advanced health care is important to take additional care about the patient health and continue to transfer the information and develop good values among the patients. E-health provides a penetrating possibility platform to transform health projection practices and decision making system that facilitate and coordinate the nursing of patients. Particular IT allows for the protected argument in order to provide patients payers regime and other applicable stakeholders who will be able to positively affect enduring treatment and people health promoting the reliable and thick share out manipulation, E-health technology is regarded as an authoritative tool to recover the condition of health care system at on sale loss and efficiency of health care system at low price out lay in alignment with the triple aim.

Currently, the world is facing an important growth of smartphone handlers (Kakria et al., 2015). Now a days animation mobile handsets are very useful and critical for everyone. Mobile phones are acting as eminent part to crack health related issues and at hand is fortune to acquire qualification in the company of users. To become aware of a patient who desires lead treatment are available with the help of WLAN/GPRS/3G network, we use Global Positioning system (GPS), Short message services (SMS) and cassette meeting. Now disparity, the patient can decide his or her physical situation by grasp person-bio indication and preserve win a resolution of once to get for doctors consultancy. Through the globe continual disease are the mainly ordinary causes of demise (Viswanathan et al., 2012). E-health is an umbrella call that connects healthcare and technology to nursing ancestors. (Van Rooij & Marsh, 2016).

Matteo (2017) presented views of different researchers and experts on using electronic health in the field of solving pulmonary disease like asthma. Stevens (2019) worked on development of eHealth apps and concluded that a better understanding of possible adverse effects could be a starting point in improving the positive impact of eHealth-based health care delivery.

Kadir (2020) worked on the role of telemedicine in healthcare during the COVID-19 pandemic in the developing countries and concluded that telemedicine play an important role in minimizing virus speed, effectively utilizing the time of health care professionals, and reducing the mental health issues also. Zheng et al. (2020) have provided the importance and role of pharmaceutical care in China perspective during COVID-19 pandemic situation. Hong et al. (2020) explained the success of using tele medicine in western China and suggested the other parts of the world to follow similarly and also concluded that practicing telemedicine was feasible, effective way during COVID -19 pandemic. Hind and Sarah (2021) have presented a rapid systematic review on the role of eHealth, telehealth, and telemedicine for chronic disease patients during COVID-19 pandemic situation.

BACKGROUND INFORMATION ON E-HEALTH

According to the World Health Organization (WHO), eHealth can be defined as "cost-effective and secure use of information and communications technologies for supporting different health and health-related fields, including providing services by the health-care units, health surveillance, health literature, and health education which includes both knowledge and research" (WHO accessed 29th March, 2021). Hence, eHealth includes all types of information and communication technology (ICT), for example, apps and websites for health promotion, screening, assessment, and therapists' video-chat sessions. Now-a days a vital importance was gained in the use of these technologies across the world since there are many positive effects of the usage of eHealth, such as reducing costs and replacing face-to-face healthcare contacts and communications especially in the COVID-19 pandemic situations. (Stevens, 2019)

E-HEALTH CHARACTERISTICS

The following are the characteristics of E-health (Sandesh, 2019).

Capability

One of the main important objective of E-health is to increase the capability in health care system and decrease the cost.

Improving the Worth of Health Care

The main important aim of E-health care is to improve the worth of health care by permitting differences between various benefactresses. E-health mostly concentrates on the excellence pledge, the main target is patient best health care in their future also.

Indication Centred

E-health contributions must be an indication centre that means their importance and capabilities are not to be accepted but confirmed by lengthy methodological processers.

Empowerment of Consumers and Patients

E-health offers best chances of patient E-health, it is health care based treatment and more over the services giving the data base medication and individual automated registers simply offered entirely everything to the patients on the internet.

Inspiration

E-health proposed inspiration for a fresh connection between the patient and doctor's patient, future health care depends on the mutual understanding and cooperation of the patient and health expert.

Education to Physicians

Different types of training programs and ongoing medication education programs helps the physicians to develop knowledge based education. Some online training programs like, health education and person protection data for patients.

Empowering

Empowering is data analysing and giving statement in a proper way among the health care organizations

Spreading

E-health is spreading a chance of patient health care additionally then its traditional limitations. These services may vary from humble request to additional multiple medicines.

Moral Values

E-health develops good moral values among the patients, this moral support helps good relationship between patient and health expert.

Justice

E-health is manageable advice to all patients it does not depend on patients age, race, gender, civilization. E-health gives equality to all the people like the people who are very poor, lack of computer knowledge and lack of computers and internet. Now a days even in this pandemic situation of Covid-19, this has also crossed the barrier of equity. Everyone is acquiring basic information of using the computers and also receiving data about E-medicine and prescriptions.

DIFFERENT CATEGORIES OF E-HEALTH AREAS

The following are the different categories of E-health areas

1. Telecare and Tele medicine
2. Experimental data classification
3. Integrated area and national data networks
4. Illness records and additional non-scientific methods are helpful for health education for people and health care organizations
5. M-health (Mobile health) and P-health (Personalized health) containing mobile apps (Cowie et al., 2013).

Many different types of apps like Apple, Google, Samsung, Endomondo, Nike, Germin, Fitbit and Withings are purchased for consumer companies to change the life style of the people, these apps play an important role to check physical activity of the human body, blood pressure, ECG, heart beat and any other health related issues with the help of connected devices. Anybody can utilise these apps to keep their health condition in a proper way (Enrico et al., 2014).

BENEFITS OF E-HEALTH

The E-health organizations helps for observing simple biological factors for example temperature of the body, oxygen percentage fluctuations, diastolic and systolic levels of heat beat, percentage of blood glucose levels etc. The improvement of the advanced technologies like wireless tools plays an important role to save the human health on online processes in this Covid-19 pandemic situation.

Management of Time

Time management is one of the important benefit in telemedicine, patients are permitted to plan their individual choice with their own like health expert. With the help of online consultancy the patient need not move from his own town or house.

Awareness in Peculiar Health

A delicate digital health care environment gives extra insight in to their health. If they wish they can share all or part of their information with a health care source or informal care as a result that they resole not cover to continually not take part to frequently tell their full check-up history. This allows the health contributor to be successful effectively to ascertain the sincere action, quickly and escape mistakes. Patients secure other check over their own up health merit to a better arrangement of their health situation.

Lower Administrative Burden

Health expect has fewer pen and paper work and able to share message fastly and simply with co-workers which will help to decrease managerial problems.

Patient Authorization

Now a days E-health offers advanced resolution, explain the complications in ageing organizations as developing size of people are aware with chronic diseases although financial plan are below stress and scarcity in health expects E-health also care patients to change precautions nearer to the people residence and to permit people by giving them control and shared duties to succeed their sickness.

Intensifying Prices

E-health and M-health are advanced technologies and these technologies are used in each and every aspect of health issues like cardiac care particularly for example controlling, analysis, risk valuation, observing, training, advising and cure the patient of advanced elucidations will confidently imprison the increasing prices of health care, present day more number of patients contact professional medical help, especially in states with huge remote areas and limited health experts and nurses.

SIGNIFICANCE OF MOBILE HEALTH APPS

- The mobile apps helps to update the doctors about the health condition of their patients.
- The health experts believe that health care apps can bring improvement in patients' health and the physicians are using the mobile technology to deliver the patient care.

LIMITATIONS OF E-HEALTH

- Economic barrier in procurement
- Price encounters
- Lack of different information technology and clinical sources
- Problem may be encompassed in acquiring computer knowledge and also using Internet
- Individual prices
- The deficiency of knowledge and usage of software
- Arranging of all health data structure, watching the period as soon as comfortable and planning of total health data structure must be standardized
- The deficiency of the primary ground work (Sandesh, 2019)

DIFFERENT TYPES OF ORGANISATIONS MODELS OF E-HEALTHCARE SYSTEMS

Wireless Body Sensor Network (WBSN) based E-healthcare Systems

There are so many causes that stay for inventing the mobile and E-health care organizations. Every day observing energetic biological constraints to the finding of an irregular experience expert by ambulatory observing system is one of the best example. The objective of mobile and E-Health care system is to improve a tele-home healthcare system which uses wearable devices, wireless statement technologies, and then multisensory data merging methods. (Hung et al., 2004).

Types of Cell Phones and Smartphones Based E-healthcare Systems

The following are some important cell phones and smartphones based on E-healthcare systems.

1. Cell phone centred patient observing system (C-SMART) developed by (Blumrosen et.al., 2011)
2. Digital phone created reduction finding system on automation stage developed by (Fang et.al., 2012)
3. Cell phones are used in Personal heart monitoring and rehabilitation system developed by (Leijdekkers & Gay, 2006) and cell phone health checking system for aging persons (iCare)

System on Chip (SoC) E-healthcare Modules

A manageable system on chip for ECG intensive care has been established by (Kim et al., 2014). This module is talented of fulfilling configurable functionality with low-power consumption.

Cloud-Based E-healthcare Systems

The idea of health-cloud has developed with the progress of mobile and e-healthcare technologies (Garkoti et al., 2014). In patient's well-being is detected using Health-Cloud has been offered. Once the place of a mobile patient changes, the related default gateway also changes and, subsequently, the optimum mapping concerning the server and the mobile node also changes (Rahul, 2016).

CHALLENGES AND SAFETY MATTERS IN E-HEALTHCARE SYSTEMS

Wearable Medical Devices WMDs and E-Healthcare

The E-healthcare systems distribute with patient-centric unfavourable health check data, anywhere precision of records is of high concern. Next chief challenges are forced in E-health showing great care.

Usability

In spite of non-trivial labours from soul (Computer- creature Interaction) explore domain, the only one of its kind food create of handler-friendly E-health monitoring systems increase a prepared of challenges. Be deficient in forthcoming interfaces/ GUI for mutually health check body and patients is one of the main reasons impeding their wider acceptance in practice (Sawand et al., 2014).

Sensor Data

The devices may be obsessed with and tale made-up or piercing numbers scheduled to unpredicted hardware disasters or defective infrastructures matters which will give information fake reading and psychoanalysis of the data (Sawand et al., 2014).

One of the main tasks and apprehensions allied with WMDs and e-healthcare systems is the affordability and expensive in helpfulness. These amenities be supposed to be ended existing to the little-revenue and central-class inhabit as well. This be supposed to be a up gesture for the price-effective e-healthcare conveniences to the drop or inadequate people.

Additionally, more than a few other issues like sensor node failure/ removal, strike on BAN/WBAN from exterior aggressor, conservational intervention like indicator fading, inadequate or hammering of power/ battery, passing of connectivity/ arrangement disappointment awaited to transceiver bankruptcy or group interruption, make contacts congestion awaited too much sensor data, and a large amount significantly, compatibility/ interoperability owed to poles apart exchange ideas standards be supposed to be carefully addressed period manipulative the e-healthcare systems (Hovakeemiaa et al., 2011; Kumar et al., 2014; Rahul, 2016).

Privacy and Protection of Patient Numbers and Data

To guarantee the security and secrecy of patients the functional information and in a row is single of the main issues in Wireless Body Area Network (WBANs). The facts precautions and secrecy issues in WBANs hold pioneer been inspected far by (Li et al., 2010). They have looked in to two critical information defence issues –guarantee and trustworthy, dispersed fact storage, and sufficient grained spread information open regulation for touchy and secret enduring remedial data. Reporters various security attacks and weakness in the wireless topologies like Bluetooth and global system for mobile communication (GSM) (Lim et al., 2010).

The functioning psychoanalysis of the scheme has been prepared by the parameters-communication fee and computation cost. Boast pooled the orthogonal matching pursuit (OMP) based encryption and compressed sensing (CS) based compression for stable image luggage compartment for cloud-based E-healthcare system.

About other protection and confidential issues and concerned solutions in wireless and in the remote patient monitoring systems are reported in (Lim et al., 2010; He & Zeadally, 2015; Lee et al., 2013; Rahul, 2016).

FUTURE WAYS AHEAD TOWARDS RESEARCH

The ever-increasing quantity of digital phones, everywhere world wide web (www) and cloud computing will little by little arise in to a new area named Wearable Internet of Things (WIoT) which is the interesting topic for researchers. This will be in charge of to greater than before ability of recognising computing and communication. Upcoming groups of WIoT contract to convert the health care region, in which persons are perfectly traced by wearable devices for adapted strength and wellness records. However to achieve multi-dimensional success, WIoT needs not only to incredulous the industrial trials of creating a lithe structure for interacting, adding, keeping and imagining, however besides want to combine its take in deceitful clarifications that stay clinically comfortable and functioning (Hiremath et al., 2014).

CONCLUSION

The advanced technologies like healthcare practices and health care technologies motivate the patients and also health experts. The health care apps helps people to lead healthier, safer and more fruitful lives. Patient centred healthcare system was developed from incorporating the technology in to the medical care. The E-health plays an important role to give good suggestion about patient's health care and care about patient's future health and give security for patient's information. These mobile apps helps people to succeed their lives very confident and happy. The E-health knowledge may help in giving good and healthy and diseases less young generation to the society.

E-health is considered as a cost-effective and efficient way of providing services and medical help to the people who are not in a position to afford more money. If it is not with in the affordable prices for the needy then it cannot be considered as a service also. But, it may also include some ethical and legal values also. The person or an agency which is providing the facilities and services in the form of e-health must have a thorough knowledge about the various things which are to be done or which should not be done, otherwise this may lead to lot of problems sometimes linked with legal issues also.

The literature lacks on the adverse effects of e-health, tele-medicine, tele-health and delivering the services to the needy in the adverse situations and pandemic situations. More emphasis and research must be carried out even to help the needy people under the various adverse situations also with less cost.

REFERENCES

Blumrosen, G., Avisdris, N., Kupfer, R., & Rubinsky, B. (2011). C-SMART: Efficient Seamless Cellular Phone Based Patient Monitoring System. *IEEE Int. Symp. on a World of Wireless, Mobile and Multimedia Networks*. 10.1109/WoWMoM.2011.5986191

Cowie, M. R., Catherine, E. C., & Panos, V. (2013). E-health innovation: Time for engagement with the cardiology community. *European Heart Journal, 34*(25), 1864–1868. doi:10.1093/eurheartj/ehs153 PMID:22733834

Enrico, G.C., Catherine, E.C., Nico, B., Przemyslaw, G., & Enno, T.V.V. (2014, September 15). The importance of e-Health in daily cardiology practice. *Cardiac Rhythm News*.

Fang, S. H., Liang, Y., & Chiu, K. M. (2012). Developing a Mobile Phone-based Fall Detection System on Android Platform. *Computing, Communications and Applications Conference*.

Garkoti, G., Peddoju, S. K., & Balasubramanian, R. (2014). Detection of Insider Attacks in Cloud based e- Healthcare Environment. *Int. Conf. on Information Technology (ICIT)*. 10.1109/ICIT.2014.43

He, D., & Zeadally, S. (2015). Authentication Protocol for an Ambient Assisted Living System. *IEEE Communications Magazine, 53*(1), 71–77. doi:10.1109/MCOM.2015.7010518

Hind, B., & Sarah, A. (2021). The role of e-Health, tele-health, and tele-medicine for chronic disease patients during COVID-19 pandemic: A rapid systematic review. *Digital Health*, 1–17.

Hiremath, S., Yang, G., & Mankodiya, K. (2014). Wearable Internet of Things: Concept, Architectural components and promises for person –Centered healthcare. *EAI 4th International conference on wireless mobile communication and health care.*

Hong, Z., Li, N., Li, D., Li, J., Li, B., Xiong, W., Lu, L., Li, W., & Zhou, D. (2020). Telemedicine during the COVID-19 pandemic: Experiences from Western China (Preprint). *Journal of Medical Internet Research, 22*(5), e19577. doi:10.2196/19577 PMID:32349962

Hovakeemiana, Y., Naik, K., & Nayak, A. (2011). A Survey on Dependability in Body Area Networks. *5th Int. Symp. on Medical Information & Communication Technology.* 10.1109/ISMICT.2011.5759786

Hung, K., Zhang, Y. T., & Tai, B. (2004). Wearable Medical Devices for Tele-Home Healthcare. *Proceedings of the 26th Annual International Conference of the IEEE.*

Kadir, M. A. (2020). Role of telemedicine in healthcare during COVID-19 pandemic in developing countries. *Telehealth Med Today., 5*(2), 1–5. doi:10.30953/tmt.v5.187

Kakria, P., Tripathi, N. K., & Kitipawang, P. (2015). A real-time health monitoring system for remote cardiac patients using smartphone and wearable sensors. *International Journal of Telemedicine and Applications, 8*, 1–11. doi:10.1155/2015/373474 PMID:26788055

Kim, H., Kim, S., Helleputte, N. V., Artes, A., & Konijnenburg, M. (2014). A Configurable and Low-Power Mixed Signal SoC for Portable ECG Monitoring Applications. *IEEE Transactions on Biomedical Circuits and Systems, 8*(2), 257–267. doi:10.1109/TBCAS.2013.2260159 PMID:24875285

Kumar, P., Porambage, P., Ylianttila, M., Gurtov, A., Lee, H. J., & Sain, M. (2014). Addressing a Secure Session- Key Scheme for Mobility Supported e-Healthcare Systems. *16th International Conference on Advanced Communication Technology.* 10.1109/ICACT.2014.6779018

Lee, S., Kim, H., & Lee, S. W. (2013). Security Concerns of Identity Authentication and Context Privacy Preservation in u Healthcare System. *14th ACIS International Conference on Software Engineering, Artificial Intelligence, Networking and Parallel/ Distributed Computing (SNPD).*

Leijdekkers, P., & Gay, V. (2006). Personal Heart Monitoring and Rehabilitation System using Smart Phones. *Int. Conf. on Mobile Business (ICMB '06)*. 10.1109/ICMB.2006.39

Li, M., Lou, W., & Ren, K. (2010). Data Security and Privacy in Wireless Body Area Networks. *IEEE Wireless Communications*, *17*(1), 51–58. doi:10.1109/MWC.2010.5416350

Lim, S., Oh, T. W., & Choi, Y. D. (2010). Tamil Lakshman, Security Issues on Wireless Body Area Network for Remote Healthcare Monitoring. *IEEE International Conference on Sensor Networks, Ubiquitous, and Trustworthy Computing (SUTC)*.

Matteo, B. (2017). Electronic health (e-health): Emerging role in Asthma. *Current Opinion in Pulmonary Medicine*, *23*(1), 21–26. doi:10.1097/MCP.0000000000000336 PMID:27763999

Rahul, K. K. (2016). Mobile and E-Health care; recent trends and future directions. *Journal of Health & Medical Economics*, *10*, 1–10.

Sandesh, A., (2019). What is E-health, its characteristics, benefits and challenges, global health. *Public Health Notes*, *5*, 1-10.

Sawand, A., Djahel, S., Zhang, Z., & Naıt-Abdessela, F. (2014). Multidisciplinary Approaches to Achieving Efficient and Trustworthy eHealth Monitoring Systems. *International Conference on Communications in China (ICCC)*. 10.1109/ICCChina.2014.7008269

Stevens, W. J. M., van der Sande, R., Beijer, L. J., Gerritsen, M. G. M., & Assendelft, W. J. J. (2019). E-Health apps replacing or complementing healthcare contacts: Scoping review on adverse effects. *Journal of Medical Internet Research*, *21*(3), e10736. doi:10.2196/10736 PMID:30821690

Van Rooij, T., & Marsh, S. (2016). E-Health: Past and future perspectives. *Personalized Medicine*, *13*(1), 57–70. doi:10.2217/pme.15.40 PMID:29749870

Viswanathan, M., Golin, C. E., Jones, C. D., Ashok, M., Blalock, S. J., Wines, R. C., Coker-Schwimmer, E. J. L., Rosen, D. L., Sista, P., & Lohr, K. N. (2012). Interventions to improve adherence to self-administered medications for chronic diseases in the United States: A systematic review. *Annals of Internal Medicine*, *157*(11), 785–795. doi:10.7326/0003-4819-157-11-201212040-00538 PMID:22964778

World Health Organization. (n.d.). *e-Health*. www.emro.who.int/health-topics/ehealth/

Yousef, W. (2012). What is E-health and why it is important? *Qatar's Technology Hotspot*, (31), 1-13.

Zheng, S.-Q., Yang, L., Zhou, P.-X., Li, H.-B., Liu, F., & Zhao, R.-S. (2020). Recommendations and guidance for providing pharmaceutical care services during COVID-19 pandemic: A China perspective. *Research in Social & Administrative Pharmacy*, *17*(1), 1819–1824. doi:10.1016/j.sapharm.2020.03.012 PMID:32249102

KEY TERMS AND DEFINITIONS

E-Health: E-health is defined as a new healthcare and service providing processes which involves the implementation and usage of information and technology for treating various health problems virtually.

E-Health Registers: E-health register is defined as a chart which maintains the complete details and health cart of a patient/patients exclusively in a digital format.

Information and Communication Technology (ICT): Information and communication technology refers to diversified set of tools and services used for storing, applying, and communicating data to the different fields when and wherever required.

Telehealth: Telehealth is simply defined as the distribution of health-related services through telecommunications technology.

Chapter 12
Improving the Management of Hospital Discharges

Ana Cecilia Coimbra
Centro ALGORITMI, Universidade do Minho, Portugal

Filipe Miranda
Centro ALGORITMI, Universidade do Minho, Portugal

Nicolas F. Lori
Universidade do Minho, Portugal

Júlio Duarte
(iD) https://orcid.org/0000-0002-5458-3390
Centro ALGORITMI, Universidade do Minho, Portugal

Luis Mendes Gomes
University of the Azores, Portugal

ABSTRACT

At the University of Porto Hospital (Centro Hospitalar Universitário do Porto [CHUP]), a tool for computerized clinical coding was developed to assist in the codification of hospital discharge. However, for this tool to be useful, it is necessary to have a process to manage the entire coding process. Thus, a platform was developed to help manage the coding of hospital dis-charge episodes. The biggest advantage of the existence of this platform is to better organize the entire coding process in order to improve the quantity and quality of work performed by CHUP's health professionals.

DOI: 10.4018/978-1-7998-9172-7.ch012

INTRODUCTION

Medical records are quite complex for computer systems to process and store, being the primary issue with such procedures not a lack of data, but rather the variety and complexity of the healthcare sector. The number of different occurrences and combinations of factors generates an enormous diversity of data. Thus, it is difficult to assess hospital productivity, therefore, the need arises to use Diagnosis Related Groups (DRGs), which in turn rely on coding systems that translate diagnoses and procedures to group episodes in groups with resembling characteristics that in turn use similar hospital resources.

In the paper "Improving the Codification of Hospital Discharges with an ICD-9-CM Single-page Application and its Transition to ICD-10-CM/PCS" (Coimbra et al., 2018) a Single-page application (SPA) was presented. The goal was to facilitate the coding process by making all the necessary data available for users to carry out the coding of each episode. It is possible to fill the fields related to the codification of diagnosis and procedures in a single page and at the same time view the general data of the patient and the discharge report. This data integration makes the coding process faster and more efficient since users do not have to consult the necessary data on several plat-forms at the same time.

However, this SPA does not bring much advantage if there is no platform that manages the episodes, that is, that differentiates between coded and non-coded episodes, among other things. The focus of this paper is to describe the workflow of the management system of the codification process.

State of the art

The Medical Coding and DRGs systems, are both powerful tools that have been employed in the modern era to satisfy financial and statistical needs (García Calderón et al., 2019). In this section are presented the main theoretic topics behind the realization of this work.

Diagnosis Related Groups

The DRGs are a very important and powerful tool in terms of financial and statistical indicators in the health sector. How a health institution is able to quantify all the resources that are allocated in all different situations that happens in a hospital? The DRGs are used for helping in that topic by helping to classify and divide the clinical episodes into groups with similar resource allocations (García Calderón et al., 2019). Epidemiological information, diagnostics, clinical features and procedures are used by the DRG system to assign episodes to an individual DRG (group) (Chok et al., 2018).

The benefit of using the DRG system is based on the premise that since each group contains episodes with similar characteristics (course of disease, length of hospital stays (LOHS) and treatment requirements) then their costs will also be similar.

It is necessary to gather a Minimum Data Set (MDS) in order to classify an inpatient episode into one of the 25 Major Diagnostic Categories (MDC) and, within these, into one of the almost 669 DGRs that are currently accessible. As a result, the MDS contains the following elements (Portalcodgh, n.d.), (Grupos de Diagnósticos Homogéneos, n.d.):

- Gender;
- Age - categorized as pediatric DGRs when the age is less than or equal to 17 years, and as adult DGRs when the age is more than 17 years ;
- Main Diagnosis - responsible diagnosis for the patient's hospitalization;
- Other diagnostics;
- Procedures - a sequence of procedures done on the patient while he or she is in the hospital;
- Birth weight (newborn);
- Destination after discharge - In addition, patients may be moved, released against medical advice, or dead.

Each DGRs group has a relative weight and a weighting coefficient that are connected with it. With this in mind, it is thus possible to assign a certain reimbursement to a DRG group and thus reduce medical expenses and related financial charges while maintaining the quality of medical services and ensuring that resources are allocated correctly (Chok et al., 2018), (Lee et al., 2019)

However, if an error in assigning a DRG to a case occurs, it can have enormous financial repercussion (García Calderón et al., 2019).

The DGR system was developed in the United States, and the version that began to be used in 1983 in the United States was used as a basis by other countries, such as Germany, France, Australia, United Kingdom and Canada; so as to develop their own version with its own episode groups and algorithm. In Portugal, the "All Patient Diagnosis Related Groups" (AP-DRG) grouper was adopted, which in turn is highly used in the United States (Grupos de Diagnósticos Homogéneos, n.d.).

ICD-10-CM

The International Classification of Diseases 10th Revision Clinical Modification (ICD-10-CM) is a medical terminology which intends to standardize all medical in-formation, so that in this way it is possible to compare clinical records anywhere in the world (Lee et al., 2019), (Hernandez-Ibarburu et al., 2019).

The ICD-10 terminology is divided into two different parts: ICD-10-CM for diagnostic codes and ICD-10-PCS for procedure codes in patients. This terminology was developed with the aim of improving the existing one (ICD-9), the main difference being the quantity and specificity of the clinical data ().

While ICD-9-CM has 14,567 diagnostic codes and 3882 procedure codes, the ICD-10-CM/PCS version has 69823 diagnostic codes and 71974 procedure codes, this was only possible by changing the format of the codes, such as changing from numeric (ICD-9-CM) to alphanumeric (ICD-10-CM/PCS). In general, ICD-10-CM/PCS is a more complex system that allows greater specificity and, consequently, a better classification of clinical episodes (Alonso et al., 2019), (Armstrong et al., 2017)

If hospital units adopt this terminology in their clinical records, it makes it easier to use DRGs since having standardized records facilitates their distribution to groups.

Hospital Morbidity Information System

The Central Administration for Health (Administração Central do Sistema de Saúde (ACSS)) and the Ministry of Health Services (Serviços Partilhados do Ministério da Saúde - SPMS) developed a new Hospital Morbidity Information System (Sistema de Informação de Morbilidade Hospitalar - SMIH) that uses ICD10-CM/PCS as a cod-ing system. The goal is the existence of a cross section across the entire National Health System (Serviço Nacional de Saúde – SNS), where clinical coding is done in ICD-10-CM/PCS of the episodes by each doctor in his working hospital, being thus an online platform based on central data (de Saúde, n.d.).

Research Methodologies

Design Research (DR) is essential to create products, services and systems capable of responding to human needs (Lee, n.d.). The difference between DR and Design Science Research (DSR) is that the first corresponds to research on or about design, while the second corresponds to research using design as a method or technique. Learning through the construction of artifacts is the characteristic that defines the DSR (Vaishnavi et al., 2012). Fig. 1 shows the DSR model that emerges from the Takeda model adaptation (Vaishnavi et al., 2012).

Figure 1. DSR Model (adapted from (Vaishnavi et al., 2012))

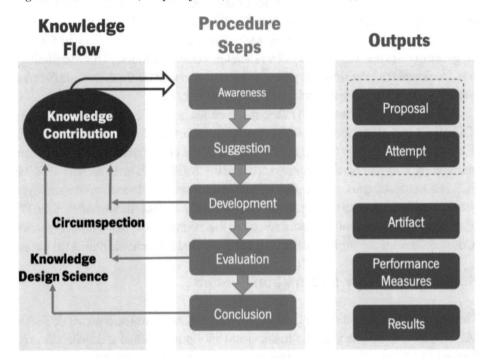

A typical DSR model follows the following methodology:

- Awareness: In this phase the problem is identified, presenting a research proposal.
- Suggestion: Considering the proposal made in the previous phase, the objectives for its development are defined. It consists of a creative phase, where in addition to existing elements, new elements can also emerge.
- Development: This phase focuses on the development and implementation of the artifact.
- Evaluation: Evaluation of the artifact, according to the criteria outlined in the first phase and the outline of improvements, if necessary.
- Conclusion: In this phase two paths can result: if the results obtained are satisfactory then the end of the research is given, otherwise, the DSR cycle is restarted.

PROOF OF CONCEPT

Proof of concept (PoC) is used to assess whether a concept or theory is valid and can be proven through the practical model. In the scope of information technology (IT), the PoC is used to assess whether the objective for which the technology was developed has been achieved or not (Sergey et al., 2015), (Schmidt, 2006)

In this paper the PoC used was SWOT analysis and it is described in section 3.4.6.

Management Platform

This section is subdivided in two parts, the first part describes the coding process management platform, and the second part describes the platform connection with the Hospital Morbidity Information System (Sistema de Informação para a Morbilidade Hospitalar (SIMH)).

"E-Codificação" Platform

The coding process management platform is called e-codificação (means e-coding in Portuguese). This platform contains all episodes that have already been discharged from the hospital.

The management platform will be used by medical coders and administrative per-sonnel who will manage and distribute episodes by coders. However, the confidential-ity of patient data is a factor that has to be taken into account, thus, the clinical in-formation of each patient can only be viewed by authorized users. With this in mind, three types of users with different access were created: administrator, administrative staff and coding physician.

The administrator, as the name implies is the platform administrator and has access to all the information.

The administrative staff manages episodes, distributing them by coders. This type of users is only able to access general information such as the process number, medical specialty in which the episode was discharged and date of discharge; without ever having access to clinical information of the patient.

On the other hand, the third type of user, the coding physician, has access to all clinical information about the episodes attributed to him, nevertheless, he/she is not able to access episodes that are attributed to other doctors.

An episode from entering in the platform until the coding is completed goes through different states. The possible states are:

- Discharge to close – episodes that are closed, but may have a lack of essential elements for coding, and therefore they cannot yet be distributed to coders;

- Discharge closed – episodes ready to be distributed;
- Pending – episodes that were flagged by the coders with any problem, whether due to lack of information or whether, for example, the impossibility to access the discharge report;
- In coding – episodes that are currently being coded by coding physicians;
- In audit – episodes that were completed by the coders, but that need to be vali-dated to be accepted as completed;
- To recode – episodes that have codification done, however this codification needs to be redone or corrected;
- To re-audit – episodes where it is not the first time that the audit is done;
- Conclude – episodes that have the codification completed;

The workflow, in terms of states of the management platform is presented in Fig. 2. In short, an episode starts with the status "Discharge to close", and if no important element is missing, it is distributed to an appropriate encoder by the type of medical specialty and type of episode (interment or ambulatory).

In the "in coding" state, the encoder does as the name indicates the codification of the episode, if it finds any problem, for example, lack of anesthesia report in the dis-charge report file, or it is not possible to view the report, the encoder sends the episode to the "Pending" folder. In this state, episodes are reprocessed, and problems are solved and sent back to the state "in coding". In case everything is alright, at the end of the codification, it goes to "In audit" status, the episodes cannot be "concluded" immediately as it is necessary to have an evaluation of the codification done.

In this state, it is confirmed if the coding was done correctly or if it contains any error in this state. If there is an error, it is sent to "recode" to the same encoder, and once finished it goes to the "to re-code" state, and then if everything is alright, it is finally finished, otherwise it goes back to recode.

Figure 2. Workflow "e-codificação"

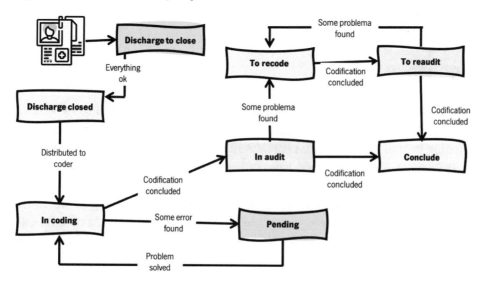

SIMH Interoperability

The ACSS and the SPMS collaborated to create the SIMH, a coding system that enables the centralization of all clinical data recorded for all Portuguese hospitals. SIMH enables the encoding of episodes using the ICD-10-CM/PCS coding system; these episodes remain accessible to the hospital, but other hospitals are unable to see each other's data; nevertheless, research and assessments by authorized authorities are feasible.

However, even though the created system has a portion where encoding can be per-formed, coders are free to utilize the SIMH method if they so choose. Developing a webservice capable of sharing information in both the SIMH-e-codificação and the SIMH-e-codificação direction was required in order for this to be possible. Having this webservice operational allows the information to be available on both the SIMH and e-codificação sides, independent of the platform selected by the coders for cod-ing.

In this way, it allows coders to maintain the system they are used to working with, (the e-codificação) and acquire interoperability with the central SIMH database because all the episodes encoded in the e-codificação are, when concluded, sent to the SIMH through the agent that was developed.

In addition to the newly encoded episodes, it was essential to transmit all of the previously e-codificação encoded episodes to SIMH. Thus, an agent was created to collect data from previously encoded and completed episodes, with which it produces a JSON file that follows the pre-defined format, which is then transmitted to SIMH through a web service.

DISCUSSION

Prior to the implementation of this system, coding was performed using an excel spreadsheet. Not only did the implementation of this system allow the coding situation to be improved, but it also permitted the coding process to be monitored.

Previously, the coder would have to search for the patient's data (age, gender, etc.) as well as the discharge report for the episode being coded, necessitating the use of several platforms simultaneously to complete the encoding process. This is no longer necessary due to the nature of the new platform, since all necessary information is shown immediately in the window where the coding is performed.

Additionally, this new approach simplifies the process of entering ICD-10-CM/PCS codes. Coders had two options in the excel version: they could either memorize the codes they often used or they could utilize an open window to assist the coding and search for the right ICD-10-CM/PCS code using the keywords. When utilizing this new platform, each field for entering codes has an auto-completion function that enables the submission of ICD-10-CM/PCS codes by just typing keywords into the field. As a consequence, it is no longer necessary to memorize all of the often-used codes, which results in the elimination of another support window. Once again, centralizing all required coding tools on one platform.

Because medical professionals are notoriously resistant to changing their routines, the adoption of new technology and techniques is constantly complicated. In this particular instance, since the new platform provided so many benefits and made the coding process easier for coders, this barrier was not seen, resulting in everyone abandoning the old excel paradigm and embracing the new platform without hesitation.

Along with the benefits previously mentioned in terms of code, the presence of a maintenance platform also adds significant value. It is useless to simplify and complete the codification in the most efficient way possible if there is no method to monitor its progression, progression that occurs since the episode is disseminated until the coding is complete. Administrative staff is thus critical, since they are responsible for distributing episodes created by coders, monitoring their progress, resolving any problems that arise, and ensuring that everything works properly.

The coders are classified by category and difficulty level, allowing for more customized episode distribution, as an orthopedic episode will not be codified by a coder who often codifies gynecological episodes. Due to the presence of the maintenance platform, this distribution of episodes by coders is simple, since basic information about the episode, such as specialty, discharge date, and module, is given. When distributing an episode, it is also possible to specify its priority as either normal or urgent, allowing for the prioritization of some episodes that need to be codified more quickly than others. The ability to quickly access the coding status of each episode makes it easier to keep track of the evolution of coding. For example, if the coders are unable to encode an episode for whatever reason, they would put it in a "pending" status until the issue is resolved by the administrative staff. Not only does this guarantee that events are not forgotten, but it also ensures that they are identified and handled quickly.

Since coding is essential to the hospital's financial sustainability, it must be done as quickly as possible. To ensure that coders are compensated fairly for their work, remuneration is based on the number of episodes coded each month and their difficulty. Once this incentive system is applied, production increases in comparison to the Excel method; nevertheless, it is essential to keep in mind that it is pointless to codify numerous episodes if they are not properly codified. To avoid this potential issue, an auditing mechanism was developed; therefore, all episodes are audited to ensure proper coding, and the episode is added to the list of episodes coded by the coder only after it has been reviewed and finished.

SWOT Analysis

A SWOT Analysis was used as a proof of concepts with the purpose of testing the viability, the utility, the quality, and the efficiency of the application. Being possible this way analyzes the strengths, weaknesses, opportunities, and threats of the application (Pereira et al., 2013).

Strengths:
- ◦ Interoperability;
- ◦ User-friendly;
- ◦ Takes into account data confidentiality;
- ◦ Decrease the human error;
- ◦ Facilitates episode distribution management to encode;
- ◦ Streamlines the coding process

Weaknesses:
- ◦ Requires internet connection.

Opportunities:
- ◦ Modernization and organizational development;
- ◦ Increasing expectation of the hospital administration to obtain methods that facilitate the hospital financing calculation;
- ◦ Provide the tool to help in the calculation of the hospital financing.

Threats:

○   Lack of acceptance to resort to new technologies by health professionals.

CONCLUSION AND FUTURE WORK

This paper presents a reliable solution for management of the coding process, so it is possible to follow all the steps that a coding episode goes through and facilitates the resolution of technical problems that may exist. For example, if an episode that is being coded has some data missing from the discharge report, the encoder will simply put it in a pending state detailing the problem encountered. Since it will appear in the pending episodes tab, it will be easily found by the administrative staff, making its resolution faster and more effective.

This tool also has the advantage of not leaving any episodes forgotten, since all episodes that are discharged are immediately loaded onto the platform.

In terms of future work, the agent that was created to guarantee the interoperability of the system with SIMH, after it is able to read all diagnostics and coded procedures, can then be adapted to be used in ETL processes so as to be later used in Data Mining processes.

REFERENCES

Alonso, V., Santos, J. V., Pinto, M., Ferreira, J., Lema, I., Lopes, F., & Freitas, A. (2019). Problems and barriers in the transition to ICD-10-CM/PCS: A qualitative study of medical coders' perceptions. *Adv. Intell. Syst. Comput.*, *932*, 72–82. doi:10.1007/978-3-030-16187-3_8

Armstrong, McDermott, Saade, & Srinivas. (2017). Coding update of the SMFM definition of low risk for cesarean delivery from ICD-9-CM to ICD-10-CM. *Am. J. Obstet. Gynecol.*, *217*(1), B2-B12.

Chok, L., Bachli, E. B., Steiger, P., Bettex, D., Cottini, S. R., Keller, E., Maggiorini, M., & Schuepbach, R. A. (2018). Effect of diagnosis related groups implementation on the intensive care unit of a Swiss tertiary hospital: A cohort study. *BMC Health Services Research*, *18*(1), 1–10. doi:10.118612913-018-2869-4 PMID:29402271

Coimbra, C., Esteves, M., Miranda, F., Portela, F., Santos, M. F., & Machado, J. (2018). Improving the Codification of Hospital Discharges with an ICD-9-CM Single-page Application and its Transition to ICD-10-CM / PCS. *International Journal on Advances in Life Sciences*, *10*(1), 23–30.

de Saúde, S. N. (n.d.). *ACSS apresenta o novo ecossistema sobre Morbilidade Hospitalar*. Available: https://www.acss.min-saude.pt/2018/06/04/acss-apresenta-o-novo-ecossistema-sobre-morbilidade-hospitalar/

García Calderón, V., Figueiras Huante, I. A., Carbajal Martínez, M., Yacaman Handal, R. E., Palami Antunez, D., Soto, M. E., & Koretzky, S. G. (2019). The impact of improving the quality of coding in the utilities of Diagnosis Related Groups system in a private healthcare institution. 14-year experience. *International Journal of Medical Informatics*, *129*(February), 248–252. doi:10.1016/j.ijmedinf.2019.06.019 PMID:31445263

Grupos de Diagnósticos Homogéneos (GDH). (n.d.). Available: http://portalcodgdh.min-saude.pt/index.php/Grupos_de_%0DDiagn%7Bó%7Dsticos_Homog%7Bé%7Dneos_(GDH)

Hernandez-Ibarburu, G., Perez-Rey, D., Alonso-Oset, E., Alonso-Calvo, R., Voets, D., Mueller, C., Claerhout, B., & Custodix, N. V. (2019). ICD-10-PCS extension with ICD-9 procedure codes to support integrated access to clinical legacy data. *International Journal of Medical Informatics*, *122*, 70–79. doi:10.1016/j.ijmedinf.2018.11.002 PMID:30623787

Lee, C., Kim, J. M., Kim, Y. S., & Shin, E. (2019). The Effect of Diagnosis-Related Groups on the Shift of Medical Services From Inpatient to Outpatient Settings: A National Claims-Based Analysis. *Asia-Pacific Journal of Public Health*, *31*(6), 499–509. doi:10.1177/1010539519872325 PMID:31516035

Lee, P. (n.d.). *Design Research: What Is It and Why Do It?* Available: https://reboot.org/2012/02/19/design-research-what-is-it-and-why-do-it/

Mills, R. E., Butler, R. R., McCullough, E. C., Bao, M. Z., & Averill, R. F. (2011). Impact of the transition to ICD-10 on medicare inpatient hospital payments. *Medicare & Medicaid Research Review*, *1*(2), 1–13. doi:10.5600/mmrr.001.02.a02 PMID:22340773

Pereira, R., Salazar, M., Abelha, A., & Machado, J. (2013). SWOT analysis of a Portuguese Electronic Health Record. *IFIP Advances in Information and Communication Technology*, *399*, 169–177. doi:10.1007/978-3-642-37437-1_14

Portalcodgh. (n.d.). Available: http://portalcodgdh.min-saude.pt/images/2/2e/CodificacaoClinica%25%0D26DesempenhoHospitalar.pdf

Schmidt, B. (2006). Proof of principle studies. *Epilepsy Research*, *68*(1), 48–52. doi:10.1016/j.eplepsyres.2005.09.019 PMID:16377153

Sergey, A. B., Alexandr, D. B., & Sergey, A. T. (2015). Proof of Concept Center— A Promising Tool for Innovative Development at Entrepreneurial Universities. *Procedia: Social and Behavioral Sciences, 166,* 240–245. doi:10.1016/j.sbspro.2014.12.518

Topaz, M., Shafran-Topaz, L., & Bowles, K. H. (2013). *ICD-9 to ICD-10: evolution, revolution, and current debates in the United States* (Vol. 10). Perspect. Health Inf. Manag.

Utter, G. H., Cox, G. L., Atolagbe, O. O., Owens, P. L., & Romano, P. S. (2018). Conversion of the Agency for Healthcare Research and Quality's Quality Indicators from ICD-9-CM to ICD-10-CM/PCS: The Process, Results, and Implications for Users. *Health Services Research, 53*(5), 3704–3727. doi:10.1111/1475-6773.12981 PMID:29846001

Vaishnavi, V., Kuechler, B., & Petter, S. (2012). *Design Science Research in Information Systems*. Academic Press.

Chapter 13
Message System to Healthcare Interoperability

Filipe Manuel Mota Miranda
Centro ALGORITMI, Universidade do Minho, Portugal

Cecilia Coimbra
Centro ALGORITMI, Universidade do Minho, Portugal

ABSTRACT

The main goal of the present case study is to infer the possibility of introducing the Apache Kafka paradigm to the exchange of healthcare information. Initially, a simple HL7 message generated in accordance with documentation was used as message origin message. Then that message should reach destination using the FHIR standard. As communication middle and handler, the Apache Kafka was implemented featuring a Confluent docker image. To map between HL7 versions, the Python language converts the original message into a JSON object. Then the Kafka API handles the socket interface between structures. Considering the charge test, the results were very positive considering a 6000-message integration under one minute and with an offset of 500 messages. Also, the systems are capable of maintaining the order of messages and recover in case of errors. So, it is possible to use Kafka to share JSON objects under FHIR standard but having in mind a prior definition of the topic, consumer, and producer configuration.

DOI: 10.4018/978-1-7998-9172-7.ch013

INTRODUCTION

In healthcare, eHealth initiatives produced transformations regarding storage, share, and reuse of data in healthcare (Digital health, 2019). Interoperability is then the capability of two or more programs/systems to exchange information over a mean and most of all understand and reuse that data to produce information (F. Rodrigues,2013).

Working in favor of interoperability for more than 30 years now, HL7 International and the purposed standards are among the most used worldwide (HL7.org, 2011). Healthcare institutions use HL7 V2, V3, or Fast Healthcare Interoperability Resources (FHIR) standards to perform all kinds of communication inside and across the organization. Some usage examples are requested patients' medical exams, retrieve administrative information, or even publish reports from previously ordered exams. The V2 is almost 30 years old and still is the most used worldwide. The FHIR most recent intends to increase semantic interoperability and reduce ambiguity. Using the best features from the previous versions, namely the Reference Information Model (RIM) a real game-changer when released on the V3 of the standard. More focused on the content, the FHIR standard opens the door open to new and innovative ways to exchange information (technical interoperability). Through the introduction of RESTful web services models to perform that job (Sousa R. et al, 2021).

As opposed to the V2 interfaces that share information using synchronous network interfaces, the old Transmission Control Protocol/Internet Protocol (TCP/IP) layer. The resultant architecture is simple, sender a receiver, and communication mean. The sender waits for a formal confirmation from the receiver indicating that the message was delivered with success or not. The so-called ACK or formal acknowledgment. Besides sockets limitation and difficult initial configurations, the existing structures are prone to errors and communication limitations. Also, the recovery from the error is very complex and perceives manual intervention.

The concept of publish/subscribe messaging system has been proliferating in the big data universe. Due to the capacity to accomplish enormous streams of data in real-time. Describes a form of communication between modules or components that are not configured with the one-to-one paradigm. The labeled information produced by the producer is shared over a common and scalable means. Then the broker delivers to the consumer ensuring the producer of the status. One of the most notorious Application Programming Interfaces (API) regarding the real-time data stream is with no doubt the Apache Kafka (Sousa, R. et al, 2021).

This case study intends to verify if it is possible to use Apache Kafka broker and adjacent concepts in the exchange of clinical information under the HL7 FHIR standard. That constitutes the main goal and the research question. Having in mind that the original message will be on HL7 V2 format and that FHIR uses JavaScript

Object Notation (JSON) format to exchange information. So, a mapping technique is necessary. That is another research question. How can we bridge between HL7 V2 and FHIR standards and at the same time maintain semantic interoperability? Dealing with clinical information implies that the system has a strong and stable communication protocol and architecture. That is another objective of the present case study. Create the architecture to modernize the way information is exchanged now in most of the healthcare facilities and at the same time maintain the levels of efficiency. Another important goal is to answer the following research question, how can we implement a system like this in FHIR when the industry uses V2 and soon will not change?

The innovation of the present case study is to introduce a big data topic (Apache Kafka) to an area that is long due to an update. Leaving the plain text sockets and Representational State Transfer (REST) endpoints and embracing an innovative way to share information. A more abstract technology (leaving the one-to-one configuration) more focused on semantic interoperability and less on the syntactic one.

The present document is organized as follows. Introduction, background explaining key concepts like big data, interoperability, HL7 and presenting at the state of the art of the respective field. Case presentation a simple section presenting main research questions and subjects that the case study should respond to. Following the results and discussion section containing the main juice of the article. To finish a brief conclusion.

BACKGROUND

Through the present section, the key topics of the case study will be detailed. At the same, a state of art will help to highlight the applicability of the fields in question.

Interoperability

Interoperability is defined by the Health Information and Management Systems Society (HIMSS) group as the ability of different information systems to access, exchange, integrate, and use data in a coordinated manner (HMS, 2019). The same organization states in the same publication "Interoperability in the Health System" that "…Health data exchange architectures, application interfaces, and standards enable data to be accessed and shared appropriately and securely across the complete spectrum of care, within all applicable settings and with relevant stakeholders, including by the individual…". Some publications define 4 others 5 or 6 interoperability levels. The most basic level is the foundation, assuring only that both systems are capable of sharing information. At the next level, structural, both systems should agree on the format syntax and organization of the information allowing field level interpretation. The semantic level intends a usage of common underlying models and data codification providing a shared understanding and meaning to the user. The last and most abstract level is organizational. Includes governance, policy, social and organizational measures to secure the communication within and between distinct organizations (F. Rodrigues, 2013). That can also be extrapolated to the continental level, like the European Commission. Through the introduction of cross-country initiatives and policies. An example of that is the eHealth initiatives and guidelines (Digital Health,2019). Worldwide organizations like HL7, SnomedCT or openEHR are dedicated to the production of internationally accepted standards featuring clinical representation, standards for data archive and exchange. Those organizations do not produce software just guidelines that Information Technology (IT) devoted to healthcare developers can and should use.

HL7 International

Founded in 1987, Health Level Seven International is an American National Standards Institute (ANSI) accredited organization dedicated to standards development. Related to exchange, integration, sharing, and retrieval of health information (HL7.org, 2011).

The first major standard from the organization was the HL7 V2. Introduced around 1980 with the objective to unify the way data was shared among heterogeneous systems. The difference in implementations was mainly caused by ad hoc message systems developed inside health care organizations that were creating gigantic islands of information}. The success of the standard was immense in such a way that to the present-day, major healthcare facilities in Portugal and around the world still use HL7 V2 based interfaces to exchange data and subsequent information (HL7.org, 2011). The major features of the standard are the simplicity, applicability, and definition of prior 80% of prior work leaving 20% of specification to be done on implementation moment (HL7.org, 2011). Figure 5 retrieved from (S. iWay, 2018) is an HL7 V2 message and is possible to perceive the simplicity and possible capabilities of the standard. The message is divided in small segments. The first line//segment represents the Message Header identifying message type and trigger event the sender system and receiver. Each of them representing a field (the smaller structure) separated by the "|" character. The second segment PID (Patient Identification) contains demographic information of the patient. Some fields are mandatory others can be omitted. Some segments can appear more than once if needed to represent the context or situation. It is important to point that a message in V2 format is order dependent (S. iWay, 2018).

The V2 simplicity is also a major drawback. Turning each implementation into a case specific one and increasing ambiguity. On top of that the standard lacks in semantic representation and lacks in consistency of the data model [20].

To circumvent that problem HL7 International presented a V3. Changing almost entirely the message paradigm and formulation. Introduced a new Extensible Markup Language (XML) format and a new way to generate messages, by constraining the so-called RIM previously developed with the intent to represent all events and scenarios in a healthcare institution. Although the learning curve for this standard was giant and at the same time the version was not compatible with the previous. Perhaps the reason why few implementations were presented to the community. One example in 2009 Bánfai et al. presented a modeling tool that encapsulates the domain-specific knowledge cleverly, as JAVA classes (Bánfai, B. et al, 2019). Shagufta et al in "Autonomous mapping of HL7 RIM and relational database schema" (Umer, S et al, 2012), purposed an automatic tool to map healthcare databases to the HL7 RIM specifications. After loading the target schema identifies the most appropriated tables and the fields using predefined rules from the Mapping Knowledge Repository.

FHIR stands for Fast Healthcare Interoperable Resources and is the most recent standard purposed by the HL7 International. Based on emerging software industry approaches and learning from the mistakes of the previous releases. Has a built-in mechanism for traceability to HL7 RIM and reducing the learning curve evident on the V3 (Bender, D., 2013). Whereas V2 has segments the FHIR has Resources. Serving as foundation bricks with a data type, common metadata, and human-readable component. Those working alone or in a group cover most use cases. The Lego (resources) building approach contra points to the V3 model that constrains the RIM. The resources are organized into models, clinical, administrative, and most important for the present study the infrastructure. That said the Message Header resource is responsible for the FHIR's V2 styled and most important to maintain the messages semantic integrity (Sousa R. et al, 2021). The Figure 1 represents a message generated following the FHIR message format. Later the message can be exchanged using RESTful web services or any other mean capable of transporting the message from system A to B. The message header encapsulates the messages enabling identification and compatibility between systems.

Figure 1. FHIR request message example retrieved from the official documentation of the standard

```
{
"resourceType": "Bundle",
"id": "10bb101f-a121-4264-a920-67be9cb82c74",
"type": "message",
"timestamp": "2015-07-14T11:15:33+10:00",
"entry":[
    {
        "fullUrl": "urn:uuid:267b18ce-3d37-4581-9baa-6fada338038b",
        "resource": {
            "resourceType": "MessageHeader",
            "id": "267b18ce-3d37-4581-9baa-6fada338038b",
            "text": {
                "status": "generated",
                "div": "<div xmlns=\"http://www.w3.org/1999/xhtml\">
                \n \n eis a request to link Patient records 654321 (Patient Donald Duck @Acme healthcare)</div>"
            },
            "eventCoding": {
                "system": "http://example.org/fhir/message-events",
                "code": "patient-link"
            },
            "source": {
                "endpoint": "http://example.org/clients/ehr-lite"
            },
            "responsible": {
                "reference": "http://acme.com/ehr/fhir/Practitioner/2323-33-4"
            },
            "focus": [
                {
                    "reference": "http://acme.com/ehr/fhir/Patient/pat1"
                },
                {
                    "reference": "http://acme.com/ehr/fhir/Patient/pat11"
                }
            ]
        }
    }
]
}
```

The FHIR approach to RESTful API as means of transportation has some differences regarding implementation to a V2 styled exchange. The message header is common to both but with different capabilities. The official documentation states that "…the REST API offers similar services (History and Subscription). On the other hand, there are differences in the capabilities offered - while a patient merge can be implemented as a series of RESTful operations performed by the client that update all resources linked to the patient, when a message command to merge patient records is processed, the server will do all the work, and is also able to merge in areas not exposed on the RESTful API. The REST API, however, provides a set of basic operations on all resources that would need special definitions in the messaging framework - definitions that are not provided…There is no expectation that RESTful systems will need to offer messaging support, or vice versa, though systems may find it useful to support both sets of functionalities to satisfy a wider range of implementers...". Reading between the lines it is not difficult to perceive that the HL7 offers RESTful implementations to modern architectures without forgetting the legacy systems (Hl7.org, 2019). That ensures a worldwide acceptance.

Sariapalle et. al presented in 2019 a prototype that uses HL7 FHIR architecture to achieve interoperability between a mobile device and an OpenEMR (online open-source healthcare database) (Saripalle, R. et al, 2019). Through a RESTful API connects a FHIR server to the client's mobile device using the JAVA HAPI open-source API for the Java programming language. The data is registered in standardized format due to the implementation of a search engine based on SNOMED CT and RXNorm Terminology. When the user submits the data, the application creates the FHIR message header and content and the messages in JSON format. Latter using the method POST the data is submitted to the server. Once on the server-side, information is inserted, retrieved, or updated on the database using the specific API. The application is in the development stage, but the results are very positive although the need for more security layers is evident. Another question is the response capability of the system if the connected users increase exponentially or the number of registries increase. A Java-based server although robust is not enough to allow a huge level of interactions and information exchange.

N. Hong et al presented in Hong, N.et al a FHIR-based EHR phenotyping framework that enables the identification of obesity based on discharge summaries supported by machine learning algorithms. The work has two major components, the conversion of discharge summaries to FHIR resources and the usage of standardized information in 4 machine learning algorithms. The paper has interesting results incorrectly classifying patients following the probability of obesity. The usage of mapping techniques can introduce semantic errors or misunderstandings. To reduce the risks, perhaps extending the system to use HL7 messages directly or SNOMED CT/ICD-10 clinical standards from the moment data are inserted on systems or even implement openEHR based forms.

To increase semantic perceptiveness of the context in each sentence perhaps a Long Short-Term Memory (LSTM) kind of recursive neural network would be a good way to go.

The FHIR standard is receiving growing interest from the scientific community. Some works are summarizing possible architectures to enable communication between mobile devices, IoT devices, and databases. One example is Ricardo J. Silva et al. "Application of HL7 FHIR for device and health information system interoperability". An interesting work that introduces a chat-bot capable of supporting patients suffering from different medical conditions. The base for information exchange is the FHIR standard serving as the background to the whole system. The author implements the system based on 3 pillars:

- Scalability based on microservices.
- Standards using FHIR.
- Conversation techniques through AIML.

It is an interesting work that approaches the HL7 information exchange to big data techniques and models (Roca, S. et al 2020).

The amount of information generated in medical contexts puts the field in big data stage. The next section will detail some big data key concepts.

BIG DATA

The world is generating data at unprecedented rates, due to technological advances and demand from applications. Collecting, storing, processing, and analyzing that, are challenges to developers and organizations around the world (Santos, M et al. 2020). Healthcare is no exception; terabits of information are generated every day making collecting data a crucial step in the big data process.

The boom of data brought to the surface the limitations of legacy systems. New and innovative solutions emerged like Hadoop distributed file system (HDFS) and computation engines (Map Reduce) for storing and processing data in batches. Both were introduced by Hadoop. Although two problems arise. First, the data needs to be in multiple systems at the same time and multiple pipelines are not an option and feed a copy of every file from Hadoop is not practical or cost-wise. The solution is a pub-sub system capable of store high volume data in hardware and allows that to be consumed multiple times. The data is persisted to disk allowing real-time and batch consumers at the same time without performance degradation. The next section will highlight Apache Kafka (Sousa R. et al, 2021) a distributed system publish/subsystem.

Publish/Subscribe Messaging Paradigm

Apache Kafka is a streaming distributed platform with three core capabilities (Garg, N., 2013):

- Publish and subscribe streams of records, like a messaging system.
- Store streams in fault-tolerant fashion.
- Process streams in real-time.

The Kafka can run as a cluster on multiple servers, storing the streams of records in categories called topics. Each record with a key, a value, and a timestamp. Figure

2 introduces the main concepts of the Apache Kafka architecture. The four key APIs that need to be implemented are:

- The producer that publishes the streams to one or more topics.
- The consumer that subscribes to one or more topics and has the responsibility to process the stream afterward.
- The broker API that stores and transforms an incoming stream into an output one. It is a stateless process that is capable of handle hundreds of thousands of reads and writes per second and TB of messages without performance impact.

Figure 2. Apache Kafka Architecture. Retrieved from Garg, N., 2013.

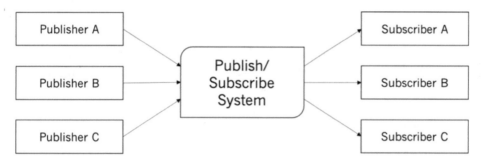

The Connector API allows building and running reusable producers or consumers that connect Kafka to real-world applications.

The communication is done with a high-performance TCP protocol. Whereas other systems only can queue the sending files. The publish-subscribe Kafka has the capability to perform both and serve as a storage system at the same time. Being a stateless system needs a mechanism to persist information. The Zookeeper is used for managing and coordinating the brokers. Notifying producers and consumers about new or failures on the broker mechanism. Besides information also handles the preparation for a new connection.

Healthcare-related in 2019 Valentina Baljak and colleagues presented a work reporting the implementation of a scalable real-time pipeline and storage architecture for physiological data monitoring. The Kafka enables the pipeline of data from raw data collected into the file system and a relational database. The work is promising but the absence of standardized data is worth notice. With HL7 V2 or even FHIR as standard, a lot of future work would have been avoided (Baljak, V. et al., 2018).

In 2019, Olivier Debauche et al in Debauche, O. et al., 2019 purposed a cloud-based monitoring system based on wireless sensors a gateway, and a Lambda cloud architecture for data processing and storage. Uses the Apache Kafka as middleware before Hadoop File System. Although not using HL7 for internal information exchange uses the HL7 FHIR HAPI Java library to perform information exports to another system.

As seen through the course of the present section much can be said regarding the interoperability international standards and big data solutions. Although interesting not all the works can reunite semantic and technical interoperability and perform with high capability.

CASE STUDY PRESENTATION

The present section intends to make a brief presentation of the case study. As stated, until the moment interoperability and HL7 International are evolving. Moving to modern approaches and implementations. Although using RESTful web services to exchange information in the most recent version FHIR most healthcare institutions still use the 30-year-old V2 version of standard with the plain text and old sockets. In accordance with [21] provides a one-size fits all approach that does not reflect the modern standards and technologies.

Generating every day enormous amounts of information is the ideal scenario/opportunity for the implementation of big data technology. The case study intends to answer the following questions:

1. Which are the main topics of HL7 FHIR standard and in which way it contributes to the increase of semantic interoperability?
2. How can Apache Kafka exchange HL7 FHIR based messages consider the protocols and case-specific adaptations?
3. How can HL7 FHIR replace the V2?
4. How to operate Apache Kafka to exchange information considering the healthcare scenarios and experiences?
5. How to handle formal acknowledgments (ACK) with Apache Kafka?
6. Which are the lessons learned and steps necessary to evolve from HL7 V2 to FHIR?

So, in order to answer the questions an architecture needs to be created in the first place. From that a protocol for communication designed that already involves the topics for the Apache Kafka broker. The conversion from HL7 V2 to FHIR is of extreme importance. Next the creation of consumer, producer and broker created and configured. Through the process a simple load test from the consumer side. A simple error recuperation test to perceive the capabilities on that front and finally a list of lessons learned for the future can be constructed.

The next section will present the developed system at the architectural level.

RESULTS

Architecture

Considering the actual context inside healthcare organizations and increased interest in semantic interoperability is urgent to update the way information is exchanged. At the moment HL7 V2 is more focused on syntactic interoperability, focused on the success or failure of the message to reach the destination. But nowadays semantic context is vital. Only FHIR can solve that problem at the moment. The present section focuses on the results achieved during the case study mainly the architecture and flow of events. System capacity and capability and finally some considerations when implementing a system like this more robust in the future.

Almost every system installed in healthcare organizations uses HL7 V2 message interfaces through TCP/IP connections. The new system must ensure communication under HL7 V2 and FHIR formats. The figure 3 presents the implemented architecture still in test local tests.

Figure 3. Proposed Architecture

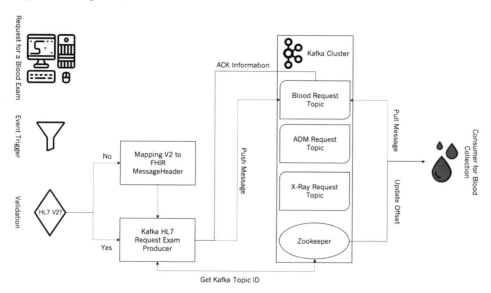

The trigger event, in this specific case a request. Starts a process in which a file is generated or in the case of FHIR standard a message is developed under the hood. If the message is already in JSON format can advance to the next stage, otherwise, the Mapping service will encapsulate the message under a Message Header and convert it to JSON. From that moment on the message is ready for the pushing stage. Through the connection, the specific producer for that kind of request asks the ZooKeeper for the TOPICID and sends the message. At this moment the Kafka broker stamps the message with an internal id, a timestamp, and metadata information and stores the message. The consumer pulls messages and takes the subscribed ones. All the systems were implemented using Python 3.6 for producer and consumer, Python FHIR open-source library, and Apache Kafka Clean open-source distribution. Running under a Linux Distro Machine on an Asus machine with 6 GB of Ram and an Intel Core I7 internal processor. Automatically the Kafka environment is responsible for acknowledging the producer if the message was delivered or not but only if the consumer says so.

Figure 4. Communication protocol between Kafka API

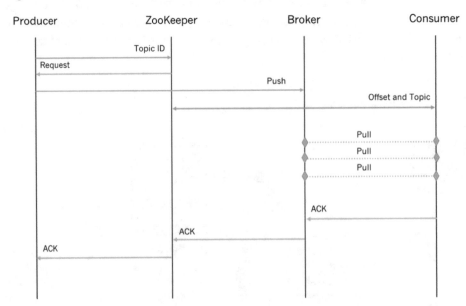

Figure 4 present the protocol communication implemented on the test system. Of course, the pull request marked as a dotted line represents constant pull information from the consumer for new messages. The broker also saves the message and logs enabling a backward search if necessary.

MAPPING TECHNIQUES

From the HL7 V2 to the FHIR standard a lot has evolved in From the HL7 V2 to the FHIR standard a lot has evolved in the semantic field. The late one has resources that the former simply can reach. So, as the purpose of the present study is ensuring that is possible to communicate HL7 messages using Kafka and big data techniques the mapping technique will be a little simplistic. A simple conversion from "|" to JSON will provide the tools needed for proof of concept. FHIR message for a simple observation contains the Message Header resource, the observation, the patient information, and the provider/ performer. All these in a simple JSON structure. Some maps are easy, a one to one from the message header (MSH) segment and OBX but the same does not happen to patient information which has no direct mapping. The PID segment from the V2 message gives a unique id and some information is used to retrieve information from a possible patient information RESTful service.

Table 1. Mapping between MSH (MessageHeader) and OBX (Observations)

Element	V2 Segment	Description
Identifier	MSH-10	Message/Control ID
Timestamp	MSH-7	Message/Date-Time
Event	MSH-9.2	Observation-provide Derived from the second component of the Message Type
Souce.name	MSH-3	Sending application name
Souce.software	MSH-3	Sending application name
Source.endpoint	MSH-24	Sending network address
Destination.name	MSH-5	Receiving application
Destination.endpoint	MSH-25	Receiving network address
valueString	OBX-5	Holds the actual value of the observation
	OBX-11	Observation result status

That is a simple mapping technique based on Python's capability to parse and generate JSON format objects. It is a simple conversion based on the prior established segment position of the original message. Off course some other techniques could be implemented. Table 1 features the result from the previously detailed mapping technique.

Information Exchange

The first result that highlights implemented work is the HL7 V2 message converter into a JSON structure, Figure 5 represents the original V2 message and Figure 6 shows the final mapped message passed through the Apache Kafka.

Figure 5. HL7 version 2 file for PID from patient. The input of the new system.

```
MSH|^~\&|EPICADT|DH|RADADT|DH|202001010915||ADT^A01|MSG000001|P|2.3
PID|||MRN12345^5^M11||Doe^Jane||19780101|F||C|||||||||123456789||
```

Figure 6. HL7 FHIR mapping result for patient identification

```
{
    "birthDate": "19780101",
    "date": "19780101",
    "gender": "F",
    "identifier": [
        {
            "type": {
                "coding": [
                    {
                        "code": "MR",
                        "system": "http://hl7.org/fhir/v2/0203"
                    }
                ]
            },
        }
    ],
    "name": {
        "family": [
            "Doe"
        ],
        "given": [
            "Jane"
        ],
        "text": [
            "Doe^Jane"
        ]
    },
    "resourceType": "Patient",
    "ssn":"123456789"
}
```

The other results that deserve highlight are the ones related to publisher and subscribers. The Kafka Confluent docker distribution has a high-level localhost dashboard. That is accessible during software running. And gives run time information from topics producers and consumers. The next figures were retrieved from the dashboard and represent the implemented solution. Figure 7 represents the topic WISE2. Important information regarding partitions, the message with a specific timestamp, and affiliated partition. Finally, the offset where the message stands.

Figure 7. Apache Kafka Confluent control center. List of topics

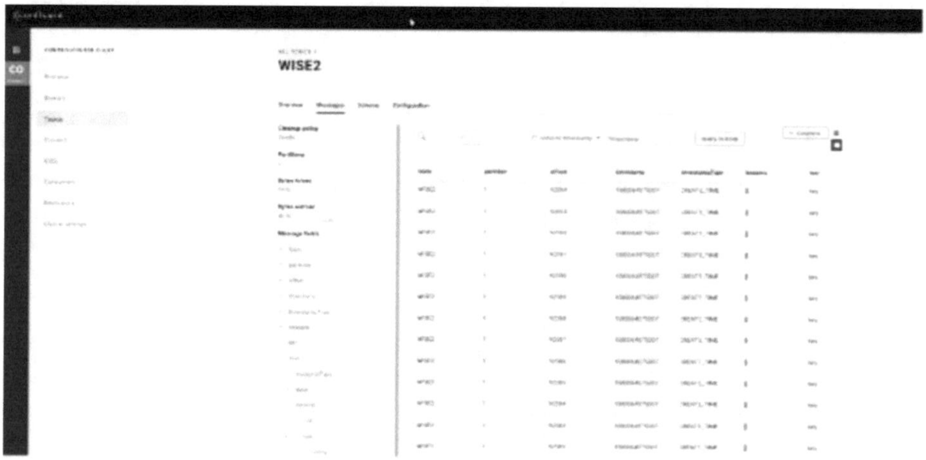

Figure 8. WISE topic specific metrics

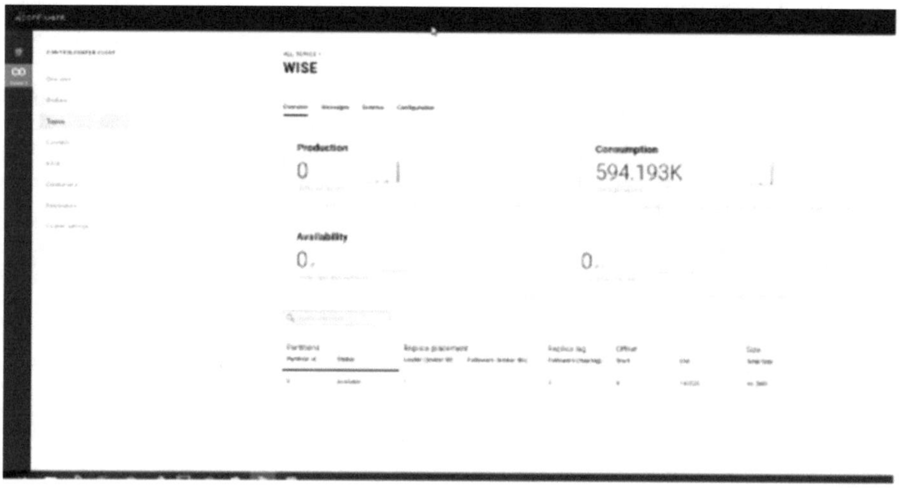

Figure 8 demonstrates central information for a specific topic. It is important to notice that it was retrieved after a breakdown test where some messages were left on the queue and consumed after that for the newly created consumers. This proves that the broker works and most important can maintain order and consistency after occurring an error. Inside healthcare facilities, the order and the correct sequence of data are extremely important.

Figure 9. Cluster Control Center metrics

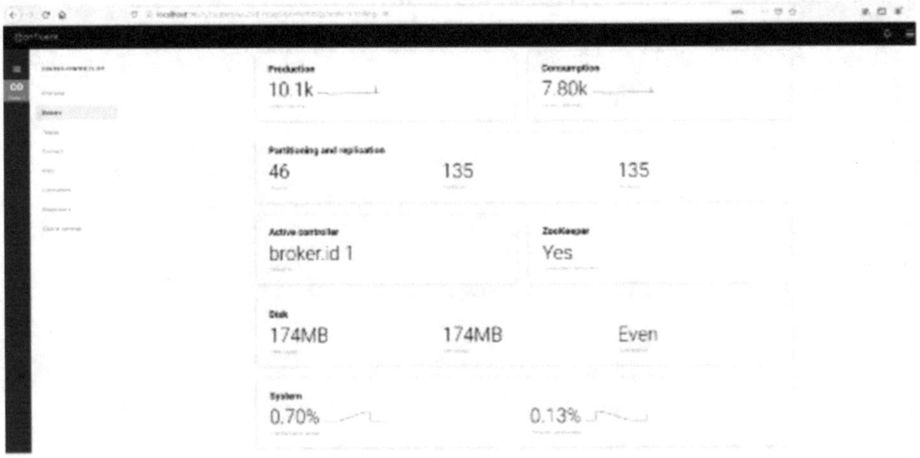

Figure 9 represents a normal broker working regarding production and consumption as well as disk space used on the process.

And finally, a brief table, Table 2, contains the information on the number of messages that a single broker and consumer are capable of handling. Using a test environment of course.

Table 2. Number of massages that brokers and consumers are capable of handling

Producer	1 Consumer	2 Consumers
6000 Messages	1:42 min	1 min
12000 Messages	3:31 min	1:38 min

On a first try, a set of 6000 was created using a while cycle on the producer size, that is converted handled and consumed by two consumer simulating to destination applications. After that, a set of 12000 messages and consumed.

LESSONS LEARNED

It is important to notice that this is a new approach to the healthcare scenario. That said it is important to retain some points for future implementations. Points to consider and look for:

- Python is the most versatile programming language and ideal for this kind of implementation. Once is capable of paring V2 messages, map to FHIR and has plugins for Apache Kafka diverse scenarios.
- How topics are organized will influence the communication protocol and all the structures to be constructed.
- It is of most importance to evolve the mapping logic to handle legacy implementations.
- The acknowledgment component will need work on the producer side once the consumer does not contact directly to the consumer.
- Instead of deciding the port number and handling IP the configuration on this case is more simple and even easier to update.
- The zookeeper and broker are extremely important and are central pieces of the system architecture.
- The important communication protocol is not very important under the Apache Kafka although extremely important with legacy architectures.
- The Apache Kafka introduction will perceive a reformulation of the legacy servers and infrastructures.

The next section will feature the discussion of the results.

DISCUSSION

The results attest that is possible to implement a big data solution to the exchange of information in a healthcare environment. More important with major impact time consumption and interface configuration. While an interface using the protocol TCP/IP needs port configuration the present one only needs a broker configuration. The presented solution is distribution-free whereas some interface systems like Iguana or Mirth are paid. The main topics under consideration when applying Kafka to

HL7 is the capability of the consumer to provide the producer with an HL7 ACK response. It is important to note that ACK messages are an important point to the standard once represent the proof that the message arrived and was integrated into the destination. In Kafka extra configuration must be done to ensure that integration to the producer. Disabling the automatic acknowledgment and adding that responsibility to the consumer base code is a possible solution that needs exploration.

Another point is the auto-retry facet. If the producer does not receive an ACK retries, but in healthcare, that scenario needs to be used wisely. If configured poorly the system could end up sending replicated information that in healthcare is not acceptable. Imagining requesting the same exam two times for the same patient at the same moment.

Sequential messages are also possible in Kafka. That is a scenario that happens a lot on the HL7 V2 once some observation results end up being a set of messages.

The Python language was a wise choice although the capabilities of the FHIR parser are limited. The JAVA HAPI library is of course more complete. A JAVA Kafka connector is also available. So, JAVA programming language is also a possibility. In the end, it is possible to approach the consumer/producer to implement the system with a more complex Multi-Agent System. Once both APIs is extended to perform work out of the initial Scopus. From Table2 is possible to perceive that Kafka producers and consumers can send huge amounts of information in a small machine with small messages. The results were accomplished in a laboratory scenario with a small JSON structure. The case where 12000 were produced and consumed is interesting to watch that producer 2 took less time to consume then consumer 1 (2x times more) perhaps some partition related block was the cause for the problem.

The architecture implemented is very simple and straight forward although can generate logs and save the exchanged messages due to the Kafka Big Data correlation. With that said machine learning and monitoring, techniques have an interesting opportunity. As figures 7, 8, and 9 state Kafka Confluent distribution offer a localhost dashboard that logs the entire operation for all the topics. The main idea is replacing the current sender and receiver ends of the v2 with topics, the producer and consumer will be case-specific to reduce the mapping Scopus from version 2 to FHIR. The mapping techniques are simple, and much more could be done. The semantic component of the FHIR is much deeper than the one on the V2. So, every scenario where actually V2 messages are exchanged needs to be carefully analyzed to perceive the simple maps and where other API is necessary to complete the information.

CONCLUSION

The present case study reports the initial steps of introducing an Apache Kafka message system to exchange healthcare information under HL7 FHIR format. To account for that the case study detailed the creation of the architecture that will be necessary, the message protocol for communication, and finally a simple implementation and load test. The load test is very simple and was introduced to validate our approach and solution capacity to sustain loads, maintain order and recover from mistakes.

It is also important to note that this represents an innovation in the actual scenario and is capable of bringing the message exchange inside and organization into a new level of organization, methodology, and capacity. This represents a leap forward in terms of load capacity. Managements of message order and error and perhaps the most important the paradigm in which messages are exchanged. Leaving a traditional one to one configuration and moving a one to many and using a broker to handle the details and specific implementation. Besides, that leaves the consumer and producer to be more modular and configurable to each case. For example, introducing mapping techniques specific to a broker job.

In conclusion is possible to use big data tools and architectures to exchange information in healthcare scenarios. The Apache Kafka is a very capable and interesting tool. The API makes the implementation very straightforward. The discussion section highlighted the main concerns and points. Following the present paper, the work will focus on ACK's detailed messages and messages in sequence. At the same time focusing on machine learning and monitoring based on collected logs. More important is the capacity to exchange information securely and cleanly without losing any data on the way. The V2 standard will be on healthcare facilities for many years so the new systems must ensure legacy compatibility. The case study presented here proved that is possible to think out of the box and maintaining the old systems working.

REFERENCES

Baljak, V., Ljubovic, A., Michel, J., Montgomery, M., & Salaway, R. (2018). A scalable realtime analytics pipeline and storage architecture for physiological monitoring big data. *Smart Health*, *9*, 275–286.

Bánfai, B., Ulrich, B., Török, Z., Natarajan, R., & Ireland, T. (2009). Implementing an HL7 version 3 modeling tool from an Ecore model. In *Medical Informatics in a United and Healthy Europe* (pp. 157–161). IOS Press.

Bender, D., & Sartipi, K. (2013, June). HL7 FHIR: An Agile and RESTful approach to healthcare information exchange. In *Proceedings of the 26th IEEE international symposium on computer-based medical systems* (pp. 326-331). IEEE.

Debauche, O., Mahmoudi, S., Manneback, P., & Assila, A. (2019). Fog IoT for Health: A new Architecture for Patients and Elderly Monitoring. *Procedia Computer Science*, *160*, 289–297.

Digital health. (2019, October 10). Retrieved December 29, 2019, from https://www.who.int/health-topics/digital-health

Garg, N. (2013). *Apache Kafka*. Packt Publishing.

HL7.org. (2011). *Health Level Seven*. The Worldwide Leader in Interoperability Standards.

HL7.org. (2019, September 1). *FHIR Overview*. Hl7 FHIR. Retrieved January 1, 2020, from https://www.hl7.org/fhir/overview.html

Hl7.org. (2019). *MessageHeader - FHIR v4.0.1*. Retrieved January 1, 2020, from https://www.hl7.org/fhir/messageheader.html

HMS. (2019). *Interoperability in Healthcare*. HIMSS - Interoperability in Healthcare. Retrieved December 29, 2019, from https://www.himss.org/resources/interoperability-healthcare

Hong, N., Wen, A., Stone, D. J., Tsuji, S., Kingsbury, P. R., Rasmussen, L. V., ... Jiang, G. (2019). Developing a FHIR-based EHR phenotyping framework: A case study for identification of patients with obesity and multiple comorbidities from discharge summaries. *Journal of Biomedical Informatics*, *99*, 103310.

iWay. (2018). *Introducing the iWay Integration Solution for EDIHL7*. Retrieved January 1, 2020, from https://iwayinfocenter.informationbuilders.com/TLs/TL_soa_ebiz_hl7/source/hl7_01intro11.htm

Roca, S., Sancho, J., García, J., & Alesanco, Á. (2020). Microservice chatbot architecture for chronic patient support. *Journal of Biomedical Informatics*, *102*, 103305.

Rodrigues. (2013). *Interoperabilidade na Saúde - Onde Estamos?* Academic Press.

Santos, M. Y., & Costa, C. (2020). *Big data: concepts, warehousing, and analytics*. River Publishers.

Saripalle, R., Runyan, C., & Russell, M. (2019). Using HL7 FHIR to achieve interoperability in patient health record. *Journal of Biomedical Informatics*, *94*, 103188.

Sousa, R., Miranda, R., Moreira, A., Alves, C., Lori, N., & Machado, J. (2021). Software Tools for Conducting Real-Time Information Processing and Visualization in Industry: An Up-to-Date Review. *Applied Sciences (Basel, Switzerland)*, *11*(11), 4800. doi:10.3390/app11114800

Umer, S., Afzal, M., Hussain, M., Latif, K., & Ahmad, H. F. (2012). Autonomous mapping of HL7 RIM and relational database schema. *Information Systems Frontiers*, *14*(1), 5–18.

Compilation of References

Aabed, K., & Lashin, M. M. (2021). An analytical study of the factors that influence COVID-19 spread. *Saudi Journal of Biological Sciences*, *28*(2), 1177–1195. doi:10.1016/j.sjbs.2020.11.067 PMID:33262677

Acharya, U. R., Fujita, H., Lih, O. S., Adam, M., Tan, J. H., & Chua, C. K. (2017). Automated detection of coronary artery disease using different durations of ECG segments with convolutional neural network. *Knowledge-Based Systems*, *132*, 62–71.

Acharya, U. R., Fujita, H., Oh, S. L., Raghavendra, U., Tan, J. H., Adam, M., ... Hagiwara, Y. (2018). Automated identification of shockable and non-shockable life-threatening ventricular arrhythmias using convolutional neural network. *Future Generation Computer Systems*, *79*, 952–959.

Acharya, U. R., Oh, S. L., Hagiwara, Y., Tan, J. H., Adam, M., Gertych, A., & San Tan, R. (2017). A deep convolutional neural network model to classify heartbeats. *Computers in Biology and Medicine*, *89*, 389–396.

Adler-milstein, J., & Pfeifer, E. (2017). Information blocking: Is it occurring and what policy strategies can address it? *The Milbank Quarterly*, *95*(1), 117–135. doi:10.1111/1468-0009.12247 PMID:28266065

Ahad, M. A., Paiva, S., & Zafar, S. (Eds.). (2021). *Sustainable and Energy Efficient Computing Paradigms for Society*. EAI/Springer Innovations in Communication and Computing. doi:10.1007/978-3-030-51070-1

Ahmad, S., Ullah, A., Shah, K., Salahshour, S., Ahmadian, A., & Ciano, T. (2020). Fuzzy fractional-order model of the novel coronavirus. *Advances in Difference Equations*, *2020*(1), 1–17. doi:10.118613662-020-02934-0 PMID:32922446

Ahmed, S., & Alhumam, A. (2021). Analyzing the Implications of COVID-19 Pandemic: Saudi Arabian Perspective. *Intelligent Automation and Soft Computing*, *27*(3), 835–851. doi:10.32604/iasc.2021.015789

Al Rahhal, M. M., Bazi, Y., AlHichri, H., Alajlan, N., Melgani, F., & Yager, R. R. (2016). Deep learning approach for active classification of electrocardiogram signals. *Information Sciences*, *345*, 340–354.

Compilation of References

Alderremy, A. A., Gómez-Aguilar, J. F., Aly, S., & Saad, K. M. (2021). A fuzzy fractional model of coronavirus (COVID-19) and its study with Legendre spectral method. *Results in Physics*, *21*, 103773. doi:10.1016/j.rinp.2020.103773 PMID:33391986

Alkan, N., & Kahraman, C. (2021). Evaluation of government strategies against COVID-19 pandemic using q-rung orthopair fuzzy TOPSIS method. *Applied Soft Computing*, *110*, 107653. doi:10.1016/j.asoc.2021.107653 PMID:34226821

Alkhammash, H. I., Otaibi, S. A., & Ullah, N. (2021). Short-and long-term predictions of novel corona virus using mathematical modeling and artificial intelligence methods. *International Journal of Modeling, Simulation, and Scientific Computing*, 2150028.

Alonso, V., Santos, J. V., Pinto, M., Ferreira, J., Lema, I., Lopes, F., & Freitas, A. (2019). Problems and barriers in the transition to ICD-10-CM/PCS: A qualitative study of medical coders' perceptions. *Adv. Intell. Syst. Comput.*, *932*, 72–82. doi:10.1007/978-3-030-16187-3_8

Alqahtani, H., Kavakli-Thorne, M., & Kumar, G. (2019). Applications of Generative Adversarial Networks (GANs): An Updated Review. *Archives of Computational Methods in Engineering*. Advance online publication. doi:10.100711831-019-09388-y

Alqahtani, M., Gumaei, A., Mathkour, H., & Maher Ben Ismail, M. (2019). A genetic-based extreme gradient boosting model for detecting intrusions in wireless sensor networks. *Sensors (Basel)*, *19*(20), 4383. doi:10.339019204383 PMID:31658774

Al-Qaness, M. A., Ewees, A. A., Fan, H., & Abd El Aziz, M. (2020a). Optimization method for forecasting confirmed cases of COVID-19 in China. *Journal of Clinical Medicine*, *9*(3), 674. doi:10.3390/jcm9030674 PMID:32131537

Al-Qaness, M. A., Ewees, A. A., Fan, H., Abualigah, L., & Abd Elaziz, M. (2020b). Marine predators algorithm for forecasting confirmed cases of COVID-19 in Italy, USA, Iran and Korea. *International Journal of Environmental Research and Public Health*, *17*(10), 3520. doi:10.3390/ijerph17103520 PMID:32443476

Al-Qaness, M. A., Saba, A. I., Elsheikh, A. H., Abd Elaziz, M., Ibrahim, R. A., Lu, S., ... Ewees, A. A. (2021). Efficient artificial intelligence forecasting models for COVID-19 outbreak in Russia and Brazil. *Process Safety and Environmental Protection*, *149*, 399–409. doi:10.1016/j.psep.2020.11.007 PMID:33204052

Alsayed, A., Sadir, H., Kamil, R., & Sari, H. (2020). Prediction of epidemic peak and infected cases for COVID-19 disease in Malaysia, 2020. *International Journal of Environmental Research and Public Health*, *17*(11), 4076. doi:10.3390/ijerph17114076 PMID:32521641

Altan, G., Kutlu, Y., & Allahverdi, N. (2016). A multistage deep belief networks application on arrhythmia classification. *International Journal of Intelligent Systems and Applications in Engineering*, 222-228.

Ammar, S., & Wright, R. (2000). Applying fuzzy-set theory to performance evaluation. *Socio-Economic Planning Sciences*, *34*(4), 285–302. doi:10.1016/S0038-0121(00)00004-5

Ammenwerth, E., Gräber, S., Herrmann, G., Bürkle, T., & König, J. (2003). Evaluation of health information systems - Problems and challenges. *International Journal of Medical Informatics*, *71*(2–3), 125–135. doi:10.1016/S1386-5056(03)00131-X PMID:14519405

Andersen, R. S., Peimankar, A., & Puthusserypady, S. (2019). A deep learning approach for real-time detection of atrial fibrillation. *Expert Systems with Applications*, *115*, 465–473.

Anter, A. M., Oliva, D., Thakare, A., & Zhang, Z. (2021). AFCM-LSMA: New intelligent model based on Lévy slime mould algorithm and adaptive fuzzy C-means for identification of COVID-19 infection from chest X-ray images. *Advanced Engineering Informatics*, *49*, 101317. doi:10.1016/j.aei.2021.101317

Apache Kafka Documentation. (n.d.). *Apache Kafka*. http://kafka.apache.org/090/documentation. html#intro_topics

Apache Kafka. (n.d.). https://kafka.apache.org/

Araújo, I. (2005). Family Roles Assessment Scale: Assessment of Psychometric Properties. *Journal of Nursing Reference*, *IV*(4), 51–59.

Ardabili, S. F., Mosavi, A., Ghamisi, P., Ferdinand, F., Varkonyi-Koczy, A. R., Reuter, U., Rabczuk, T., & Atkinson, P. M. (2020). Covid-19 outbreak prediction with machine learning. *Algorithms*, *13*(10), 249. doi:10.3390/a13100249

Arjovsky, M., Chintala, S., & Bottou, L. (2017). *Wasserstein GAN*. https://arxiv.org/abs/1701.07875

Armstrong, McDermott, Saade, & Srinivas. (2017). Coding update of the SMFM definition of low risk for cesarean delivery from ICD-9-CM to ICD-10-CM. *Am. J. Obstet. Gynecol.*, *217*(1), B2-B12.

Asadi, S., Nilashi, M., Abumalloh, R. A., Samad, S., Ahani, A., Ghabban, F., ... Supriyanto, E. (2021). Evaluation of Factors to Respond to the COVID-19 Pandemic Using DEMATEL and Fuzzy Rule-Based Techniques. *International Journal of Fuzzy Systems*, 1–17.

Auffray, C., Charron, D., & Hood, L. (2010). Predictive, preventive, personalized and participatory medicine: Back to the future. *Genome Medicine*, *2*(8), 1–3. doi:10.1186/gm178 PMID:20804580

Azziz, R., Carmina, E., Dewailly, D., Diamanti-Kandarakis, E., Escobar-Morreale, H. F., Futterweit, W., Janssen, O. E., Legro, R. S., Norman, R. J., Taylor, A. E., & Witchel, S. F. (2009). The Androgen Excess and PCOS Society criteria for the polycystic ovary syndrome: The complete task force report. *Fertility and Sterility*, *91*(2), 456–488. doi:10.1016/j.fertnstert.2008.06.035 PMID:18950759

Babylon Health. (2013). *About*. Babylon Health. https://www.babylonhealth.com/about/

Balen, A., & Rajkowha, M. (2003). Polycystic ovary syndrome—A systemic disorder? *Best Practice & Research. Clinical Obstetrics & Gynaecology*, *17*(2), 263–274. doi:10.1016/S1521-6934(02)00119-0 PMID:12758099

Baljak, V., Ljubovic, A., Michel, J., Montgomery, M., & Salaway, R. (2018). A scalable realtime analytics pipeline and storage architecture for physiological monitoring big data. *Smart Health*, *9*, 275–286.

Banerjee, S., & Singh, G. K. (2021). A new approach of ECG steganography and prediction using deep learning. *Biomedical Signal Processing and Control*, *64*, 102151.

Bánfai, B., Ulrich, B., Török, Z., Natarajan, R., & Ireland, T. (2009). Implementing an HL7 version 3 modeling tool from an Ecore model. In *Medical Informatics in a United and Healthy Europe* (pp. 157–161). IOS Press.

Barbarito, F., Pinciroli, F., Mason, J., Marceglia, S., Mazzola, L., & Bonacina, S. (2012). Implementing standards for the interoperability among healthcare providers in the public regionalized Healthcare Information System of the Lombardy Region. *Journal of Biomedical Informatics*, *45*(4), 736–745. doi:10.1016/j.jbi.2012.01.006 PMID:22285983

Barrière, D. A., Magalhães, R., Novais, A., Marques, P., Selingue, E., Geffroy, F., Marques, F., Cerqueira, J., Sousa, J. C., Boumezbeur, F., Bottlaender, M., Jay, T. M., Cachia, A., Sousa, N., & Mériaux, S. (2019). The SIGMA rat brain templates and atlases for multimodal MRI data analysis and visualization. *Nature Communications*, *2019*(1), 1–13. doi:10.103841467-019-13575-7 PMID:31836716

Bartz, C. (2010). International Council of Nurses and person-centered care. *International Journal of Integrated Care*, *10*(5), 24–26. doi:10.5334/ijic.480 PMID:20228907

Bates, D. W., Saria, S., Ohno-Machado, L., Shah, A., & Escobar, G. (2014). Big data in health care: Using analytics to identify and manage high-risk and high-cost patients. *Health Affairs*, *33*(7), 1123–1131. doi:10.1377/hlthaff.2014.0041 PMID:25006137

Baumgartner, C. F., Koch, L. M., Tezcan, K. C., Ang, J. X., & Konukoglu, E. (2018). Visual Feature Attribution Using Wasserstein GANs. *Proceedings of the IEEE Computer Society Conference on Computer Vision and Pattern Recognition*, 8309–8319. 10.1109/CVPR.2018.00867

Baz, A., & Alhakami, H. (2021). Fuzzy based decision making approach for evaluating the severity of COVID-19 pandemic in cities of kingdom of saudi arabia. *Computers, Materials, & Continua*, 1155-1174.

Beaver, K. (2002). *Healthcare Information Systems*. CRC Press. doi:10.1201/9781420031409

Behnood, A., Golafshani, E. M., & Hosseini, S. M. (2020). Determinants of the infection rate of the COVID-19 in the US using ANFIS and virus optimization algorithm (VOA). *Chaos, Solitons, and Fractals*, *139*, 110051. doi:10.1016/j.chaos.2020.110051 PMID:32834605

Belle, A., Thiagarajan, R., Soroushmehr, S. M., Navidi, F., Beard, D. A., & Najarian, K. (2015). Big data analytics in healthcare. *BioMed Research International*. PMID:26229957

Bender, D., & Sartipi, K. (2013, June). HL7 FHIR: An Agile and RESTful approach to healthcare information exchange. In *Proceedings of the 26th IEEE international symposium on computer-based medical systems* (pp. 326-331). IEEE.

Bengio, Y., & LeCun, Y. (2007). Scaling learning algorithms towards AI. *Large-Scale Kernel Machines, 34*(5), 1-41.

Bergstra, J., Bastien, F., Breuleux, O., Lamblin, P., Pascanu, R., Delalleau, O., & Bengio, Y. (2011). Theano: Deep learning on gpus with python. In *NIPS 2011, BigLearning Workshop, Granada, Spain* (Vol. 3, pp. 1–48). Citeseer.

Bernstam, E. V., Hersh, W. R., Sim, I., Eichmann, D., Silverstein, J. C., Smith, J. W., & Becich, M. J. (2010). Unintended consequences of health information technology: A need for biomedical informatics. *Journal of Biomedical Informatics, 43*(5), 828–830. doi:10.1016/j.jbi.2009.05.009 PMID:19508898

Best Free Mobile Apps for Pharmacists. (2021, March 5). *Pharmacy Times*. Retrieved 2021, from https://www.pharmacytimes.com/view/best-free-mobile-apps-for-pharmacists

Bhatia, M., & Sood, S. K. (2016). Temporal Informative Analysis in Smart-ICU Monitoring: M-HealthCare Perspective. *Journal of Medical Systems, 40*(8), 190. Advance online publication. doi:10.100710916-016-0547-9 PMID:27388507

Bhatt, H., Mehta, S., & D'mello, L. R. (2015). Use of ID3 decision tree algorithm for placement prediction. *International Journal of Computer Science and Information Technologies, 6*(5), 4785–4789.

Bindha, P. G., Rajalaxmi, R. R., & Poorani, S. (2019). *Predicting the Presence of Poly Cystic Ovarian Syndrome using Classification Techniques*. Academic Press.

Black, M. (1961). *The Social Theories of Talcott Parsons: A Critical Examination*. Prentice Hall.

Blackstone, E. A., Fuhr, J. P. Jr, & Pociask, S. (2014). The health and economic effects of counterfeit drugs. *American Health & Drug Benefits, 7*(4), 216–224. PMID:25126373

Blumrosen, G., Avisdris, N., Kupfer, R., & Rubinsky, B. (2011). C-SMART: Efficient Seamless Cellular Phone Based Patient Monitoring System. *IEEE Int. Symp. on a World of Wireless, Mobile and Multimedia Networks*. 10.1109/WoWMoM.2011.5986191

Bocek, T., Rodrigues, B. B., Strasser, T., & Stiller, B. (2017). Blockchains everywhere - a use-case of blockchains in the pharma supply-chain. *2017 IFIP/IEEE Symposium on Integrated Network and Service Management (IM)*. https://doi:10.23919/inm.2017.7987376

Borji, A. (2021). *Pros and Cons of GAN Evaluation Measures: New Developments*. https://arxiv.org/abs/2103.09396

Borji, A. (2019). Pros and cons of GAN evaluation measures. *Computer Vision and Image Understanding, 179*, 41–65. doi:10.1016/j.cviu.2018.10.009

Bose, S. (2018). A comparative study: Java vs Kotlin programming in Android application development. *International Journal of Advanced Research in Computer Science, 9*(3), 41–45. https://doi.org/10.26483/ijarcs.v9i3.5978

Bouwmans, T., Javed, S., Sultana, M., & Jung, S. K. (2019). Deep neural network concepts for background subtraction: A systematic review and comparative evaluation. *Neural Networks*, *117*, 8–66.

Braga, A., Portela, F., Santos, M. F., Abelha, A., Machado, J., Silva, Á., & Rua, F. (2016). Data mining to predict the use of vasopressors in intensive medicine patients. *Jurnal Teknologi*, *78*(6–7), 1–6. doi:10.11113/jt.v78.9075

Braga, A., Portela, F., Santos, M. F., Machado, J., Abelha, A., Silva, Á., & Rua, F. (2015). Step Towards a Patient Timeline in Intensive Care Units. *Procedia Computer Science*, *64*, 618–625. doi:10.1016/j.procs.2015.08.575

Burr, V. (1998). *Gender and Social Psychology*. Routledge.

Çakıt, E., & Karwowski, W. (2017). Predicting the occurrence of adverse events using an adaptive neuro-fuzzy inference system (ANFIS) approach with the help of ANFIS input selection. *Artificial Intelligence Review*, *48*(2), 139–155. doi:10.100710462-016-9497-3

Çakıt, E., & Karwowski, W. (2017b). Estimating electromyography responses using an adaptive neuro-fuzzy inference system with subtractive clustering. *Human Factors and Ergonomics in Manufacturing & Service Industries*, *27*(4), 177–186. doi:10.1002/hfm.20701

Çakıt, E., Karwowski, W., Bozkurt, H., Ahram, T., Thompson, W., Mikusinski, P., & Lee, G. (2014). Investigating the relationship between adverse events and infrastructure development in an active war theater using soft computing techniques. *Applied Soft Computing*, *25*, 204–214. doi:10.1016/j.asoc.2014.09.028

Çakıt, E., Karwowski, W., & Servi, L. (2020). Application of soft computing techniques for estimating emotional states expressed in Twitter® time series data. *Neural Computing & Applications*, *32*(8), 3535–3548. doi:10.100700521-019-04048-5

Castillo, O., & Melin, P. (2020). Forecasting of COVID-19 time series for countries in the world based on a hybrid approach combining the fractal dimension and fuzzy logic. *Chaos, Solitons, and Fractals*, *140*, 110242. doi:10.1016/j.chaos.2020.110242 PMID:32863616

Catalyst, N. (2018, January 1). *Healthcare Big Data and the Promise of Value-Based Care*. NEJM Catalyst. https://catalyst.nejm.org/doi/full/10.1056/CAT.18.0290

Chadwick, R. (2017). What's in a Name: Conceptions of Personalized Medicine and Their Ethical Implications. *LatoSensu. Revue de La Société de Philosophie Des Sciences*, *4*(2), 5–11. doi:10.20416/lsrsps.v4i2.893

Chakraborty, S., & Mali, K. (2021a). SuFMoFPA: A superpixel and meta-heuristic based fuzzy image segmentation approach to explicate COVID-19 radiological images. *Expert Systems with Applications*, *167*, 114142. doi:10.1016/j.eswa.2020.114142 PMID:34924697

Chakraborty, S., & Mali, K. (2021b). SUFMACS: A machine learning-based robust image segmentation framework for covid-19 radiological image interpretation. *Expert Systems with Applications*, *178*, 115069. doi:10.1016/j.eswa.2021.115069 PMID:33897121

Chan, R. W., Lau, J. Y. C., Lam, W. W., & Lau, A. Z. (2019). Magnetic Resonance Imaging. In R. Narayan (Ed.), *Encyclopedia of Biomedical Engineering* (pp. 574–587). Elsevier. doi:10.1016/B978-0-12-801238-3.99945-8

Chatfield, K., Simonyan, K., Vedaldi, A., & Zisserman, A. (2014). *Return of the devil in the details: Delving deep into convolutional nets.* arXiv preprint arXiv:1405.3531.

Chawla, N. V., Bowyer, K. W., Hall, L. O., & Kegelmeyer, W. P. (2002). SMOTE: Synthetic minority over-sampling technique. *Journal of Artificial Intelligence Research, 16,* 321–357. doi:10.1613/jair.953

Chen, T., Wang, Y. C., & Chiu, M. C. (2020, December). Assessing the robustness of a factory amid the COVID-19 pandemic: A fuzzy collaborative intelligence approach. In Healthcare (Vol. 8, No. 4, p. 481). Multidisciplinary Digital Publishing Institute.

Chen, Y., Shi, F., Christodoulou, A. G., Xie, Y., Zhou, Z., & Li, D. (2018). Efficient and accurate MRI super-resolution using a generative adversarial network and 3D multi-level densely connected network. Lecture Notes in Computer Science (Including Subseries Lecture Notes in Artificial Intelligence and Lecture Notes in Bioinformatics), 11070 LNCS, 91–99. doi:10.1007/978-3-030-00928-1_11

Chen, X. W., & Lin, X. (2014). Big data deep learning: Challenges and perspectives. *IEEE Access: Practical Innovations, Open Solutions, 2,* 514–525.

Chen, X., Kingma, D. P., Salimans, T., Duan, Y., Dhariwal, P., Schulman, J., Sutskever, I., & Abbeel, P. (2017). Variational lossy autoencoder. *5th International Conference on Learning Representations, ICLR 2017 - Conference Track Proceedings,* 1–17.

Cheraghi, M. A., Reza, A., Nasrabadi, N., Nejad, E. M., Salari, A., Ehsani, S. R., & Kheyli, K. (2011). *Medication Errors Among Nurses in Intensive Care Units.* ICU.

Chok, L., Bachli, E. B., Steiger, P., Bettex, D., Cottini, S. R., Keller, E., Maggiorini, M., & Schuepbach, R. A. (2018). Effect of diagnosis related groups implementation on the intensive care unit of a Swiss tertiary hospital: A cohort study. *BMC Health Services Research, 18*(1), 1–10. doi:10.118612913-018-2869-4 PMID:29402271

Chou, E. T., & Carrino, J. A. (2007). Magnetic Resonance Imaging. In S. D. Waldman & J. I. Bloch (Eds.), *Pain Management* (pp. 106–117). W.B. Saunders. doi:10.1016/B978-0-7216-0334-6.50014-5

Chowdhury, A. A., Hasan, K. T., & Hoque, K. K. S. (2021). Analysis and Prediction of COVID-19 Pandemic in Bangladesh by Using ANFIS and LSTM Network. *Cognitive Computation, 13*(3), 761–770. doi:10.100712559-021-09859-0 PMID:33868501

Chua, L. O. (1998). *CNN: A paradigm for complexity* (Vol. 31). World Scientific.

Chui, K. T., Liu, R. W., Zhao, M., & De Pablos, P. O. (2020). Predicting students' performance with school and family tutoring using generative adversarial network-based deep support vector machine. *IEEE Access: Practical Innovations, Open Solutions*, 8, 86745–86752. doi:10.1109/ACCESS.2020.2992869

Chung, J., Gulcehre, C., Cho, K., & Bengio, Y. (2014). *Empirical evaluation of gated recurrent neural networks on sequence modeling*. arXiv preprint arXiv:1412.3555.

Cleary, J. O. S. H., & Guimarães, A. R. (2014). Magnetic Resonance Imaging. In L. M. McManus & R. N. Mitchell (Eds.), *Pathobiology of Human Disease* (pp. 3987–4004). Academic Press. doi:10.1016/B978-0-12-386456-7.07609-7

Coimbra, C., Esteves, M., Miranda, F., Portela, F., Santos, M. F., & Machado, J. (2018). Improving the Codification of Hospital Discharges with an ICD-9-CM Single-page Application and its Transition to ICD-10-CM/PCS. *International Journal on Advances in Life Sciences*, 10(1), 23–30.

Collins, R. (2020). Accessing UK Biobank Data. *Scientia*, (October), 1–50.

Combs, V. (2020, November 5). *Humana uses Azure and Kafka to make healthcare less frustrating for doctors and patients*. TechRepublic. https://www.techrepublic.com/article/humana-uses-azure-and-kafka-to-make-healthcare-less-frustrating-for-doctors-and-patients/

Committee on the Review of Omics-Based Tests for Predicting Patient Outcomes in Clinical Trials, Board on Health Care Services, Board on Health Sciences Policy, and Institute of Medicine. (2012). *Evolution of Translational Omics: Lessons Learned and the Path Forward* (C. M. Micheel, S. J. Nass, & G. S. Omenn, Eds.). National Academies Press. doi:10.17226/13297

Confluent. (2020). *Humana Adopts Event Streaming and Interoperability Using Confluent. Confluent*. https://www.confluent.io/customers/humana/

Cordon, O., Herrera, F., Hoffmann, F., & Magdalena, L. (2001). *Genetic Fuzzy Systems: Evolutionary Tuning and Learning of Fuzzy Knowledge Bases. In Advances in Fuzzy Systems - Applications and Theory* (Vol. 19). World Scientific. doi:10.1142/4177

Coronavirus Disease. (COVID-19) situation report – 43. (2020). *World Health Organization*. Available from: https://www.who.int/docs/default-source/coronaviruse/situation-reports/20200303-sitrep-43-covid-19.pdf?sfvrsn=76e425ed_2

Costa, C. M., Menárguez-Tortosa, M., & Fernández-Breis, J. T. (2011). Clinical data interoperability based on archetype transformation. *Journal of Biomedical Informatics*, 44(5), 869–880. doi:10.1016/j.jbi.2011.05.006 PMID:21645637

Costa, P., Galdran, A., Meyer, M. I., Niemeijer, M., Abràmoff, M., Mendonça, A. M., & Campilho, A. (2018). End-to-End Adversarial Retinal Image Synthesis. *IEEE Transactions on Medical Imaging*, 37(3), 781–791. doi:10.1109/TMI.2017.2759102 PMID:28981409

Cowie, M. R., Catherine, E. C., & Panos, V. (2013). E-health innovation: Time for engagement with the cardiology community. *European Heart Journal*, 34(25), 1864–1868. doi:10.1093/eurheartj/ehs153 PMID:22733834

Cruz-Correia, R. J., Rodrigues, P. P., Freitas, A., Almeida, F. C., Chen, R., & Costa-Pereira, A. (2009). Data quality and integration issues in electronic health records. In *Information Discovery on Electronic Health Records*. doi:10.1201/9781420090413-c4

Cruz, R., Guimarães, T., Peixoto, H., & Santos, M. F. (2021). Architecture for Intensive Care Data Processing and Visualization in Real-time. *Procedia Computer Science*, *184*, 923–928. doi:10.1016/j.procs.2021.03.115

Cutler, A., Cutler, D. R., & Stevens, J. R. (2012). Random forests. In *Ensemble machine learning* (pp. 157–175). Springer. doi:10.1007/978-1-4419-9326-7_5

D'souza, S., Nazareth, D., Vaz, C., & Shetty, M. (2021). Blockchain and AI in Pharmaceutical Supply Chain. *SSRN Electronic Journal*. doi:10.2139/ssrn.3852034

D'Urso, P., De Giovanni, L., & Vitale, V. (2021). Spatial robust fuzzy clustering of COVID 19 time series based on B-splines. *Spatial Statistics*, 100518. doi:10.1016/j.spasta.2021.100518 PMID:34026473

Dash, S., Shakyawar, S. K., Sharma, M., & Kaushik, S. (2019). Big data in healthcare: Management, analysis and future prospects. *Journal of Big Data*, *6*(1), 54. Advance online publication. doi:10.118640537-019-0217-0

de la Torre, C., Wagner, B., & Rousos, M. (2019). *NET Microservices: Architecture for Containerized. NET Applications*. Microsoft Corporation. https://docs.microsoft.com/en-us/dotnet/architecture/microservices/

De Mauro, A., Greco, M., & Grimaldi, M. (2016). A formal definition of Big Data based on its essential features. *Library Review*, *65*(3), 122–135. doi:10.1108/LR-06-2015-0061

de Saúde, S. N. (n.d.). *ACSS apresenta o novo ecossistema sobre Morbilidade Hospitalar*. Available: https://www.acss.min-saude.pt/2018/06/04/acss-apresenta-o-novo-ecossistema-sobre-morbilidade-hospitalar/

Dean, J., Corrado, G., Monga, R., Chen, K., Devin, M., Mao, M., ... Ng, A. (2012). Large scale distributed deep networks. *Advances in Neural Information Processing Systems*, 25.

Debauche, O., Mahmoudi, S., Manneback, P., & Assila, A. (2019). Fog IoT for Health: A new Architecture for Patients and Elderly Monitoring. *Procedia Computer Science*, *160*, 289–297.

Denny, A., Raj, A., Ashok, A., Ram, C. M., & George, R. (2019, October). i-HOPE: Detection And Prediction System For Polycystic Ovary Syndrome (PCOS) Using Machine Learning Techniques. In TENCON 2019-2019 IEEE Region 10 Conference (TENCON) (pp. 673-678). IEEE.

Dhiraj, K. (2019). *Top 5 advantages and disadvantages of Decision Tree Algorithm*. Available in: https://dhirajkumarblog.medium.com/top-5-advantages-and-disadvantages-of-decision-tree-algorithm-428ebd199d9a di Muzio, M., de Vito, C., Tartaglini, D., & Villari, P. (2017). Knowledge, behaviours, training and attitudes of nurses during preparation and administration of intravenous medications in intensive care units (ICU). A multicenter Italian study. *Applied Nursing Research, 38*, 129–133. doi:10.1016/j.apnr.2017.10.002 PMID:29241505

Dick, R. S., Steen, E. B., & Detmer, D. E. (1997). *The computer-based patient record: an essential technology for health care*. National Academies Press.

Digital health. (2019, October 10). Retrieved December 29, 2019, from https://www.who.int/health-topics/digital-health

dos Santos Gomes, D. C., & de Oliveira Serra, G. L. (2021). Machine Learning Model for Computational Tracking and Forecasting the COVID-19 Dynamic Propagation. *IEEE Journal of Biomedical and Health Informatics, 25*(3), 615–622. doi:10.1109/JBHI.2021.3052134 PMID:33449891

Dragoni, N., Giallorenzo, S., Lafuente, A. L., Mazzara, M., Montesi, F., Mustafin, R., & Safina, L. (2017). Microservices: Yesterday, Today, and Tomorrow. *Present and Ulterior Software Engineering*, 195–216. doi:10.1007/978-3-319-67425-4_12

Drews, F. A. (2008). *Patient Monitors in Critical Care: Lessons for Improvement. In Advances in Patient Safety: New Directions and Alternative Approaches* (Vol. 3). Performance and Tools.

Dua, D., & Graff, C. (2017). *UCI machine learning repository*. Academic Press.

Duarte, J., Salazar, M., Quintas, C., Santos, M., Neves, J., Abelha, A., & Machado, J. (2010). Data Quality Evaluation of Electronic Health Records in the Hospital Admission Process. *2010 IEEE/ACIS 9th International Conference on Computer and Information Science*, 201–206. 10.1109/ICIS.2010.97

Duran, C., Sobieszczyk, P. S., & Rybicki, F. J. (2013). Chapter 13 - Magnetic Resonance Imaging. In M. A. Creager, J. A. Beckman, & J. Loscalzo (Eds.), *Vascular Medicine: A Companion to Braunwald's Heart Disease* (2nd ed., pp. 166–183). W.B. Saunders.

Dutta, P., & Borah, G. (2021). Multicriteria decision making approach using an efficient novel similarity measure for generalized trapezoidal fuzzy numbers. *Journal of Ambient Intelligence and Humanized Computing*, 1–23. doi:10.100712652-021-03347-x PMID:34178177

Eddy, D. M. (1984). Variations in physician practice: The role of uncertainty. *Health Affairs, 3*(2), 74–89. doi:10.1377/hlthaff.3.2.74 PMID:6469198

Ehteshami, A., Sadoughi, F., Ahmadi, M., & Kashefi, P. (2013). Intensive care information system impacts. *Acta Informatica Medica, 21*(3), 185–191. doi:10.5455/aim.2013.21.185-191 PMID:24167389

El Hayek, S., Bitar, L., Hamdar, L. H., Mirza, F. G., & Daoud, G. (2016). Poly cystic ovarian syndrome: An updated overview. *Frontiers in Physiology, 7*, 124. doi:10.3389/fphys.2016.00124 PMID:27092084

Enrico, G.C., Catherine, E.C., Nico, B., Przemyslaw, G., & Enno, T.V.V. (2014, September 15). The importance of e-Health in daily cardiology practice. *Cardiac Rhythm News*.

Erdenebayar, U., Kim, Y. J., Park, J. U., Joo, E. Y., & Lee, K. J. (2019). Deep learning approaches for automatic detection of sleep apnea events from an electrocardiogram. *Computer Methods and Programs in Biomedicine*, *180*, 105001.

Erhan, D., Courville, A., Bengio, Y., & Vincent, P. (2010, March). Why does unsupervised pre-training help deep learning? In *Proceedings of the thirteenth international conference on artificial intelligence and statistics* (pp. 201-208). JMLR Workshop and Conference Proceedings.

ESHRE. (2004). Revised 2003 consensus on diagnostic criteria and long-term health risks related to polycystic ovary syndrome. *Fertility and Sterility*, *81*(1), 19–25. doi:10.1016/j.fertnstert.2003.10.004 PMID:14711538

Eysenbach, G. (2001). What is e-health? *Journal of Medical Internet Research*, *3*(2), e20. doi:10.2196/jmir.3.2.e20 PMID:11720962

Fajardo, A. (2021, December 8). 8 Best Healthcare Apps for Patients | Top Mobile Apps in 2021 - Rootstrap. *Rootstrap - Call Rootstrap Today*. Retrieved 2021, from https://www.rootstrap.com/blog/healthcare-apps/

Fan, D., Li, Y., Liu, W., Yue, X. G., & Boustras, G. (2021). Weaving public health and safety nets to respond the COVID-19 pandemic. *Safety Science*, *134*, 105058. doi:10.1016/j.ssci.2020.105058 PMID:33110294

Fang, S. H., Liang, Y., & Chiu, K. M. (2012). Developing a Mobile Phone-based Fall Detection System on Android Platform. *Computing, Communications and Applications Conference*.

Farhadi, J., Attarodi, G., Dabanloo, N. J., Mohandespoor, M., & Eslamizadeh, M. (2018, September). Classification of atrial fibrillation using stacked auto encoders neural networks. In *2018 Computing in cardiology conference (CinC)* (Vol. 45, pp. 1-3). IEEE.

Faust, O. (2018). Documenting and predicting topic changes in Computers in Biology and Medicine: A bibliometric keyword analysis from 1990 to 2017. *Informatics in Medicine Unlocked*, *11*, 15–27.

Faust, O., Hagiwara, Y., Hong, T. J., Lih, O. S., & Acharya, U. R. (2018). Deep learning for healthcare applications based on physiological signals: A review. *Computer Methods and Programs in Biomedicine*, *161*, 1–13.

Faust, O., Shenfield, A., Kareem, M., San, T. R., Fujita, H., & Acharya, U. R. (2018). Automated detection of atrial fibrillation using long short-term memory network with RR interval signals. *Computers in Biology and Medicine*, *102*, 327–335.

Feng, R., Zheng, X., Gao, T., Chen, J., Wang, W., Chen, D. Z., & Wu, J. (2021). Interactive Few-Shot Learning: Limited Supervision, Better Medical Image Segmentation. *IEEE Transactions on Medical Imaging*, *40*(10), 2575–2588. doi:10.1109/TMI.2021.3060551 PMID:33606628

Ferreira, D., Silva, S., Abelha, A., & Machado, J. (2020). Recommendation system using autoencoders. *Applied Sciences (Basel, Switzerland)*, *10*(16), 5510. doi:10.3390/app10165510

Fischer, A., & Igel, C. (2012, September). An introduction to restricted Boltzmann machines. In *Iberoamerican congress on pattern recognition* (pp. 14–36). Springer.

Flores, Glusman, & Brogaard, Price, & Hood. (2013). P4 Medicine: How Systems Medicine Will Transform the Healthcare Sector and Society. *Personalized Medicine*, *10*(6), 565–576. doi:10.2217/pme.13.57

Foroozandeh, M., & Eklund, A. (2020). *Synthesizing brain tumor images and annotations by combining progressive growing GAN and SPADE*. ArXiv Preprint ArXiv:2009.05946.

Fromme, E. K., Eilers, K. M., Mori, M., Hsieh, Y. C., & Beer, T. M. (2004). How accurate is clinician reporting of chemotherapy adverse effects? A comparison with patient-reported symptoms from the Quality-of-Life Questionnaire C30. *Journal of Clinical Oncology*, *22*(17), 3485–3490. doi:10.1200/JCO.2004.03.025 PMID:15337796

Fullér, R. (1999). *Introduction to Neuro-Fuzzy Systems*. Physica-Verlag.

Gan, S. K. E., Koshy, C., Nguyen, P. V., & Haw, Y. X. (2016). An overview of clinically and healthcare-related apps in Google and Apple app stores: Connecting patients, drugs, and clinicians. *Scientific Phone Apps and Mobile Devices*, *2*(1), 8. Advance online publication. doi:10.118641070-016-0012-7

García Calderón, V., Figueiras Huante, I. A., Carbajal Martínez, M., Yacaman Handal, R. E., Palami Antunez, D., Soto, M. E., & Koretzky, S. G. (2019). The impact of improving the quality of coding in the utilities of Diagnosis Related Groups system in a private healthcare institution. 14-year experience. *International Journal of Medical Informatics*, *129*(February), 248–252. doi:10.1016/j.ijmedinf.2019.06.019 PMID:31445263

Garcia-Garcia, A., Orts-Escolano, S., Oprea, S., Villena-Martinez, V., Martinez-Gonzalez, P., & Garcia-Rodriguez, J. (2018). A survey on deep learning techniques for image and video semantic segmentation. *Applied Soft Computing*, *70*, 41–65.

Garde, S., Knaup, P., Hovenga, E. J. S., & Heard, S. (2007). Towards semantic interoperability for electronic health records. *Methods of Information in Medicine*, *46*(03), 332–343. doi:10.1160/ME5001 PMID:17492120

Garg, N. (2013). *Apache Kafka*. Packt Publishing.

Garkoti, G., Peddoju, S. K., & Balasubramanian, R. (2014). Detection of Insider Attacks in Cloud based e- Healthcare Environment. *Int. Conf. on Information Technology (ICIT)*. 10.1109/ICIT.2014.43

GeeksforGeeks. (2020, November 13). *Creating dApps using the Truffle Framework*. https://www.geeksforgeeks.org/creating-dapps-using-the-truffle-framework/

Genay, S., Décaudin, B., Ethgen, S., Barthélémy, C., Odou, P., & Lebuffe, G. (2013). Impact of noradrenaline infusion set on mean arterial pressure: A retrospective clinical study. *Annales Francaises d'Anesthesie et de Reanimation, 32*(11), e159–e162. Advance online publication. doi:10.1016/j.annfar.2013.08.011 PMID:24138772

Ghosh, D., & Vogt, A. (2012, July). Outliers: An evaluation of methodologies. In Joint statistical meetings (Vol. 2012). Academic Press.

Ghosh, B., & Biswas, A. (2021). Status evaluation of provinces affected by COVID-19: A qualitative assessment using fuzzy system. *Applied Soft Computing, 109*, 107540. doi:10.1016/j. asoc.2021.107540 PMID:34093096

Gibson-Helm, M., Teede, H., Dunaif, A., & Dokras, A. (2017). Delayed diagnosis and a lack of information associated with dissatisfaction in women with polycystic ovary syndrome. *The Journal of Clinical Endocrinology and Metabolism, 102*(2), 604–612. PMID:27906550

Gmb, H. R. 2021. *Deep Learning - RapidMiner Documentation.* Available at: https://docs. rapidminer.com/latest/studio/operators/modeling/predictive/neural_nets/deep_learning.html

Gold, J., McGrath, K., & Mohan, V. (2017). *Perceptions of Data Quality and Accuracy During ICU Round.* Academic Press.

Goldberger, A. L., Amaral, L. A., Glass, L., Hausdorff, J. M., Ivanov, P. C., Mark, R. G., ... & Stanley, H. E. (2000). PhysioBank, PhysioToolkit, and PhysioNet: components of a new research resource for complex physiologic signals. *Circulation, 101*(23), e215-e220.

Goldberger, A., Amaral, L., Glass, L., Hausdorff, J., Ivanov, P. C., Mark, R., Mietus, J. E., Moody, G. B., Peng, C.-K., & Stanley, H. E. (2000). PhysioBank, PhysioToolkit, and PhysioNet: Components of a new research resource for complex physiologic signals. *Circulation, 101*(23), e215–e220. doi:10.1161/01.CIR.101.23.e215 PMID:10851218

Goodfellow, I. J., Pouget-Abadie, J., Mirza, M., Xu, B., Warde-Farley, D., Ozair, S., Courville, A., & Bengio, Y. (2014). Generative adversarial nets. *Advances in Neural Information Processing Systems, 3*(January), 2672–2680.

Goodfellow, I., Bengio, Y., & Courville, A. (2016). *Deep learning.* MIT press.

Gramacho, M. (1971). Cuidados intensivos. *Revista de Enfermagem, 18*(1). PMID:5211521

Grandia, L. (2017). Healthcare information systems: a look at the past, present, and future. *Health Catalyst*, 1–4.

Graupe, D. (2013). *Principles of artificial neural networks* (Vol. 7). World Scientific. doi:10.1142/8868

Greenhalgh, T., & Papoutsi, C. (2018). *Studying complexity in health services research: Desperately seeking an overdue paradigm shift.* Academic Press.

Grupos de Diagnósticos Homogéneos (GDH). (n.d.). Available: http://portalcodgdh.min-saude. pt/index.php/Grupos_de_%0DDiagn%7Bó%7Dsticos_Homog%7Bé%7Dneos_(GDH)

Gubbi, J., Buyya, R., Marusic, S., & Palaniswami, M. (2013). Internet of Things (IoT): A vision, architectural elements, and future directions. *Future Generation Computer Systems, 29*(7), 1645–1660. doi:10.1016/j.future.2013.01.010

Gui, J., Sun, Z., Wen, Y., Tao, D., & Ye, J. (2020). *A Review on Generative Adversarial Networks: Algorithms, Theory, and Applications.* https://arxiv.org/abs/2001.06937

Gulrajani, I., Ahmed, F., Arjovsky, M., Dumoulin, V., & Courville, A. (2017). *Improved training of wasserstein GANs.* Advances in Neural Information Processing Systems.

Guo, L., Sim, G., & Matuszewski, B. (2019). Inter-patient ECG classification with convolutional and recurrent neural networks. *Biocybernetics and Biomedical Engineering, 39*(3), 868–879.

Guo, Y., Liu, Y., Georgiou, T., & Lew, M. S. (2018). A review of semantic segmentation using deep neural networks. *International Journal of Multimedia Information Retrieval, 7*(2), 87–93.

Han, C., Hayashi, H., Rundo, L., Araki, R., Shimoda, W., Muramatsu, S., Furukawa, Y., Mauri, G., & Nakayama, H. (2018). GAN-based synthetic brain MR image generation. *Proceedings - International Symposium on Biomedical Imaging,* 734–738. 10.1109/ISBI.2018.8363678

Hand, D. J., & Adams, N. M. (2014). Data mining. *Wiley StatsRef: Statistics Reference Online,* 1-7.

Hanson, S. M. (2005). *Family Health Nursing: Theory, Practice and Research.* Lusodidacta.

Hao, X., Zhang, G., & Ma, S. (2016). Deep learning. *International Journal of Semantic Computing, 10*(03), 417–439. doi:10.1142/S1793351X16500045 PMID:28113886

Hao, Y., Xu, T., Hu, H., Wang, P., & Bai, Y. (2020). Prediction and analysis of corona virus disease 2019. *PLoS One, 15*(10), e0239960. doi:10.1371/journal.pone.0239960 PMID:33017421

Hassan, F. E. M., & Sahal, R. (2020). Real-Time Healthcare Monitoring System using Online Machine Learning and Spark Streaming. *International Journal of Advanced Computer Science and Applications, 11*(9). Advance online publication. doi:10.14569/IJACSA.2020.0110977

Hassan, N., Ahmad, T., Ashaari, A., Awang, S. R., Mamat, S. S., Mohamad, W. M. W., & Fuad, A. A. A. (2021). A fuzzy graph approach analysis for COVID-19 outbreak. *Results in Physics, 25,* 104267. doi:10.1016/j.rinp.2021.104267 PMID:33968605

Haynes, R. B., & Goodman, S. N. (2015). An Interview with David Sackett, 2014–2015. *Clinical Trials. Journal of the Society for Clinical Trials, 12*(5), 540–551. doi:10.1177/1740774515597895

He, D., & Zeadally, S. (2015). Authentication Protocol for an Ambient Assisted Living System. *IEEE Communications Magazine, 53*(1), 71–77. doi:10.1109/MCOM.2015.7010518

He, K., Zhang, X., Ren, S., & Sun, J. (2016). Deep residual learning for image recognition. In *Proceedings of the IEEE conference on computer vision and pattern recognition* (pp. 770-778). IEEE.

Hernandez-Ibarburu, G., Perez-Rey, D., Alonso-Oset, E., Alonso-Calvo, R., Voets, D., Mueller, C., Claerhout, B., & Custodix, N. V. (2019). ICD-10-PCS extension with ICD-9 procedure codes to support integrated access to clinical legacy data. *International Journal of Medical Informatics*, *122*, 70–79. doi:10.1016/j.ijmedinf.2018.11.002 PMID:30623787

Heusser, M. (2020, August 19). *Orchestration vs. choreography in microservices architecture.* SearchAppArchitecture. https://searchapparchitecture.techtarget.com/tip/Orchestration-vs-choreography-in-microservices-architecture

Hind, B., & Sarah, A. (2021). The role of e-Health, tele-health, and tele-medicine for chronic disease patients during COVID-19 pandemic: A rapid systematic review. *Digital Health*, 1–17.

Hinton, G. E., & Salakhutdinov, R. R. (2006). Reducing the dimensionality of data with neural networks. *Science, 313*(5786), 504-507.

Hinton, G. E., & Salakhutdinov, R. R. (2006). Reducing the dimensionality of data with neural networks. *Science*, *313*(5786), 504–507. doi:10.1126cience.1127647 PMID:16873662

Hiremath, S., Yang, G., & Mankodiya, K. (2014). Wearable Internet of Things: Concept, Architectural components and promises for person –Centered healthcare. *EAI 4th International conference on wireless mobile communication and health care.*

HL7.org. (2011). *Health Level Seven.* The Worldwide Leader in Interoperability Standards.

Hl7.org. (2019). *MessageHeader - FHIR v4.0.1.* Retrieved January 1, 2020, from https://www.hl7.org/fhir/messageheader.html

HL7.org. (2019, September 1). *FHIR Overview.* Hl7 FHIR. Retrieved January 1, 2020, from https://www.hl7.org/fhir/overview.html

HMS. (2019). *Interoperability in Healthcare.* HIMSS - Interoperability in Healthcare. Retrieved December 29, 2019, from https://www.himss.org/resources/interoperability-healthcare

Hochreiter, S., & Schmidhuber, J. (1997). Long short-term memory. *Neural Computation*, *9*(8), 1735–1780.

Hodach, R., Chase, A., Fortini, R., Delaney, C., & Hodach, R. (2014). *Population health management: A roadmap for provider-based automation in a new era of healthcare.* Institute for Health Technology Transformation. Http://Ihealthtran. Com/Pdf/PHMReport. Pdf

Hofmann, M., & Klinkenberg, R. (Eds.). (2016). *RapidMiner: Data mining use cases and business analytics applications.* CRC Press. doi:10.1201/b16023

Hong, N., Wen, A., Stone, D. J., Tsuji, S., Kingsbury, P. R., Rasmussen, L. V., ... Jiang, G. (2019). Developing a FHIR-based EHR phenotyping framework: A case study for identification of patients with obesity and multiple comorbidities from discharge summaries. *Journal of Biomedical Informatics*, *99*, 103310.

Hong, S., Zhou, Y., Shang, J., Xiao, C., & Sun, J. (2020). Opportunities and challenges of deep learning methods for electrocardiogram data: A systematic review. *Computers in Biology and Medicine*, *122*, 103801.

Hong, Z., Li, N., Li, D., Li, J., Li, B., Xiong, W., Lu, L., Li, W., & Zhou, D. (2020). Telemedicine during the COVID-19 pandemic: Experiences from Western China (Preprint). *Journal of Medical Internet Research*, *22*(5), e19577. doi:10.2196/19577 PMID:32349962

Hou, B., Yang, J., Wang, P., & Yan, R. (2019). LSTM-based auto-encoder model for ECG arrhythmias classification. *IEEE Transactions on Instrumentation and Measurement*, *69*(4), 1232–1240.

Hovakeemiana, Y., Naik, K., & Nayak, A. (2011). A Survey on Dependability in Body Area Networks. *5th Int. Symp. on Medical Information & Communication Technology*. 10.1109/ISMICT.2011.5759786

Huang, J., Gretton, A., Borgwardt, K., Schölkopf, B., & Smola, A. (2006). Correcting sample selection bias by unlabeled data. *Advances in Neural Information Processing Systems*, 19.

Huff, S. M., Rocha, R. A., Bray, B. E., Warner, H. R., & Haug, P. J. (1995). An event model of medical information representation. *Journal of the American Medical Informatics Association: JAMIA*, *2*(2), 116–134. doi:10.1136/jamia.1995.95261905 PMID:7743315

Humana (HUM). (2021). *Forbes*. https://www.forbes.com/companies/humana/?sh=5fce4cf04390

Hung, K., Zhang, Y. T., & Tai, B. (2004). Wearable Medical Devices for Tele-Home Healthcare. *Proceedings of the 26th Annual International Conference of the IEEE.*

Iandola, F., Moskewicz, M., Karayev, S., Girshick, R., Darrell, T., & Keutzer, K. (2014). *Densenet: Implementing efficient convnet descriptor pyramids*. arXiv preprint arXiv:1404.1869.

Isin, A., & Ozdalili, S. (2017). Cardiac arrhythmia detection using deep learning. *Procedia Computer Science*, *120*, 268–275.

iWay. (2018). *Introducing the iWay Integration Solution for EDIHL7*. Retrieved January 1, 2020, from https://iwayinfocenter.informationbuilders.com/TLs/TL_soa_ebiz_hl7/source/hl7_01intro11.htm

Jalaber, C., Lapotre, T., Morcet-Delattre, T., Ribet, F., Jouneau, S., & Lederlin, M. (2020). Chest CT in COVID-19 pneumonia: A review of current knowledge. *Diagnostic and Interventional Imaging*, *101*(7-8), 431–437. doi:10.1016/j.diii.2020.06.001 PMID:32571748

Jang, J. S. R. (1993). ANFIS: Adaptive-network-based fuzzy inference system. *IEEE Transactions on Systems, Man, and Cybernetics*, *23*(5), 665–685. doi:10.1109/21.256541

Janzen, B., & Hellsten, L. (2018). Does the psychosocial quality of unpaid family work contribute to educational disparities in mental health among employed partnered mothers? *International Archives of Occupational and Environmental Health*, *91*(5), 633–641. doi:10.100700420-018-1310-y PMID:29691657

Jayatilleke, B. G., Ranawaka, G. R., Wijesekera, C., & Kumarasinha, M. C. (2018). Development of mobile application through design-based research. *Asian Association of Open Universities Journal, 13*(2), 145–168. doi:10.1108/aaouj-02-2018-0013

Jenkinson, M. (2009). Image Registration and Motion Correction. *Image Processing, 28*(3), 2009–2009.

Jenkinson, M., Beckmann, C. F., Behrens, T. E. J., Woolrich, M. W., & Smith, S. M. (2012). Fsl. *NeuroImage, 62*(2), 782–790. doi:10.1016/j.neuroimage.2011.09.015 PMID:21979382

Jorland, G., Opinel, A., & Weisz, G. (Eds.). (2005). Body Counts: Medical Quantification in Historical and Sociological Perspective [La Quantification Medicale, Perspectives Historiques et Sociologiques]. McGill Queen's University Press.

JSON and BSON. (n.d.). *MongoDB*. https://www.mongodb.com/json-and-bson

Kadir, M. A. (2020). Role of telemedicine in healthcare during COVID-19 pandemic in developing countries. *Telehealth Med Today., 5*(2), 1–5. doi:10.30953/tmt.v5.187

Kadry, S. (2014). On the Evolution of Information Systems. Academic Press.

Kaggle.com. (2021). *Kaggle: Your Machine Learning and Data Science Community*. Available at: https://www.kaggle.com

Kaieski, N., da Costa, C. A., da Rosa Righi, R., Lora, P. S., & Eskofier, B. (2020). Application of artificial intelligence methods in vital signs analysis of hospitalized patients: A systematic literature review. In *Applied Soft Computing Journal* (Vol. 96). Elsevier Ltd. doi:10.1016/j.asoc.2020.106612

Kakas, A., Kowalski, R., & Toni, F. (1998). The role of abduction in logic programming. In D. Gabbay, C. Hogger, & I. Robinson (Eds.), *Handbook of Logic in Artificial Intelligence and Logic Programming* (Vol. 5, pp. 235–324). Oxford University Press. doi:10.1093/oso/9780198537922.003.0007

Kakria, P., Tripathi, N. K., & Kitipawang, P. (2015). A real-time health monitoring system for remote cardiac patients using smartphone and wearable sensors. *International Journal of Telemedicine and Applications, 8*, 1–11. doi:10.1155/2015/373474 PMID:26788055

Kalender, W. A. (2006). X-ray computed tomography. *Physics in Medicine and Biology, 51*(13), R29–R43. doi:10.1088/0031-9155/51/13/R03 PMID:16790909

Kamaleswaran, R., Mahajan, R., & Akbilgic, O. (2018). A robust deep convolutional neural network for the classification of abnormal cardiac rhythm using single lead electrocardiograms of variable length. *Physiological Measurement, 39*(3), 035006.

Karras, T., Aila, T., Laine, S., & Lehtinen, J. (2018). Progressive growing of GANs for improved quality, stability, and variation. *6th International Conference on Learning Representations, ICLR 2018 - Conference Track Proceedings*, 1–26.

Kern, C. (2012). *Hospitals Need To Renew Their Digital Strategies To Reclaim Patient Engagement.* Retrieved 2021, from https://www.healthitoutcomes.com/doc/hospitals-need-renew-digital-strategies-patient-engagement-0001

Kim, H., Kim, S., Helleputte, N. V., Artes, A., & Konijnenburg, M. (2014). A Configurable and Low-Power Mixed Signal SoC for Portable ECG Monitoring Applications. *IEEE Transactions on Biomedical Circuits and Systems, 8*(2), 257–267. doi:10.1109/TBCAS.2013.2260159 PMID:24875285

Kingma, D. P., & Ba, J. L. (2015). Adam: A method for stochastic optimization. *3rd International Conference on Learning Representations, ICLR 2015 - Conference Track Proceedings,* 1–15.

Kingma, D. P., & Welling, M. (2014a). Auto-encoding variational bayes. *2nd International Conference on Learning Representations, ICLR 2014 - Conference Track Proceedings,* 1–14.

Kingma, D. P., & Welling, M. (2014b). Stochastic Gradient VB and the Variational Auto-Encoder. *2nd International Conference on Learning Representations, ICLR 2014 - Conference Track Proceedings,* 1–14.

Kiranyaz, S., Ince, T., & Gabbouj, M. (2015). Real-time patient-specific ECG classification by 1-D convolutional neural networks. *IEEE Transactions on Biomedical Engineering, 63*(3), 664–675.

Kodali, N., Abernethy, J., Hays, J., & Kira, Z. (2017). *On Convergence and Stability of GANs.* https://arxiv.org/abs/1705.07215

Kose, U., Deperlioglu, O., Alzubi, J., & Patrut, B. (2021). *Deep Learning for Medical Decision Support Systems.* Springer. https://link.springer.com/content/pdf/10.1007/978-981-15-6325-6.pdf

Kostecka-Jurczyk, D. (2019). Tying on the mobile apps market and competition rules. *Ekonomia, 25*(3), 43–54. doi:10.19195/2084-4093.25.3.4

Kottarathil, P. (2021). *Polycystic ovary syndrome (PCOS).* Available at: https://www.kaggle.com/prasoonkottarathil/polycystic-ovary-syndrome-pcos

Kramer, M. A. (1991). Nonlinear principal component analysis using autoassociative neural networks. *AIChE Journal. American Institute of Chemical Engineers, 37*(2), 233–243. doi:10.1002/aic.690370209

Krizhevsky, A., Sutskever, I., & Hinton, G. E. (2012). Imagenet classification with deep convolutional neural networks. *Advances in Neural Information Processing Systems, 25.*

Kruse, C. S., Goswamy, R., Raval, Y. J., & Marawi, S. (2016). Challenges and opportunities of Big Data in health care: A systematic review. *JMIR Medical Informatics, 4*(4), e5359. doi:10.2196/medinform.5359 PMID:27872036

Kumar, N., & Kumar, H. (2021). A novel hybrid fuzzy time series model for prediction of COVID-19 infected cases and deaths in India. *ISA Transactions.* Advance online publication. doi:10.1016/j.isatra.2021.07.003 PMID:34253340

Kumar, N., & Susan, S. (2021). Particle swarm optimization of partitions and fuzzy order for fuzzy time series forecasting of COVID-19. *Applied Soft Computing*, *110*, 107611. doi:10.1016/j.asoc.2021.107611 PMID:34518764

Kumar, P., Porambage, P., Ylianttila, M., Gurtov, A., Lee, H. J., & Sain, M. (2014). Addressing a Secure Session- Key Scheme for Mobility Supported e-Healthcare Systems. *16th International Conference on Advanced Communication Technology*. 10.1109/ICACT.2014.6779018

Kwon, G., Han, C., & Kim, D. (2019). Generation of 3D Brain MRI Using Auto-Encoding Generative Adversarial Networks. Lecture Notes in Computer Science (Including Subseries Lecture Notes in Artificial Intelligence and Lecture Notes in Bioinformatics), 11766 LNCS, 118–126. doi:10.1007/978-3-030-32248-9_14

Labati, R. D., Muñoz, E., Piuri, V., Sassi, R., & Scotti, F. (2019). Deep-ECG: Convolutional neural networks for ECG biometric recognition. *Pattern Recognition Letters*, *126*, 78–85.

Lamine, E., Guédria, W., Rius Soler, A., Ayza Graells, J., Fontanili, F., Janer-García, L., & Pingaud, H. (2017). An Inventory of Interoperability in Healthcare Ecosystems: Characterization and Challenges. *Enterprise Interoperability: INTEROP-PGSO Vision*, *1*, 167–198. doi:10.1002/9781119407928.ch9

Landrigan, C. P., Rothschild, J. M., Cronin, J. W., Kaushal, R., Burdick, E., Katz, J. T., Lilly, C. M., Stone, P. H., Lockley, S. W., Bates, D. W., & Czeisler, C. A. (2004). Effect of reducing interns' work hours on serious medical errors in intensive care units. *The New England Journal of Medicine*, *351*(18), 1838–1848. doi:10.1056/NEJMoa041406 PMID:15509817

Laney, D. (2001). 3D data management: Controlling data volume, velocity and variety. *META Group Research Note, 6*(70), 1.

Larochelle, H., Mandel, M., Pascanu, R., & Bengio, Y. (2012). Learning algorithms for the classification restricted Boltzmann machine. *Journal of Machine Learning Research*, *13*(1), 643–669.

Latonero, M. (2018, Oct.). Governing artificial intelligence: Upholding human rights & dignity. *Data & Society*.

Laudon, K. C., & Laudon, J. P. (2011). *Essentials of management information systems*. Academic Press.

Le Gall, J.-R., Lemeshow, S., & Saulnier, F. (1993). A new Simplified Acute Physiology Score (SAPS II) based on a European/North American multicenter study. *Journal of the American Medical Association*, *270*(24), 2957–2963. doi:10.1001/jama.1993.03510240069035 PMID:8254858

LeCun, Y., & Bengio, Y. (1995). Convolutional networks for images, speech, and time series. The handbook of brain theory and neural networks, 3361(10).

Lee, P. (n.d.). *Design Research: What Is It and Why Do It?* Available: https://reboot.org/2012/02/19/design-research-what-is-it-and-why-do-it/

Lee, C., Kim, J. M., Kim, Y. S., & Shin, E. (2019). The Effect of Diagnosis-Related Groups on the Shift of Medical Services From Inpatient to Outpatient Settings: A National Claims-Based Analysis. *Asia-Pacific Journal of Public Health*, *31*(6), 499–509. doi:10.1177/1010539519872325 PMID:31516035

Lee, S., Kim, H., & Lee, S. W. (2013). Security Concerns of Identity Authentication and Context Privacy Preservation in u Healthcare System. *14th ACIS International Conference on Software Engineering, Artificial Intelligence, Networking and Parallel/Distributed Computing (SNPD)*.

Leijdekkers, P., & Gay, V. (2006). Personal Heart Monitoring and Rehabilitation System using Smart Phones. *Int. Conf. on Mobile Business (ICMB '06)*. 10.1109/ICMB.2006.39

Leon, L. I. R., & Mayrin, J. V. (2020). *Polycystic Ovarian Disease*. StatPearls.

Lewis, J., & Fowler, M. (2014, March 25). *Microservices*. https://martinfowler.com/articles/microservices.html

Lih, O. S., Jahmunah, V., San, T. R., Ciaccio, E. J., Yamakawa, T., Tanabe, M., ... Acharya, U. R. (2020). Comprehensive electrocardiographic diagnosis based on deep learning. *Artificial Intelligence in Medicine*, *103*, 101789.

Li, M., Lou, W., & Ren, K. (2010). Data Security and Privacy in Wireless Body Area Networks. *IEEE Wireless Communications*, *17*(1), 51–58. doi:10.1109/MWC.2010.5416350

Lim, S., Oh, T. W., & Choi, Y. D. (2010). Tamil Lakshman, Security Issues on Wireless Body Area Network for Remote Healthcare Monitoring. *IEEE International Conference on Sensor Networks, Ubiquitous, and Trustworthy Computing (SUTC)*.

Liu, M., & Kim, Y. (2018, July). Classification of heart diseases based on ECG signals using long short-term memory. In *2018 40th Annual International Conference of the IEEE Engineering in Medicine and Biology Society (EMBC)* (pp. 2707-2710). IEEE.

Liu, J., Chang, H., Forrest, J. Y. L., & Yang, B. (2020). Influence of artificial intelligence on technological innovation: Evidence from the panel data of china's manufacturing sectors. *Technological Forecasting and Social Change*, *158*, 120142. doi:10.1016/j.techfore.2020.120142

Liu, X., Wang, H., Li, Z., & Qin, L. (2021). Deep learning in ECG diagnosis: A review. *Knowledge-Based Systems*, *227*, 107187.

Li, Y., Pang, Y., Wang, J., & Li, X. (2018). Patient-specific ECG classification by deeper CNN from generic to dedicated. *Neurocomputing*, *314*, 336–346.

Li, Z., Wang, Y., & Yu, J. (2017). Reconstruction of thin-slice medical images using generative adversarial network. *International Workshop on Machine Learning in Medical Imaging*, 325–333. 10.1007/978-3-319-67389-9_38

Loshchilov, I., & Hutter, F. (2019). Decoupled weight decay regularization. *7th International Conference on Learning Representations, ICLR 2019*.

Lown, B., Klein, M. D., & Hershberg, P. I. (1969). Coronary and precoronary care. *The American Journal of Medicine*, *46*(5), 705–724.

Lukasiewicz, J. (1920). On 3-valued Logic. In Polish Logic. Oxford U.P.

Luo, J., & Huang, J. (2019). Generative adversarial network: An overview. *Yi Qi Yi Biao Xue Bao. Yiqi Yibiao Xuebao*, *40*(3), 74–84. doi:10.19650/j.cnki.cjsi.J1804413

Luo, K., Li, J., Wang, Z., & Cuschieri, A. (2017). Patient-specific deep architectural model for ECG classification. *Journal of Healthcare Engineering*.

Ly, K. T. (2021). A COVID-19 forecasting system using adaptive neuro-fuzzy inference. *Finance Research Letters*, *41*, 101844. doi:10.1016/j.frl.2020.101844 PMID:34131413

Magalhães, R., Barrière, D. A., Novais, A., Marques, F., Marques, P., Cerqueira, J., Sousa, J. C., Cachia, A., Boumezbeur, F., Bottlaender, M., Jay, T. M., Mériaux, S., & Sousa, N. (2018). The dynamics of stress: A longitudinal MRI study of rat brain structure and connectome. *Molecular Psychiatry*, *23*(10), 1998–2006. doi:10.1038/mp.2017.244 PMID:29203852

Mahmoudi, M. R., Baleanu, D., Mansor, Z., Tuan, B. A., & Pho, K. H. (2020). Fuzzy clustering method to compare the spread rate of Covid-19 in the high risks countries. *Chaos, Solitons, and Fractals*, *140*, 110230. doi:10.1016/j.chaos.2020.110230 PMID:32863611

Majumder, S., Kar, S., & Samanta, E. (2020). A fuzzy rough hybrid decision making technique for identifying the infected population of COVID-19. *Soft Computing*, 1–11. PMID:33250663

Makhzani, A., & Frey, B. (2013). *K-sparse autoencoders*. arXiv preprint arXiv:1312.5663.

Maksimovic, Z. (2017). *MongoDB 3 Succinctly*. Syncfusion Inc. https://s3.amazonaws.com/ebooks.syncfusion.com/downloads/MongoDB_3_Succinctly/MongoDB_3_Succinctly.pdf

Maltese, F., Adda, M., Bablon, A., Hraeich, S., Guervilly, C., Lehingue, S., Wiramus, S., Leone, M., Martin, C., Vialet, R., Thirion, X., Roch, A., Forel, J. M., & Papazian, L. (2016). Night shift decreases cognitive performance of ICU physicians. *Intensive Care Medicine*, *42*(3), 393–400. doi:10.100700134-015-4115-4 PMID:26556616

Mamdani, E. H., & Assilian, S. (1975). An experiment in linguistic synthesis with a fuzzy logic controller. *International Journal of Man-Machine Studies*, *7*(1), 1–13. doi:10.1016/S0020-7373(75)80002-2

Mangla, M., Sharma, N., & Mittal, P. (2021). A fuzzy expert system for predicting the mortality of COVID'19. *Turkish Journal of Electrical Engineering and Computer Sciences*, *29*(3), 1628–1642. doi:10.3906/elk-2008-27

Manigandan, S., Wu, M. T., Ponnusamy, V. K., Raghavendra, V. B., Pugazhendhi, A., & Brindhadevi, K. (2020). A systematic review on recent trends in transmission, diagnosis, prevention and imaging features of COVID-19. *Process Biochemistry*.

Marks, H. M. (2000). The Progress of Experiment: Science and Therapeutic Reform in the United States, 1900–1990. In Cambridge History of Medicine. Cambridge Univ. Press.

Martínez-Costa, C., Menárguez-Tortosa, M., & Fernández-Breis, J. T. (2010). An approach for the semantic interoperability of ISO EN 13606 and OpenEHR archetypes. *Journal of Biomedical Informatics*, *43*(5), 736–746. doi:10.1016/j.jbi.2010.05.013 PMID:20561912

Martins, B., Ferreira, D., Neto, C., Abelha, A., & Machado, J. (2021). Data Mining for Cardiovascular Disease Prediction. *Journal of Medical Systems*, *45*(1), 1–8. doi:10.100710916-020-01682-8 PMID:33404894

Marty, A. T. (1996). Textbook of Critical Care. *Critical Care Medicine*, *24*(5), 901–902. doi:10.1097/00003246-199605000-00039

Mathieu, M., Couprie, C., & LeCun, Y. (2016). Deep multi-scale video prediction beyond mean square error. *4th International Conference on Learning Representations, ICLR 2016 - Conference Track Proceedings, 2015*, 1–14.

Matteo, B. (2017). Electronic health (e-health): Emerging role in Asthma. *Current Opinion in Pulmonary Medicine*, *23*(1), 21–26. doi:10.1097/MCP.0000000000000336 PMID:27763999

Ma, Y., Smith, D., Hof, P. R., Foerster, B., Hamilton, S., Blackband, S. J., Yu, M., & Benveniste, H. (2008). In vivo 3D digital atlas database of the adult C57BL/6J mouse brain by magnetic resonance microscopy. *Frontiers in Neuroanatomy*, *2*(APR), 1–10. doi:10.3389/neuro.05.001.2008 PMID:18958199

McDonald, C. J. (1997). The barriers to electronic medical record systems and how to overcome them. *Journal of the American Medical Informatics Association: JAMIA*, *4*(3), 213–221. doi:10.1136/jamia.1997.0040213 PMID:9147340

Melin, P., Sánchez, D., Monica, J. C., & Castillo, O. (2021). Optimization using the firefly algorithm of ensemble neural networks with type-2 fuzzy integration for COVID-19 time series prediction. *Soft Computing*, 1–38. doi:10.100700500-020-05549-5 PMID:33456340

Mian, M., Teredesai, A., Hazel, D., Pokuri, S., & Uppala, K. (2014). In-Memory Analysis for Healthcare Big Data. *IEEE International Congress on Big Data*.

Mijwel, M. M. (2018). *Artificial neural networks advantages and disadvantages*. Retrieved from LinkedIn https//www. linkedin. com/pulse/artificial-neuralnet Work

Mills, R. E., Butler, R. R., McCullough, E. C., Bao, M. Z., & Averill, R. F. (2011). Impact of the transition to ICD-10 on medicare inpatient hospital payments. *Medicare & Medicaid Research Review*, *1*(2), 1–13. doi:10.5600/mmrr.001.02.a02 PMID:22340773

Minematsu, T., Shimada, A., Uchiyama, H., & Taniguchi, R. I. (2018). Analytics of deep neural network-based background subtraction. *Journal of Imaging*, *4*(6), 78.

Min, S., Lee, B., & Yoon, S. (2017). Deep learning in bioinformatics. *Briefings in Bioinformatics*, *18*(5), 851–869.

Miranda, M., Duarte, J., Abelha, A., Machado, J. M., & Neves, J. (2009). *Interoperability and healthcare*. Academic Press.

Miranda, M., Salazar, M., Portela, F., Santos, M., Abelha, A., Neves, J., & Machado, J. (2012). Multi-agent systems for hl7 interoperability services. *Procedia Technology*, *5*, 725–733. doi:10.1016/j.protcy.2012.09.080

Mishra, A. R., Rani, P., Krishankumar, R., Ravichandran, K. S., & Kar, S. (2021). An extended fuzzy decision-making framework using hesitant fuzzy sets for the drug selection to treat the mild symptoms of Coronavirus Disease 2019 (COVID-19). *Applied Soft Computing*, *103*, 107155. doi:10.1016/j.asoc.2021.107155 PMID:33568967

Miyato, T., Kataoka, T., Koyama, M., & Yoshida, Y. (2018). Spectral normalization for generative adversarial networks. *6th International Conference on Learning Representations, ICLR 2018 - Conference Track Proceedings*.

Mnih, V., Larochelle, H., & Hinton, G. E. (2012). *Conditional restricted boltzmann machines for structured output prediction*. arXiv preprint arXiv:1202.3748.

Moher, D., Liberati, A., Tetzlaff, J., & Altman, D. G. (2009). Preferred reporting items for systematic reviews and meta-analyses: The PRISMA statement. *PLoS Medicine*, *6*(7), e1000097. doi:10.1371/journal.pmed.1000097 PMID:19621072

Monge García, M. I., Santos, A., Diez Del Corral, B., Guijo González, P., Gracia Romero, M., Gil Cano, A., & Cecconi, M. (2018). Noradrenaline modifies arterial reflection phenomena and left ventricular efficiency in septic shock patients: A prospective observational study. *Journal of Critical Care*, *47*, 280–286. doi:10.1016/j.jcrc.2018.07.027 PMID:30096635

MongoDB - Overview. (n.d.). *Tutorials Point*. https://www.tutorialspoint.com/mongodb/mongodb_overview.htm

Moody, G. B., & Mark, R. G. (1996). A Database to Support Development and Evaluation of Intelligent Intensive Care Monitoring. *Computers in Cardiology*, *23*, 657–660.

Moody, G. B., & Mark, R. G. (2001). The impact of the MIT-BIH arrhythmia database. *IEEE Engineering in Medicine and Biology Magazine*, *20*(3), 45–50. doi:10.1109/51.932724 PMID:11446209

Moreno-Conde, A., Moner, D., da Cruz, W. D., Santos, M. R., Maldonado, J. A., Robles, M., & Kalra, D. (2015). Clinical information modeling processes for semantic interoperability of electronic health records: Systematic review and inductive analysis. *Journal of the American Medical Informatics Association: JAMIA*, *22*(4), 925–934. doi:10.1093/jamia/ocv008 PMID:25796595

Mosa, A. S. M., Yoo, I., & Sheets, L. (2012). A Systematic Review of Healthcare Applications for Smartphones. *BMC Medical Informatics and Decision Making*, *12*(1). https://doi.org/10.1186/1472-6947-12-67

Murat, F., Yildirim, O., Talo, M., Baloglu, U. B., Demir, Y., & Acharya, U. R. (2020). Application of deep learning techniques for heartbeats detection using ECG signals-analysis and review. *Computers in Biology and Medicine*, *120*, 103726.

Murat, F., Yildirim, O., Talo, M., Demir, Y., Tan, R. S., Ciaccio, E. J., & Acharya, U. R. (2021). Exploring deep features and ECG attributes to detect cardiac rhythm classes. *Knowledge-Based Systems*, *232*, 107473.

Murdoch, T. B., & Detsky, A. S. (2013). The Inevitable Application of Big Data to Health Care. *Journal of the American Medical Association*, *309*(13), 1351. doi:10.1001/jama.2013.393 PMID:23549579

Mydukuri, R. V., Kallam, S., Patan, R., Al-Turjman, F., & Ramachandran, M. (2021). Deming least square regressed feature selection and Gaussian neuro-fuzzy multi-layered data classifier for early COVID prediction. *Expert Systems: International Journal of Knowledge Engineering and Neural Networks*, 12694. doi:10.1111/exsy.12694 PMID:34230740

Myles, A. J., Feudale, R. N., Liu, Y., Woody, N. A., & Brown, S. D. (2004). An introduction to decision tree modeling. *Journal of Chemometrics: A Journal of the Chemometrics Society*, *18*(6), 275-285.

Nalepa, J., Marcinkiewicz, M., & Kawulok, M. (2019). Data Augmentation for Brain-Tumor Segmentation: A Review. *Frontiers in Computational Neuroscience*, *13*(December), 1–18. doi:10.3389/fncom.2019.00083 PMID:31920608

Narkhede, N., Shapira, G., & Palino, T. (2017). *Kafka: The definitive guide: Real-time data and stream processing at scale*. O'Reilly Media.

Natarajan, P., Krishnan, N., Kenkre, N. S., Nancy, S., & Singh, B. P. (2012). Tumor detection using threshold operation in MRI brain images. *2012 IEEE International Conference on Computational Intelligence and Computing Research, ICCIC 2012*. 10.1109/ICCIC.2012.6510299

Nauck, D., Klawonn, F., & Kruse, R. (1997). *Foundations of Neuro-Fuzzy Systems*. John Wiley & Sons, Inc.

Neto, C., Brito, M., Lopes, V., Peixoto, H., Abelha, A., & Machado, J. (2019). Application of data mining for the prediction of mortality and occurrence of complications for gastric cancer patients. *Entropy (Basel, Switzerland)*, *21*(12), 1163. doi:10.3390/e21121163

Neto, C., Peixoto, H., Abelha, V., Abelha, A., & Machado, J. (2017). Knowledge discovery from surgical waiting lists. *Procedia Computer Science*, *121*, 1104–1111. doi:10.1016/j.procs.2017.11.141

Neves, J. (1984). A logic interpreter to handle time and negation in logic databases. In R. Muller, & J. Pottmyer (Eds.), *Proceedings of the 1984 annual conference of the ACM on the 5th Generation Challenge* (pp. 50–54). Association for Computing Machinery. 10.1145/800171.809603

Neves, J., Maia, N., Marreiros, G., Neves, M., Fernandes, A., Ribeiro, J., Araújo, I., Araújo, N., Ávidos, L., Ferraz, F., Capita, A., Lori, N., Alves, V., & Vicente, H. (2019). Entropy and Organizational Performance. In H. Pérez García, L. Sánchez González, M. Castejón Limas, H. Quintián Pardo, & E. Corchado Rodríguez (Eds.), Lecture Notes in Computer Science: Vol. 11734. *Hybrid Artificial Intelligent Systems* (pp. 206–217). Springer. doi:10.1007/978-3-030-29859-3_18

Neves, J., Maia, N., Marreiros, G., Neves, M., Fernandes, A., Ribeiro, J., Araújo, I., Araújo, N., Ávidos, L., Ferraz, F., Capita, A., Lori, N., Alves, V., & Vicente, H. (2021). Employees Balance and Stability as Key Points in Organizational Performance. *Logic Journal of the IGPL*, jzab010. Advance online publication. doi:10.1093/jigpal/jzab010

Neves, J., Vicente, H., Esteves, M., Ferraz, F., Abelha, A., Machado, J., Machado, J., Neves, J., Ribeiro, J., & Sampaio, L. (2018). A deep-big data approach to health care in the AI age. *Mobile Networks and Applications*, *23*(4), 1123–1128. doi:10.100711036-018-1071-6

Newman, A. (2020, September 30). *Is your microservice a distributed monolith?* Gremelin. https://www.gremlin.com/blog/is-your-microservice-a-distributed-monolith/

Niemeijer, M., Abràmoff, M. D., & van Ginneken, B. (2006). Image structure clustering for image quality verification of color retina images in diabetic retinopathy screening. *Medical Image Analysis*, *10*(6), 888–898. doi:10.1016/j.media.2006.09.006 PMID:17138215

NITRD (Networking and Information Technology Research and Development), National Coordination Office (NC), & National Science Foundation. (2019). Notice of Workshop on Artificial Intelligence & Wireless Spectrum: Opportunities and Challenges. Notice of workshop. *Federal Register*, *84*(145), 36625–36626.

Noble, R., & Nobilia, F. (2019, May 14). *One Key to Rule them All*. Confluent Kafka Summit London 2019. https://www.confluent.io/kafka-summit-lon19/one-key-to-rule-them-all/

Nurmaini, S., Darmawahyuni, A., Sakti Mukti, A. N., Rachmatullah, M. N., Firdaus, F., & Tutuko, B. (2020). Deep learning-based stacked denoising and autoencoder for ECG heartbeat classification. *Electronics (Basel)*, *9*(1), 135.

Ohri, A. (2021, March 19). *Types Of Big Data: Simplified*. Jigsaw Academy. https://www.jigsawacademy.com/blogs/big-data-analytics/types-of-big-data#Semi-Structured-Data

Pandey, P., & Litoriya, R. (2020). Securing E-health Networks from Counterfeit Medicine Penetration Using Blockchain. *Wireless Personal Communications*, *117*(1), 7–25. https://doi.org/10.1007/s11277-020-07041-7

Panganiban, E. B., Paglinawan, A. C., Chung, W. Y., & Paa, G. L. S. (2021). ECG diagnostic support system (EDSS): A deep learning neural network based classification system for detecting ECG abnormal rhythms from a low-powered wearable biosensors. *Sensing and Bio-Sensing Research*, *31*, 100398.

Compilation of References

Parsazadeh, N., Ali, R., & Rezaei, M. (2018). A framework for cooperative and interactive mobile learning to improve online information evaluation skills. *Computers & Education*, *120*, 75–89. doi:10.1016/j.compedu.2018.01.010

Peixoto, H., Guimarães, T., & Santos, M. F. (2020). A New Architecture for Intelligent Clinical Decision Support for Intensive Medicine. *Procedia Computer Science*, *170*, 1035–1040. https://doi.org/10.1016/j.procs.2020.03.077

Penedo, J., Ribeiro, A., Lopes, H., Pimentel, J., Pedrosa, J., Vasconcelos e Sá, R., & Moreno, R. (2013). Avaliação da Situação Nacional das Unidades de Cuidados Intensivos. In *SNS - Serviço Nacional de Saúde*. Governo de Portugal, Ministério da Saúde. https://www.sns.gov.pt/wp-content/uploads/2016/05/Avalia%C3%A7%C3%A3o-nacional-da-situa%C3%A7%C3%A3o-das-unidades-de-cuidados-intensivos.pdf

Peng, C. Y. J., Lee, K. L., & Ingersoll, G. M. (2002). An introduction to logistic regression analysis and reporting. *The Journal of Educational Research*, *96*(1), 3–14. doi:10.1080/00220670209598786

Pereira, J. (2005). *Modelos de Data Mining para multi-previsão: aplicação à medicina intensiva*. Academic Press.

Pereira, A., Marins, F., Rodrigues, B., Portela, F., Santos, M. F., Machado, J., Rua, F., Silva, Á., & Abelha, A. (2015). Improving quality of medical service with mobile health software. *Procedia Computer Science*, *63*, 292–299. doi:10.1016/j.procs.2015.08.346

Pereira, R., Duarte, J., Salazar, M., Santos, M., Abelha, A., & Machado, J. (2012). Usability of an electronic health record. *2012 IEEE International Conference on Industrial Engineering and Engineering Management*, 1568–1572. 10.1109/IEEM.2012.6838010

Pereira, R., Salazar, M., Abelha, A., & Machado, J. (2013). SWOT analysis of a Portuguese Electronic Health Record. *IFIP Advances in Information and Communication Technology*, *399*, 169–177. doi:10.1007/978-3-642-37437-1_14

Pham, Q. V., Nguyen, D. C., Huynh-The, T., Hwang, W. J., & Pathirana, P. N. (2020). *Artificial intelligence (AI) and big data for coronavirus (COVID-19) pandemic: A survey on the state-of-the-arts*. Academic Press.

Pharmaceuticals in the environment: a growing problem. (2015). *The Pharmaceutical Journal*. doi:10.1211/PJ.2015.20067898

Pinter, G., Felde, I., Mosavi, A., Ghamisi, P., & Gloaguen, R. (2020). COVID-19 pandemic prediction for Hungary; a hybrid machine learning approach. *Mathematics*, *8*(6), 890. doi:10.3390/math8060890

Pipberger, H. V., Arms, R. J., & Stallmann, F. W. (1961). Automatic Screening of Normal and Abnormal Electrocardiograms by Means of a Digital Electronic Computer. *Proceedings of the Society for Experimental Biology and Medicine*, *106*(1), 130–132.

Portalcodgh. (n.d.). Available: http://portalcodgdh.min-saude.pt/images/2/2e/CodificacaoClinica%25%0D26DesempenhoHospitalar.pdf

Portela, F., Gago, P., Santos, M. F., Machado, J., Abelha, A., Silva, Á., & Rua, F. (2013). Implementing a pervasive real-time intelligent system for tracking critical events with intensive care patients. *International Journal of Healthcare Information Systems and Informatics*, *8*(4), 1–16. doi:10.4018/ijhisi.2013100101

Prabakaran, G., Vaithiyanathan, D., & Kumar, H. (2021). *Fuzzy Decision Support System for the Outbreak of COVID-19 and Improving the People Livelihood*. Academic Press.

Prabhu, V., Kannan, A., Ravuri, M., Chablani, M., Sontag, D., Amatriain, X., & Tech, G. (2019). Few-Shot Learning for Dermatological Disease Diagnosis. *Proceedings of Machine Learning Research*, *106*(Icd), 1–15. http://www.dermnet.com/

Pramanik, P. K. D., & Choudhury, P. (2018). IoT Data Processing: The Different Archetypes and their Security & Privacy Assessments. In *Internet of Things (IoT) Security: Fundamentals, Techniques and Applications*. River Publishers. doi:10.4018/978-1-5225-4044-1.ch007

Pranckevičius, T., & Marcinkevičius, V. (2017). Comparison of naive bayes, random forest, decision tree, support vector machines, and logistic regression classifiers for text reviews classification. *Baltic Journal of Modern Computing*, *5*(2), 221. doi:10.22364/bjmc.2017.5.2.05

Radford, A., Metz, L., & Chintala, S. (2016). Unsupervised representation learning with deep convolutional generative adversarial networks. *4th International Conference on Learning Representations, ICLR 2016 - Conference Track Proceedings*, 1–16.

Radhakrishnan, T., Karhade, J., Ghosh, S. K., Muduli, P. R., Tripathy, R. K., & Acharya, U. R. (2021). AFCNNet: Automated detection of AF using chirplet transform and deep convolutional bidirectional long short term memory network with ECG signals. *Computers in Biology and Medicine*, *137*, 104783.

Raghupathi, W., & Raghupathi, V. (2014). Big data analytics in healthcare: Promise and potential. *Health Information Science and Systems*, *2*(1), 1–10. doi:10.1186/2047-2501-2-3 PMID:25825667

Rahul, J., & Sharma, L. D. (2022). Artificial intelligence-based approach for atrial fibrillation detection using normalised and short-duration time-frequency ECG. *Biomedical Signal Processing and Control*, *71*, 103270.

Rahul, J., Sora, M., & Sharma, L. D. (2021). Dynamic thresholding based efficient QRS complex detection with low computational overhead. *Biomedical Signal Processing and Control*, *67*, 102519.

Rahul, J., Sora, M., Sharma, L. D., & Bohat, V. K. (2021). An improved cardiac arrhythmia classification using an RR interval-based approach. *Biocybernetics and Biomedical Engineering*, *41*(2), 656–666.

Rahul, K. K. (2016). Mobile and E-Health care; recent trends and future directions. *Journal of Health & Medical Economics*, *10*, 1–10.

Rajalakshmi, K., Chandra Mohan, S., & Babu, S. D. (2011). Decision Support System in Healthcare Industry. *International Journal of Computers and Applications*, *26*(9), 42–44. doi:10.5120/3129-4310

Rallapalli, S., Aggarwal, S., & Singh, A. P. (2021). Detecting SARS-CoV-2 RNA prone clusters in a municipal wastewater network using fuzzy-Bayesian optimization model to facilitate wastewater-based epidemiology. *The Science of the Total Environment, 778*, 146294. doi:10.1016/j.scitotenv.2021.146294 PMID:33714094

Ramaraj, E. (2021). A novel deep learning based gated recurrent unit with extreme learning machine for electrocardiogram (ECG) signal recognition. *Biomedical Signal Processing and Control, 68*, 102779.

Ramon, J., Fierens, D., Güiza, F., Meyfroidt, G., Blockeel, H., Bruynooghe, M., & Van Den Berghe, G. (2007). Mining data from intensive care patients. *Advanced Engineering Informatics, 21*(3), 243–256. doi:10.1016/j.aei.2006.12.002

Rangayyan, R. M. (2015). *Biomedical signal analysis*. John Wiley & Sons.

Rasti-Meymandi, A., & Ghaffari, A. (2022). A deep learning-based framework For ECG signal denoising based on stacked cardiac cycle tensor. *Biomedical Signal Processing and Control, 71*, 103275.

Rathore, B., & Gupta, R. (2021). A fuzzy based hybrid decision-making framework to examine the safety risk factors of healthcare workers during COVID-19 outbreak. *Journal of Decision Systems*, 1–34.

Razavi-Termeh, S. V., Sadeghi-Niaraki, A., & Choi, S. M. (2021). Coronavirus disease vulnerability map using a geographic information system (GIS) from 16 April to 16 May 2020. *Physics and Chemistry of the Earth, Parts A/B/C*, 103043.

Reid, J. A., & Kenny, G. N. C. (1984). Data collection in the intensive care unit. *Journal of Microcomputer Applications, 7*(3), 257–269. doi:10.1016/0745-7138(84)90058-7

Rezende, D. J., Mohamed, S., & Wierstra, D. (2014). Stochastic backpropagation and approximate inference in deep generative models. *31st International Conference on Machine Learning, ICML 2014, 4*, 3057–3070.

Richardson, C., & Smith, F. (2016). *Microservices From Design to Deployment*. NGINX, Inc. https://www.nginx.com/resources/library/designing-deploying-microservices/

Rish, I. (2001, August). An empirical study of the naive Bayes classifier. In IJCAI 2001 workshop on empirical methods in artificial intelligence (Vol. 3, No. 22, pp. 41-46). Academic Press.

Rivers, P. A., & Glover, S. H. (2008b). Health care competition, strategic mission, and patient satisfaction: Research model and propositions. *Journal of Health Organization and Management, 22*(6), 627–641. doi:10.1108/14777260810916597 PMID:19579575

Robinson, J. A. (1965). A Machine-Oriented Logic Based on the Resolution Principle. *Journal of the Association for Computing Machinery, 12*(1), 23–41. doi:10.1145/321250.321253

Roca, S., Sancho, J., García, J., & Alesanco, Á. (2020). Microservice chatbot architecture for chronic patient support. *Journal of Biomedical Informatics, 102*, 103305.

Rodrigues, M. F. (2018). *Brain Semantic Segmentation: A DL approach in Human and Rat MRI studies.* http://hdl.handle.net/1822/64177

Rodrigues. (2013). *Interoperabilidade na Saúde - Onde Estamos?* Academic Press.

Rosca, M., Lakshminarayanan, B., Warde-Farley, D., & Mohamed, S. (2017). *Variational Approaches for Auto-Encoding Generative Adversarial Networks.* https://arxiv.org/abs/1706.04987

Russell, W. M. S., & Burch, R. L. (1959). *The principles of humane experimental technique.* Methuen.

Saadatnejad, S., Oveisi, M., & Hashemi, M. (2019). LSTM-based ECG classification for continuous monitoring on personal wearable devices. *IEEE Journal of Biomedical and Health Informatics, 24*(2), 515–523.

Sadegh-Zadeh, K. (2015). Clinical Decision Support Systems. In Philosophy and Medicine (Vol. 119). doi:10.1007/978-94-017-9579-1_20

Saif, S., Das, P., & Biswas, S. (2021). *A Hybrid Model based on mBA-ANFIS for COVID-19 Confirmed Cases Prediction and Forecast. Journal of The Institution of Engineers. Series B.*

Samanlioglu, F., & Kaya, B. E. (2020). Evaluation of the COVID-19 pandemic intervention strategies with hesitant F-AHP. *Journal of Healthcare Engineering.* doi:10.1155/2020/8835258 PMID:32850105

Samsudin, M. R., Sulaiman, R., Guan, T. T., Yusof, A. M., & Yaacob, M. F. C. (2021). Mobile Application Development Trough ADDIE Model. *International Journal of Academic Research in Progressive Education and Development, 10*(2), 1017–1027.

Sánchez, I., & Vilaplana, V. (2018). Brain MRI super-resolution using 3D generative adversarial networks. *ArXiv, Midl,* 1–8.

Sandesh, A., (2019). What is E-health, its characteristics, benefits and challenges, global health. *Public Health Notes, 5,* 1-10.

Sanjaya, H. (2020, March 11). *Monolith vs Microservices.* Hengky Sanjaya Blog. https://medium.com/hengky-sanjaya-blog/monolith-vs-microservices-b3953650dfd

Santos, M. F., Portela, F., Vilas-Boas, M., Machado, J., Abelha, A., Neves, J., Silva, A., & Rua, F. (2009). Information architecture for intelligent decision support in intensive medicine. *WSEAS Transactions on Computers, 8*(5), 810–819.

Santos, M. Y., & Costa, C. (2020). *Big data: concepts, warehousing, and analytics.* River Publishers.

Saripalle, R., Runyan, C., & Russell, M. (2019). Using HL7 FHIR to achieve interoperability in patient health record. *Journal of Biomedical Informatics, 94,* 103188.

Satish, C. N., Chew, X., & Khaw, K. W. (2020). *Polycystic Ovarian Syndrome (PCOS) classification and feature selection by machine learning techniques.* Academic Press.

Savalia, S., & Emamian, V. (2018). Cardiac arrhythmia classification by multi-layer perceptron and convolution neural networks. *Bioengineering (Basel, Switzerland)*, 5(2), 35.

Sawand, A., Djahel, S., Zhang, Z., & Naıt-Abdessela, F. (2014). Multidisciplinary Approaches to Achieving Efficient and Trustworthy eHealth Monitoring Systems. *International Conference on Communications in China (ICCC)*. 10.1109/ICCChina.2014.7008269

Sax, M. J. (2018). Apache Kafka. *Encyclopedia of Big Data Technologies*, 1–8. doi:10.1007/978-3-319-63962-8_196-1

Sayan, M., Sarigul Yildirim, F., Sanlidag, T., Uzun, B., Uzun Ozsahin, D., & Ozsahin, I. (2020). Capacity evaluation of diagnostic tests for COVID-19 using multicriteria decision-making techniques. *Computational and Mathematical Methods in Medicine*. doi:10.1155/2020/1560250 PMID:32802146

Scaling Horizontally vs. Scaling Vertically. (2020, July 24). *Section*. https://www.section.io/blog/scaling-horizontally-vs-vertically/

Schaffer, C. (1993). Selecting a classification method by cross-validation. *Machine Learning*, 13(1), 135–143.

Schmidt, B. (2006). Proof of principle studies. *Epilepsy Research*, 68(1), 48–52. doi:10.1016/j.eplepsyres.2005.09.019 PMID:16377153

Schuster, M., & Paliwal, K. K. (1997). Bidirectional recurrent neural networks. *IEEE Transactions on Signal Processing*, 45(11), 2673–2681.

Scikit-learn. (2021). *feature_selection: f_classif*. Available at: https://scikit-learn.org/stable/modules/generated/sklearn.feature_selection.f_classif.html

Sergey, A. B., Alexandr, D. B., & Sergey, A. T. (2015). Proof of Concept Center— A Promising Tool for Innovative Development at Entrepreneurial Universities. *Procedia: Social and Behavioral Sciences*, 166, 240–245. doi:10.1016/j.sbspro.2014.12.518

Shah, S. (2016, February 18). *Why patient engagement is so challenging to achieve*. Retrieved August 2, 2018, from https://www.ibmbigdatahub.com/blog/why-patient-engagement-so-challenging-achieve

Shaker, A. M., Tantawi, M., Shedeed, H. A., & Tolba, M. F. (2020). Generalization of Convolutional Neural Networks for ECG Classification Using Generative Adversarial Networks. *IEEE Access: Practical Innovations, Open Solutions*, 8, 35592–35605. doi:10.1109/ACCESS.2020.2974712

Sharma, L. D., & Sunkaria, R. K. (2018a). Stationary wavelet transform based technique for automated external defibrillator using optimally selected classifiers. *Measurement*, 125, 29–36.

Sharma, L. D., & Sunkaria, R. K. (2018b). Inferior myocardial infarction detection using stationary wavelet transform and machine learning approach. *Signal, Image and Video Processing*, 12(2), 199–206.

Sharma, L. D., & Sunkaria, R. K. (2020). Myocardial infarction detection and localization using optimal features based lead specific approach. *IRBM*, *41*(1), 58–70.

Sharma, M. K., Dhiman, N., & Mishra, V. N. (2021). Mediative fuzzy logic mathematical model: A contradictory management prediction in COVID-19 pandemic. *Applied Soft Computing*, *105*, 107285. doi:10.1016/j.asoc.2021.107285 PMID:33723486

Shin, H.-C., Tenenholtz, N. A., Rogers, J. K., Schwarz, C. G., Senjem, M. L., Gunter, J. L., Andriole, K. P., & Michalski, M. (2018). Medical image synthesis for data augmentation and anonymization using generative adversarial networks. *International Workshop on Simulation and Synthesis in Medical Imaging*, 1–11. 10.1007/978-3-030-00536-8_1

Silva, Á., Cortez, P., Santos, M. F., Gomes, L., & Neves, J. (2008). Rating organ failure via adverse events using data mining in the intensive care unit. *Artificial Intelligence in Medicine*, *43*(3), 179–193. doi:10.1016/j.artmed.2008.03.010 PMID:18486459

Silva, C., Oliveira, D., Peixoto, H., Machado, J., & Abelha, A. (2018, May). Data mining for prediction of length of stay of cardiovascular accident inpatients. In *International Conference on Digital Transformation and Global Society* (pp. 516-527). Springer. 10.1007/978-3-030-02843-5_43

Simonyan, K., & Zisserman, A. (2014). *Very deep convolutional networks for large-scale image recognition*. arXiv preprint arXiv:1409.1556.

Smith, L. N. (2017). Cyclical learning rates for training neural networks. *Proceedings - 2017 IEEE Winter Conference on Applications of Computer Vision*, 464–472. 10.1109/WACV.2017.58

Sodmann, P., Vollmer, M., Nath, N., & Kaderali, L. (2018). A convolutional neural network for ECG annotation as the basis for classification of cardiac rhythms. *Physiological Measurement*, *39*(10), 104005.

Song, L., Sun, D., Wang, Q., & Wang, Y. (2019). Automatic classification method of arrhythmia based on discriminative deep belief networks. *Sheng wu yi xue gong cheng xue za zhi= Journal of biomedical engineering= Shengwu yixue gongchengxue zazhi, 36*(3), 444-452.

Sousa, R., Miranda, R., Moreira, A., Alves, C., Lori, N., & Machado, J. (2021). Software Tools for Conducting Real-Time Information Processing and Visualization in Industry: An Up-to-Date Review. *Applied Sciences (Basel, Switzerland)*, *11*(11), 4800. doi:10.3390/app11114800

Standardization, I. O. (2011). *Health informatics-Requirements for an electronic health record architecture*. Author.

Stevenson, A., & Frenay, J. (2019, December 16). *Big Data LDN 2019: Freeing up engineering and infrastructure resources to scale with DataOps*. YouTube. https://www.youtube.com/watch?v=J7bEunZXkxc

Stevens, W. J. M., van der Sande, R., Beijer, L. J., Gerritsen, M. G. M., & Assendelft, W. J. J. (2019). E-Health apps replacing or complementing healthcare contacts: Scoping review on adverse effects. *Journal of Medical Internet Research, 21*(3), e10736. doi:10.2196/10736 PMID:30821690

Stiegelmeier, E. W., & Bressan, G. M. (2021). A fuzzy approach in the study of COVID-19 pandemic in Brazil. *Research on Biomedical Engineering*, *37*(2), 263–271. doi:10.100742600-021-00144-5

Stroetman, V., Kalra, D., Lewalle, P., Rector, A., Rodrigues, J., Stroetman, K., Surjan, G., Ustun, B., Virtanen, M., & Zanstra, P. (2009). *Semantic interoperability for better health and safer healthcare*. Academic Press.

Sucaria, D. (2021, April 23). *Microservices Architecture - orchestrator, choreography, hybrid... Which approach to use?* Diego Sucaria. https://diegosucaria.info/microservices-architecture-orchestrator-choreography-hybrid-which-approach-to-use/

Sujadevi, V. G., Soman, K. P., & Vinayakumar, R. (2017, September). Real-time detection of atrial fibrillation from short time single lead ECG traces using recurrent neural networks. In *The International Symposium on Intelligent Systems Technologies and Applications* (pp. 212-221). Springer.

Sun, Y., Yuan, P., & Sun, Y. (2020). MM-GAN: 3D MRI data augmentation for medical image segmentation via generative adversarial networks. *Proceedings - 11th IEEE International Conference on Knowledge Graph, ICKG 2020*, 227–234. 10.1109/ICBK50248.2020.00041

Sung, F., Yang, Y., & Zhang, L. (2018). Relation Network for Few-Shot Learning. *Cvpr*, 1199–1208.

Sun, L., Wang, Y., He, J., Li, H., Peng, D., & Wang, Y. (2020). A stacked LSTM for atrial fibrillation prediction based on multivariate ECGs. *Health Information Science and Systems*, *8*(1), 1–7.

Suter, P., Armaganidis, A., Beaufils, F., Bonfill, X., Burchardi, H., Cook, D., Fagot-Largeault, A., Thijs, L., Vesconi, S., Williams, A., Le Gall, J. R., & Chang, R. (1994). Predicting outcome in ICU patients. *Intensive Care Medicine*, *20*(5), 390–397. doi:10.1007/BF01720917 PMID:7930037

Sviri, S., Hashoul, J., Stav, I., & van Heerden, P. (2014). Does high-dose vasopressor therapy in medical intensive care patients indicate what we already suspect? *Journal of Critical Care*, *29*(1), 157–160. doi:10.1016/j.jcrc.2013.09.004 PMID:24140297

Sylim, P., Liu, F., Marcelo, A., & Fontelo, P. (2018). Blockchain Technology for Detecting Falsified and Substandard Drugs in Distribution: Pharmaceutical Supply Chain Intervention. *JMIR Research Protocols*, *7*(9), e10163. https://doi.org/10.2196/10163

Taji, B., Chan, A. D., & Shirmohammadi, S. (2017). False alarm reduction in atrial fibrillation detection using deep belief networks. *IEEE Transactions on Instrumentation and Measurement*, *67*(5), 1124–1131.

Takalo-Mattila, J., Kiljander, J., & Soininen, J. P. (2018, August). Inter-patient ECG classification using deep convolutional neural networks. In *2018 21st Euromicro Conference on Digital System Design (DSD)* (pp. 421-425). IEEE.

Tanaka, F. H. K. dos S., & Aranha, C. (2019). *Data augmentation using GANs*. ArXiv Preprint ArXiv:1904.09135.

Tan, J. H., Hagiwara, Y., Pang, W., Lim, I., Oh, S. L., Adam, M., ... Acharya, U. R. (2018). Application of stacked convolutional and long short-term memory network for accurate identification of CAD ECG signals. *Computers in Biology and Medicine*, *94*, 19–26.

Thurner, S., Hanel, R., & Klimek, P. (2018). *Introduction to the theory of complex systems*. Oxford University Press. doi:10.1093/oso/9780198821939.001.0001

Tokui, S., Oono, K., Hido, S., & Clayton, J. (2015, December). Chainer: a next-generation open source framework for deep learning. In *Proceedings of workshop on machine learning systems (LearningSys) in the twenty-ninth annual conference on neural information processing systems (NIPS)* (*Vol. 5*, pp. 1-6). Academic Press.

Tong, Y., Sun, Y., Zhou, P., Shen, Y., Jiang, H., Sha, X., & Chang, S. (2021). Locating abnormal heartbeats in ECG segments based on deep weakly supervised learning. *Biomedical Signal Processing and Control*, *68*, 102674.

Topaz, M., Shafran-Topaz, L., & Bowles, K. H. (2013). *ICD-9 to ICD-10: evolution, revolution, and current debates in the United States* (Vol. 10). Perspect. Health Inf. Manag.

Tseng, K. K., Wang, C., Xiao, T., Chen, C. M., Hassan, M. M., & de Albuquerque, V. H. C. (2021). Sliding large kernel of deep learning algorithm for mobile electrocardiogram diagnosis. *Computers & Electrical Engineering*, *96*, 107521.

Tuncer, T., Ozyurt, F., Dogan, S., & Subasi, A. (2021). A novel Covid-19 and pneumonia classification method based on F-transform. *Chemometrics and Intelligent Laboratory Systems*, *210*, 104256. doi:10.1016/j.chemolab.2021.104256 PMID:33531722

Umer, S., Afzal, M., Hussain, M., Latif, K., & Ahmad, H. F. (2012). Autonomous mapping of HL7 RIM and relational database schema. *Information Systems Frontiers*, *14*(1), 5–18.

United Healthcare uses Hadoop to Detect Health Care Fraud, Waste and Abuse. (2018). Retrieved April 20, 2018, from https://mapr.com/customers/unitedhealthcare/

Upadhyay, H. K., Juneja, S., Maggu, S., Dhingra, G., & Juneja, A. (2021). Multi-criteria analysis of social isolation barriers amid COVID-19 using fuzzy AHP. *World Journal of Engineering*.

Utter, G. H., Cox, G. L., Atolagbe, O. O., Owens, P. L., & Romano, P. S. (2018). Conversion of the Agency for Healthcare Research and Quality's Quality Indicators from ICD-9-CM to ICD-10-CM/PCS: The Process, Results, and Implications for Users. *Health Services Research*, *53*(5), 3704–3727. doi:10.1111/1475-6773.12981 PMID:29846001

Vaishnavi, V., Kuechler, B., & Petter, S. (2012). *Design Science Research in Information Systems*. Academic Press.

Van Rooij, T., & Marsh, S. (2016). E-Health: Past and future perspectives. *Personalized Medicine*, *13*(1), 57–70. doi:10.2217/pme.15.40 PMID:29749870

Vedaei, S. S., Fotovvat, A., Mohebbian, M. R., Rahman, G. M., Wahid, K. A., Babyn, P., Marateb, H. R., Mansourian, M., & Sami, R. (2020). COVID-SAFE: An IoT-based system for automated health monitoring and surveillance in post-pandemic life. *IEEE Access: Practical Innovations, Open Solutions, 8,* 188538–188551. doi:10.1109/ACCESS.2020.3030194 PMID:34812362

Veloso, R., Portela, F., Santos, M. F., Machado, J., da Silva Abelha, A., Rua, F., & Silva, Á. (2017). Categorize readmitted patients in intensive medicine by means of clustering data mining. *International Journal of E-Health and Medical Communications, 8*(3), 22–37. doi:10.4018/IJEHMC.2017070102

Veloso, R., Portela, F., Santos, M. F., Silva, Á., Rua, F., Abelha, A., & Machado, J. (2014). A Clustering Approach for Predicting Readmissions in Intensive Medicine. *Procedia Technology, 16,* 1307–1316. doi:10.1016/j.protcy.2014.10.147

Vidal, R., Bruna, J., Giryes, R., & Soatto, S. (2017). *Mathematics of deep learning.* arXiv preprint arXiv:1712.04741.

Vincent, P., Larochelle, H., Lajoie, I., Bengio, Y., Manzagol, P. A., & Bottou, L. (2010). Stacked denoising autoencoders: Learning useful representations in a deep network with a local denoising criterion. *Journal of Machine Learning Research, 11*(12).

Visa, S., Ramsay, B., Ralescu, A. L., & Van Der Knaap, E. (2011). Confusion matrix-based feature selection. *MAICS, 710,* 120–127.

Viswanathan, M., Golin, C. E., Jones, C. D., Ashok, M., Blalock, S. J., Wines, R. C., Coker-Schwimmer, E. J. L., Rosen, D. L., Sista, P., & Lohr, K. N. (2012). Interventions to improve adherence to self-administered medications for chronic diseases in the United States: A systematic review. *Annals of Internal Medicine, 157*(11), 785–795. doi:10.7326/0003-4819-157-11-201212040-00538 PMID:22964778

Wang, X., Chen, C., Du, Y., Zhang, Y., & Wu, C. (2021, February). Analysis of Policies Based on the Multi-Fuzzy Regression Discontinuity, in Terms of the Number of Deaths in the Coronavirus Epidemic. In Healthcare (Vol. 9, No. 2, p. 116). Multidisciplinary Digital Publishing Institute.

Wang, F., Liu, H., & Cheng, J. (2018). Visualizing deep neural network by alternately image blurring and deblurring. *Neural Networks, 97,* 162–172.

Wang, H. F., Jin, J. F., Feng, X. Q., Huang, X., Zhu, L. L., Zhao, X. Y., & Zhou, Q. (2015). Quality improvements in decreasing medication administration errors made by nursing staff in an academic medical center hospital: A trend analysis during the journey to Joint Commission International accreditation and in the post-accreditation era. *Therapeutics and Clinical Risk Management, 11,* 393–406. doi:10.2147/TCRM.S79238 PMID:25767393

Wang, Q., Cao, W., Guo, J., Ren, J., Cheng, Y., & Davis, D. N. (2019). DMP_MI: An effective diabetes mellitus classification algorithm on imbalanced data with missing values. *IEEE Access: Practical Innovations, Open Solutions, 7,* 102232–102238. doi:10.1109/ACCESS.2019.2929866

Wang, Y., Kung, L., & Byrd, T. A. (2018). Big data analytics: Understanding its capabilities and potential benefits for healthcare organizations. *Technological Forecasting and Social Change*, *126*, 3–13. doi:10.1016/j.techfore.2015.12.019

Wang, Y., Yao, Q., Kwok, J. T., & Ni, L. M. (2020). Generalizing from a Few Examples: A Survey on Few-shot Learning. *ACM Computing Surveys*, *53*(3), 1–34. doi:10.1145/3386252

Wenterodt, T., & Herwig, H. (2014). The Entropic Potential Concept: A New Way to Look at Energy Transfer Operations. *Entropy (Basel, Switzerland)*, *16*(4), 2071–2084. doi:10.3390/e16042071

West, J. H., Belvedere, L. M., Andreasen, R., Frandsen, C., Hall, P. C., & Crookston, B. T. (2017). Controlling Your "App" site: How Diet and Nutrition-Related Mobile Apps Lead to Behavior Change. *JMIR mHealth and uHealth*, *5*(7), e95. doi:10.2196/mhealth.7410 PMID:28694241

What is a Document Database? (n.d.). *MongoDB*. https://www.mongodb.com/document-databases

White House. (2019). Executive Order on Maintaining American Leadership in Artificial Intelligence. *Executive Orders: Infrastructure & Technology*. https://www.whitehouse.gov/presidential-actions/executive-order-maintaining-american-leadership-a

Whitten, J. L., Bentley, L. D., & Dittman, K. C. (1989). *Systems analysis and design methods*. Irwin Homewood.

WHO Factsheet. (2018, January 31). *Substandard and falsified medical products*. Retrieved December 16, 2021, from https://www.who.int/news-room/fact-sheets/detail/substandard-and-falsified-medical-products

Wilkinson, M. D., Dumontier, M., Aalbersberg, I. J., Appleton, G., Axton, M., Baak, A., Blomberg, N., Boiten, J. W., da Silva Santos, L. B., Bpeoplene, P. E., & Bouwman, J. (2016). The FAIR Guiding Principles for scientific data management and stewardship. *Scientific Data*, 3.

Wilmer, A., Louie, K., Dodek, P., Wong, H., & Ayas, N. (2010). Incidence of medication errors and adverse drug events in the ICU: A systematic review. In Quality and Safety in Health Care (Vol. 19, Issue 5). doi:10.1136/qshc.2008.030783

Wilson, T. D. (2001). Information overload: Implications for healthcare services. *Health Informatics Journal*, *7*(2), 112–117. doi:10.1177/146045820100700210

Wirtz, B. W., Weyerer, J. C., & Geyer, C. (2019). Artificial intelligence and the public sector—Applications and challenges. *International Journal of Public Administration*, *42*(7), 596–615. doi:10.1080/01900692.2018.1498103

Witchel, S. F., Oberfield, S. E., & Peña, A. S. (2019). Polycystic ovary syndrome: Pathophysiology, presentation, and treatment with emphasis on adolescent girls. *Journal of the Endocrine Society*, *3*(8), 1545–1573. doi:10.1210/js.2019-00078 PMID:31384717

Witten, I. H., Frank, E., Hall, M. A., & Pal, C. J. (2005). Practical machine learning tools and techniques. Morgan Kaufmann.

Compilation of References

World Health Organization. (n.d.). *e-Health*. www.emro.who.int/health-topics/ehealth/

Wu, H. C., Wang, Y. C., & Chen, T. C. T. (2020). Assessing and comparing COVID-19 intervention strategies using a varying partial consensus fuzzy collaborative intelligence approach. *Mathematics*, *8*(10), 1725. doi:10.3390/math8101725

Xia, Y., Wulan, N., Wang, K., & Zhang, H. (2018). Detecting atrial fibrillation by deep convolutional neural networks. *Computers in Biology and Medicine*, *93*, 84–92.

Yang, J., Bai, Y., Lin, F., Liu, M., Hou, Z., & Liu, X. (2018). A novel electrocardiogram arrhythmia classification method based on stacked sparse auto-encoders and softmax regression. *International Journal of Machine Learning and Cybernetics*, *9*(10), 1733–1740.

Yildirim, Ö. (2018). A novel wavelet sequence based on deep bidirectional LSTM network model for ECG signal classification. *Computers in Biology and Medicine*, *96*, 189–202.

Yi, X., & Babyn, P. (2018). Sharpness-Aware Low-Dose CT Denoising Using Conditional Generative Adversarial Network. *Journal of Digital Imaging*, *31*(5), 655–669. doi:10.100710278-018-0056-0 PMID:29464432

Yousef, W. (2012). What is E-health and why it is important? *Qatar's Technology Hotspot*, (31), 1-13.

Yu, Y. H., Chasman, D. I., Buring, J. E., Rose, L., & Ridker, P. M. (2015). Cardiovascular risks associated with incident and prevalent periodontal disease. *Journal of Clinical Periodontology*, *42*(1), 21–28. doi:10.1111/jcpe.12335 PMID:25385537

Zadeh, L. A. (1965). Fuzzy Sets. *Information and Control*, *8*(3), 338–353. doi:10.1016/S0019-9958(65)90241-X

Zadeh, L. A. (1968). Fuzzy algorithm. *Information and Control*, *12*(2), 94–102. doi:10.1016/S0019-9958(68)90211-8

Zadeh, L. A. (1973). Outline of a new approach to the analysis of complex systems and decision processes. *IEEE Transactions on Systems, Man, and Cybernetics*, *3*(1), 28–44. doi:10.1109/TSMC.1973.5408575

Zadeh, L. A. (1994). Soft computing and fuzzy logic. *IEEE Software*, *11*(6), 48–56. doi:10.1109/52.329401

Zadrozny, B. (2004, July). Learning and evaluating classifiers under sample selection bias. In *Proceedings of the twenty-first international conference on Machine learning* (p. 114). Academic Press.

Zaheeruddin & Garima. (2006). A neuro-fuzzy approach for prediction of human work efficiency in noisy environment. *Applied Soft Computing, 6*(3), 283-294.

Zhai, X., & Tin, C. (2018). Automated ECG classification using dual heartbeat coupling based on convolutional neural network. *IEEE Access: Practical Innovations, Open Solutions*, 6, 27465–27472.

Zhang, X. D. (2020). *A Matrix Algebra Approach to Artificial Intelligence*. Springer.

Zhao, M., Wang, L., Chen, J., Nie, D., Cong, Y., Ahmad, S., Ho, A., Yuan, P., Fung, S. H., Deng, H. H., & ... (2018). Craniomaxillofacial bony structures segmentation from MRI with deep-supervision adversarial learning. *International Conference on Medical Image Computing and Computer-Assisted Intervention*, 720–727. 10.1007/978-3-030-00937-3_82

Zhao, Z. Q., Zheng, P., Xu, S. T., & Wu, X. (2019). Object detection with deep learning: A review. *IEEE Transactions on Neural Networks and Learning Systems*, 30(11), 3212–3232.

Zheng, S.-Q., Yang, L., Zhou, P.-X., Li, H.-B., Liu, F., & Zhao, R.-S. (2020). Recommendations and guidance for providing pharmaceutical care services during COVID-19 pandemic: A China perspective. *Research in Social & Administrative Pharmacy*, 17(1), 1819–1824. doi:10.1016/j.sapharm.2020.03.012 PMID:32249102

Zhong, W., Liao, L., Guo, X., & Wang, G. (2018). A deep learning approach for fetal QRS complex detection. *Physiological Measurement*, 39(4), 045004.

Zivkovic, M., Bacanin, N., Venkatachalam, K., Nayyar, A., Djordjevic, A., Strumberger, I., & Al-Turjman, F. (2021). COVID-19 cases prediction by using hybrid machine learning and beetle antennae search approach. *Sustainable Cities and Society*, 66, 102669. doi:10.1016/j.scs.2020.102669 PMID:33520607

About the Contributors

José Machado is an Associate Professor with Habilitation in the Department of Informatics, Universidade do Minho. He got his PhD in Informatics, in 2002, and Habilitation in 2011. He is the Director of the ALGORITMI research centre, member of the Computer Science and Technology (CST) group and header of the lab Knowledge Engineering (KE). His research interests span the domain of Biomedical Informatics, Electronic Health Records, Interoperability, Databases, Business Intelligence and Applied Artificial Intelligence. He is the Editor in chief of BiomedInformatics (MDPI) and associate editor of IJRQEH (IGI Global). He is the chair of the IEEE CIS Portugal Chapter.

Regina Sousa is a Ph.D. student in Biomedical Engineering with technical skills in Artificial Intelligence, Business Intelligence, Big Data, Healthcare Information Systems, among others. She collaborated in a professional project with TecMinho in the years 2017 and 2018 called DermoID -Núcleo de Investigação e Desenvolvimento de Dermocosméticos. In 2018 she was a trainer of children's computer programming in the company HappyCode Braga. In 2019 she joined geoatributo as a software analyst where she prevailed until the end of the year. She took leave from the profession to start her Ph.D. in Biomedical Engineering in the Medical Informatics Branch. In Jan 2020 he won a research fellowship in the Factory of the Future: Smart Facturing project where he still collaborates. In Nov 2020 experienced the first activity as a guest lecturer in the course of Asian Institute of Technology (AIT) - Data Modeling and Management in the School of Engineering and Technology (SET) Asian Institute of Technology (AIT), Thailand. In Jan 2021 she was a lecturer at Instituto Piaget Vila Nova de Gaia in the Information Systems course.

* * *

António Abelha graduated in Systems and Informatics Engineering, University of Minho, in 1992, MSc in Informatics Management from the same institution in 1997 and PhD in Informatics from the same institution since 2004. He is currently guiding 10 PhD in Biomedical Engineering or Informatics. He supervised 3 PhD thesis with success, and more than 40 MSc thesis, several participation in doctoral juries, published over 250 articles in journals and international meetings, many of which already indexed in Scopus.

Inês Afonso is a student of the Integrated Master's in Engineering and Management of Information Systems at the University of Minho. While she is finishing her degree, she is also working as tech analyst at Deloitte. She is currently finishing her master's thesis on "Data mining classification models for automatic problem identification in intensive medicine". During her 5 years of college, she found a passion for research, particularly in the area of Data Science. In order to improve her skills and add value to her research project, she took an online course with the theme "Python for Data Science and Machine Learning Bootcamp".

Achyut Agrawal is a prefinal year student at VIT pursuing Electrical and Electronics Engineering. AI and Robotics enthusiast. Love to research and innovate in various domains, technical as well as non-technical. Founder and COO of a startup ' Checked It'.

Victor Alves is Assistant Professor of the Department of Informatics, School of Engineering, University of Minho. He got his PhD in Computer Science in 2002. He teaches and taught several curricular units in the topics of Programing Paradigms, Medical Informatics, Artificial Intelligence, Knowledge Engineering, Intelligent Systems, Medical Imaging Informatics, Informatic Engineering Projects in different and related fields of Computer Engineering. His main expertise lies in the Medical Imaging Informatics field, mainly in modeling of the imaging modalities and their interpretation by synergistic human-machine methods for clinical benefits and applications not only in the computer-aided diagnosis/detection research context but in the broader context of ambient intelligence.

Suvarna Latha Anchapakala obtained her M.Sc. degree in Botany from Nagarjuna University, Guntur, A.P, India in 2001. She took her M.Phil. and Ph.D degrees from S.V. University, Tirupati, A.P, in 2004 and 2014 respectively. Now she is working as Assistant Professor at Department of Biosciences and Sericulture, Division of Botany, Sri Padmavati Mahila Visvavidyalayam, Tirupati, A.P. She has 16 years of teaching experience in teaching Botany at PG level. Dr. A. Suvarna Latha published 28 research papers in reputed National and International Journals and published one book and 2 book chapters. She has participated and presented papers in various National and International Conferences, Seminars and attended 30 Workshops and 4 training programmes.

Malavika B. has pursued BSc computer science from University of Calicut in 2019, Palakkad and at present she is pursuing MCA at Hindusthan College of Arts and science Coimbatore. Her area of interest is cyber security.

Erman Çakıt received his Ph.D. in Industrial Engineering from the University of Central Florida, Orlando, USA, in 2013. He is currently working as an associate professor at the Department of Industrial Engineering, Gazi University, Turkey. His research interests include applications of human factors / ergonomics and safety using machine learning and applied statistics.

M. Krishna Chaitanya is currently pursuing Ph.D in the School of Electronics Engineering at VIT-AP University. He received M.Tech in the year 2008 from Kakatiya Institute of Technology and Science, Warangal, Telangana, India. His research areas include Biomedical Signal Processing, Deep Learning, Machine learning and ECG Signal Filtering.

Ana Cecília Sousa Rocha Coimbra finished the PhD in Biomedical Engineering at the Universidade do Minho in 2021.The field of information technology has always captivated her attention and was one of the elements that led her to choosing Biomedical Engineering. After an initial encounter with programming, namely the Java language, in my first year of university, curiosity grew and was developed an affinity for medical informatics. Various programming languages such as Python, Java, Logic Programming, HTML, and XML were used in the first year of the Master's in Medical Informatics program. Plus, also dealing with the processing of enormous volumes of data in order to work with it (using the PLSQL language and Oracle tools) and draw conclusions. The aim of her doctoral research, which was produced in collaboration with the Centro Hospitalar Universitário do Porto, was to improve clinical problem lists using artificial intelligence technologies. The key objective was to use data mining techniques to create a predictive model of the primary diagnosis based on secondary diagnoses. Her entire academic experience aimed at contributing to the development of both learning capacity and adaptability, since work was done with various languages and platforms. Thus, several unique technologies and methodologies were developed along ther academic path, resulting in the publishing of several scientific articles in international conferences.

Bharathi Depuru has been working as Professor, Department of Biosciences and Sericulture and Dean, Academic affairs, Sri Padmavati Mahila Visvavidyalayam, Tirupati. She has 33 years of teaching and 38 years of research experience. She has guided 3 M. Phil and 9 Ph.D students. She acted as Dean, School of Sciences and Dean of Examinations of Sri Padmavati Mahila Visvavidyalayam, Tirupati. She worked as Head, Department of Sericulture and Zoology, Sri Padmavati Mahila Visvavidyalayam, Tirupati. She has completed 4 projects. To her credit Prof. D. Bharathi has published 148 research papers in reputed National and International Journals and published 4 books. She has presented 90 papers in National and International conferences, seminars and workshops. She has visited China, Japan, Thailand, Nepal, Srilanka and Australia and presented papers in the conferences, chaired sessions and acted as keynote speaker. She received Best Teacher Award from Andhra Pradesh State Government for the Year 2008. She received Best Research Award in 2017 from Sri Padmavati Mahila Visvavidyalayam. She was appointed as Member of Executive council of Sri Padmavati Mahila University, Tirupati. Her research areas are Biochemistry, Physiology, Biotechnology and Biomedicine. She is the referee to several Journals. Dr. D. Bharathi has been selected for Chinese Govt. Scholarship for Post-Doctoral Research in Sericulture for a period of one year from September 2000- July 2001 through Ministry of HRD, New Delhi, India. To her credit she has been nominated as Honorary foreign member of Sericulture Society of Zhejiang University, P.R.China 2000. She is the adjudicator of Ph.D Thesis of several Universities. She is the Member in Black Caspian Seas & Central Asia Association (BACSA), Samboliiski Str., Bulgaria and Non Official member in the Advisory Committee of Forest Dept- Wildlife, Govt. of Andhra Pradesh at S.V. Zoological Park, Tirupati. She received 5 National Awards.

Júlio Duarte is currently working as Junior Researcher at Centro Algoritmi in the University of Minho. Invited Assistant Professor, teaching Technology and Information Systems, Data Storage and Access and Clinical Systems Integration. Long-held interests in electronic health record, medical information systems, interoperability, and integration in healthcare domain.

Diana Ferreira is a Biomedical Engineer with a master's degree in Medical Informatics and experience in several areas of information technology focusing on health information systems and artificial intelligence. She is a researcher at the ALGORITMI research center, in the Knowledge Engineering Group (KEG), at the University of Minho, where she also works as a guest assistant professor. She is currently pursuing a PhD in Biomedical Engineering, having recently acquired the support and funding of the Fundação para a Ciência e Tecnologia (FCT). She participated as a Research Fellow in 3 research projects, two of which were the result of a collaboration between Bosch and the University of Minho, and the third was an European project. She has published several scientific articles in national and international conferences, books, and specialized journals, and has participated in several conferences in person and virtually, both as a presenter and organizer.

Luís Gomes completed his PhD in Informatics (specialty in Computer Science) at the University of the Azores (Portugal). He has been an assistant professor at the Department of Informatics at the Faculty of Sciences and Technology of the University of the Azores since 2000. And, since 2014, he has been an integrated member of the R&D center CST / Algoritmi of the University of Minho (Portugal). His research interests are associated with Computing Theory (Computability and Complexity), Artificial Intelligence and Information Systems. He is co-author of several articles published by international conferences. He has co-organized several international conferences and workshops on computability, artificial intelligence, and information systems. He also belongs to some scientific committees of international conferences on information systems.

Hélia Guerra is Auxiliary Professor at the Faculty of Sciences and Technology of the University of Azores, Ponta Delgada, Portugal, where she has been since 1993. She holds a PhD in Computer Science (2004), a MSc in Informatics (1997), and a BSc in Mathematics/Informatics (1992). She is a researcher at Algoritmi Centre (Computer Science and Technologies R&D line) of the University of Minho and a founding member and the coordinator of the eHealth R&D unit of the University of Azores. Her research interests span the domain of information systems, software engineering, artificial intelligence, and health informatics. She has been involved in several organizations of international conferences and has several publications in conference proceedings, chapter books and journals.

Tiago Guimarães is currently in the fourth year of his Ph.D. in Biomedical Engineering. He is an invited assistant professor at the Department of Information Systems, University of Minho, Portugal. He is a Research Collaborator and Member of the IDS R&D Group at ALGORITMI Centre, with the current research interests: Blockchain; Blockchain Analytics; Intelligent Decision Support Systems; Business Intelligence and Analytics.

Francini Hak is a PhD student in the area of Information Systems and Technologies, and a Research Collaborator in the Algoritmi Research Center. She also works as Invited Professor at University of Minho in Portugal.

Deden Witarsyah Jacob currently works at School of Industrial and System Engineering, Telkom University. Deden does researches in Information Systems, IT Project Management, e-Government, open data, and artificial intelligence. His current project is 'open data'. He finished Master Degree in Electrical and Computer Engineering at Curtin University of Technology, Australia. Last, for doctoral degree, Deden continued his education in Twente University Netherlands and Universiti

Tun Hussein Onn Malaysia. He joined in Cybernetics Research Group and Head of Open Data Research Center since 2018 until present.

A. V. Senthil Kumar is working as a Director & Professor in the Department of Research and PG in Computer Applications, Hindusthan College of Arts and Science, Coimbatore since 05/03/2010. He has to his credit 11 Book Chapters, 250 papers in International Journals, 15 papers in National Journals, 25 papers in International Conferences, 5 papers in National Conferences, and edited 8 books (IGI Global, USA). He is an Editor-in-Chief for International Journal titled "International Journal of Data Mining and Emerging Technologies", "International Journal of Image Processing and Applications", "International Journal of Advances in Knowledge Engineering & Computer Science", "International Journal of Advances in Computers and Information Engineering" and "International Journal of Research and Reviews in Computer Science". Key Member for India, Machine Intelligence Research Lab (MIR Labs). He is an Editorial Board Member and Reviewer for various International Journals.

B. Hemavathi Latha obtained her M.Sc. degree in Zoology from Gulbarga University, Gulbarga, Karnataka, India in 1998. She took her Ph.D degrees from S.V. University, Tirupati, A.P, in 2006. Now she is working as Assistant Professor at Department of Biosciences and Sericulture, Division of Zoology, Sri Padmavati Mahila Visvavidyalayam, Tirupati, A.P. She has 20 years of teaching experience in teaching Zoology at P.G level. Dr. B.Hemavathi published 15 research papers in reputed National and International Journals and published 3 book chapters. She has participated and presented papers in various National and International Conferences, Seminars and attended 30 Workshops and 12 training programmes.

Nicolas F. Lori graduated in Physics by the University of Coimbra in 1993, completed a PhD degree in Physics by Washington University in St. Louis in 2001 and completed a PhD degree in Informatics by University of Minho in 2020. NF Lori published over 35 papers in international peer review journals (such as PNAS and Journal of Magnetic Resonance Imaging) with over 2000 citations; with only a small fraction of the papers published with the PhD supervisor. NF Lori completed the (co-)supervision of 6 master degree students. He was PI in a 180.000 € national project grant, and co-Investigator on several national projects totaling over 1.400.000 €. He has been in over 40 international abstracts. He was 2 years a graduate teaching assistant and 4 years a research assistant at the WashingtonUniversity in St Louis Physics Department (USA); 2 years a Post-doctoral researcher on diffusion MRI at the "Commission for the Atomic Energy" in Orsay-Ville (France); 18 months a Post-doctoral research associate on diffusion MRI at Neuroimaging Laboratories,

Mallinckrodt Institute of Radiology, Washington University School of Medicine, Saint Louis, USA; 2 years as a tenure track Assistant Professor in Antonio Damasio's group, first at the Department of Neurology of the University of Iowa in Iowa City (USA), and then at the Department of Occupational Science and Occupational Therapy of the University of Southern California in Los Angeles (USA); and is now an "Investigador Auxiliar (Ciencia 2007)" at IBILI in the University of Coimbra. Fulbright fellow during PhD, and was then vice-President of Fulbrighters Portugal. He was also Director of the Laboratory for Neuroimaging in Neuroscience of INECO-INCYT at Rosario (Santa Fe, Argentina), and a Researcher at the ICVS/3Bs (Research Group: NERD) of University of Minho in Braga/Guimarães (Portugal), and at the Centre Algoritmi (Research Group: CST; Lab: ISLAB) of the University of Minho in Braga/Guimarães (Portugal). He was then a researcher at "Instituto de Engenharia de Sistemas e Computadores Investigação e Desenvolvimento" (INESC-ID) in Lisbon (Portugal). He is now a researcher at the Centre Algoritmi of the University of Minho in Braga (Portugal).

Joana Machado is Master in Pharmacy and PhD student in Biomedical Engineering-Medical Informatics since 2019, at the University of Minho. Member of the Knowledge Engineering Group of the ALGORITMI research center.

Ricardo Magalhães is a Biomedical Engineer and PhD in Health Sciences who works with medical imaging.

Marcelo Marreiros is an MSc student in Biomedical Engineering at the University of Minho in Portugal that focuses on the development of viable solutions for biomedical problems, mostly in healthcare, to improve human experience and quality of life. His main areas of interest are artificial intelligence, business intelligence, decision support systems, and hospital information systems.

Filipe Miranda is a senior data engineer from 2022-present Data engineer from 2019-2022. PhD at Uminho University 2018-2021.

Cristiana Neto completed the Master in Biomedical Engineering (Medical Informatics) in 2018 at the University of Minho and is currently enrolled in the Doctoral Program in Biomedical Engineering since 2019, at the same institution. She is a researcher at the ALGORITMI Center (University of Minho), where she participated in several research projects, two of them partnerships between the University of Minho and Bosch Car Multimedia Portugal. Cristiana Neto also works as an assistant professor at the University of Minho. She currently holds a grant from the Fundação para a Ciência e Tecnologia (FCT) as part of her PhD. During her journey, she published several articles in specialized magazines, book chapters and participated in several conferences, as a presenter and organizer. Her work focuses on several areas of computer science, such as hospital information systems, machine learning and interoperability.

José Neves is Full Professor of Computer Science at Minho University, Portugal, and Emeritus Professor since 2019 at the same university. He also integrates the faculty of CESPU (Cooperative of Higher Education Polytechnic and University, CRL). He received his Ph.D. in Computer Science from Heriot Watt University, Scotland, in 1983. His current research interests relate to the areas of Logic Programming, Knowledge Representation and Reasoning, Evolutionary Intelligence and Machine Learning. Lately it has been focusing on the area of Computational Sustainability, namely on the relationship between the disciplines of Psychology, Economics, Computer Science, Mathematical Logic and Philosophy and their contributions to Decision Making in Business Environments.

Daniela Oliveira has a PhD in Biomedical Engineering from the University of Minho, specializing in patient-oriented clinical software development and standardized and open approaches. In addition to software development, she specializes in data analysis and knowledge discovery, oriented to different contexts and realities, in healthcare context. She is also an Invited Professor at the Informatics Department of the University of Minho.

Maria Passos is a student of the Integrated Master's in Engineering and Management of Information Systems at the University of Minho. Being on a very diversified course, she could take several career paths, however, she has always shown interest and passion for the area of Data Science. She is now finalising her master's thesis with the topic "Decision and optimization models on therapies, orders and procedures for intensive medicine". It should be noted that throughout her dissertation she was proactive and decided to take two online courses that gave her a background for her work. The courses were: "Python for Data Science and Machine Learning Bootcamp" and "Artificial Intelligence: Optimization Algorithms in Python". On a professional level she is now working at Deloitte as Tech Analyst in Strategy, Analytics and M&A Data Science.

Hugo Peixoto is an Assistent Researcher at Algoritmi Research Center at University of Minho, Portugal. Previously work as an IT Director at Centro Hospitalar de Entre o Douro e Vouga, and as an IT Specialist at Centro Hospitalar do Tâmega e Sousa (CHTS) in Penafiel where he is engaged in the development of several projects in the area of Electronic Medical Processes and Interoperability. Also, he is currently invited assistant professor at University of Minho, Braga, Portugal. Hugo Peixoto holds a PhD in Biomedical Engineering from the University of Minho, Portugal, with a thesis focused on Interoperability Strategies in HealthCare Environment. In addition, he holds a Master´s degree in the field on Medical Informatics, during which he had the opportunity to collaborate with the research team of the Informatics Department of the University of Freiburg, Germany. Since 2009, he is member of the research team of Information Systems Technologies in the Algoritmi Center in the University of Minho. In addition, he holds a position of Invited Auxiliary Professor of Knowledge Extraction and Electronic Health Records of the Biomedical Engineering Course at University of Minho. He also took part in the organization of several international workshops (including the FiCloud 2017), he is a reviewer on international conferences and a member of the scientific committee of several international conferences.

Jagdeep Rahul received his undergraduate degree in Electronics & Communication from Bundelkhand University, India in 2009. He completed his Master of Technology from ABV-IIITM, India in 2012. He received Ph.D. in Computer Science and Engineering from Rajiv Gandhi University. He has been working as Assistant Professor at Rajiv Gandhi University (A Central University) since 2015. His research areas of interest are biomedical signal processing, machine learning, deep learning, and ECG analysis. He has published many research articles in SCI/ Scopus journals.

Jorge Ribeiro was born in 1975, in Braga, Portugal and is Adjunct Professor of the School of Technology and Management Polytechnic of the Institute of Viana do Castelo – Portugal, since 2006. He teaches topics in the Artificial Intelligence, Decision Support Systems, Systems Integration and Enterprise Information Systems field. Is member of the Artificial Intelligence Group of the Informatics Department of the University of Minho - Portugal. He received graduate degree in 2002 and the MSc degree in computer science (2007) from the University of Minho-Portugal where was also teacher in ICT from 2002 to 2005. He received the PhD in 2011 at the Department of Electronic and Computation of the University of Santiago de Compostela, Spain. He has been an author and co-author of some papers in the field of Data Mining, Software Engineering, Knowledge Representation, Evolutionary Systems and Geographic Information Systems. He is project manager and programmer in Information Technology and Software Development projects implemented on national and international entities.

Amarjit Roy received the M. Tech degree from NIT Silchar in 2014, and the Ph.D. degree from NIT Silchar in Electronics and Communication Engineering.

After that, he joined as an Assistant Professor in BML Munjal University in 2017. In July 2020, he joined as an Assistant Professor Sr. Grade 1 in VIT AP University. His research interests include Image noise removal, soft computing, biomedical image processing etc. He has published many papers in journals such as IEEE, Elsevier, Springer, etc.

Manuel Filipe Santos is associate professor with habilitation at the Department of Information Systems, UMinho, teaching undergraduate and graduate classes of Business Intelligence and Decision Support Systems. He is the head of Intelligent Data Systems lab and the coordinator of the Information Systems and Technology group of the R&D ALGORITMI Centre, with the current research interests: Business Intelligence; Intelligent Decision Support Systems; Data Mining and Machine Learning (Learning Classifier Systems); and Grid Data Mining. He is part of the steering committees of the master's course in Engineering and Management of Information Systems and the Doctoral Program in Information Systems and Technology.

Rui Santos is a Software Engineer who joined ISEC in 2016 and finished Informatics Engineering degree in 2019. After that, he proceeded to a master in Informatics Engineering at University of Minho in Braga. With background and interests in Big Data, Microservices in the healthcare domain.

Lakhan Dev Sharma (Member, IEEE) received the M.Tech. degree from the Atal Bihari Vajpayee-Indian Institute of Information Technology and Management, Gwalior, India, in 2012, and the Ph.D. degree from Dr. B. R. Ambedkar National Institute of Technology Jalandhar, India, in 2018. He has been serving as a Sr. Assistant Professor with the School of Electronics Engineering, VIT-AP University, Amaravati, India. He has teaching experience at various technical institutes and university levels. His research interests include biomedical signal and image processing, machine learning, and deep learning.

Álvaro Silva is senior consultant at the Centro Hospitalar e Universitário do Porto's Intensive Care Unit. He is also a full professor at the School of Medicine and Biomedical Sciences, where he lectures the curricular unit of Medicine I, and was member of the board of the Health Regulator Entity in Portugal. He completed his Ph.D. in Medical Science in 2008 and has since been involved in a number of research initiatives, both as a team member and as the primary investigator. He also mentors master students and PhD theses, having written over a hundred publications.

André Ferreira is a Biomedical Engineer (Master's degree from the University of Minho) who has worked in Deep Learning and Medical Imaging. He was an intern at NeuroSpin - Institut des sciences du vivant Frédéric Joliot, where he learned how to use different tools to acquire and process MRI scans.

Inês Tavares is a Tech Analyst for Deloitte. She is passionate about research, mainly in the areas of Data Analytics and Data Mining. Inês is currently finishing her master's thesis in Engineering and Management of Information Systems at the University of Minho, whose subject is Data mining Association Models for Relating Problems with Semiologic Data in Intensive Medicine. In 2020 she was a part of a project in the area of BI and Data Mining within the course unit of Systems for Business and Organization Intelligence in partnership with the School of Psychology at the University of Minho, with the production of an article for an international conference. She considers herself a hardworking and persevering person with leadership skills and team spirit. In her spare time, she really enjoys exercising, cooking and spending time with family and friends.

Kavitha V. achieved her PhD degree in Computer Science. She has published 7 Book Chapters in several Book Publications, 67 research papers in various International Journals, 32 research papers in several International as well as National Conferences. She is an reviewer for 4 International Journals. She has 18 years of teaching experience and 15 yrs of Research experience.

Henrique Vicente went to the University of Lisbon, where he studied Chemistry and obtained his degrees in 1988. He joined the University of Évora in 1989 and received his PhD in Chemistry in 2005. He is now Auxiliary Professor at the Department of Chemistry and Biochemistry at the University of Évora. He is a researcher at the REQUIMTE/LAQV (University of Évora) and at Algoritmi Research Center (University of Minho). His current interests include Water Quality Control, Lakes and Reservoirs Management, Data Mining, Knowledge Discovery from Databases, Knowledge Representation and Reasoning Systems, Evolutionary Intelligence, and Intelligent Information Systems.

Index

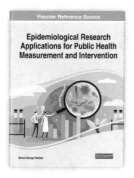
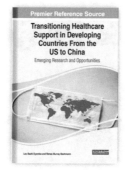
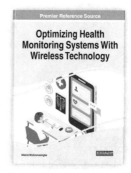
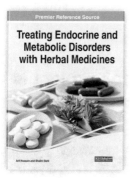
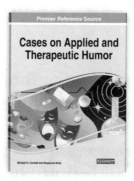
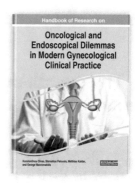
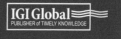

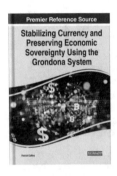
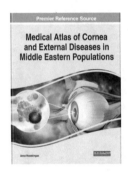
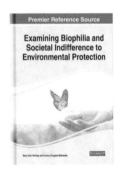
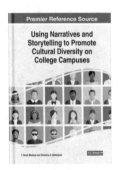

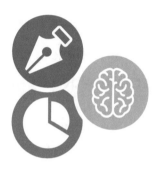
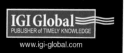

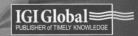

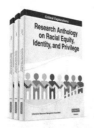
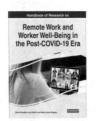
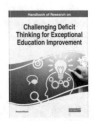

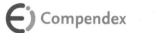

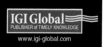

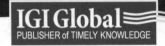
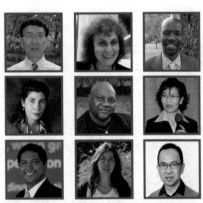
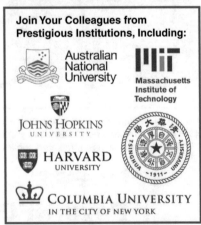

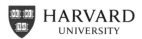
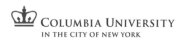
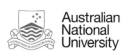
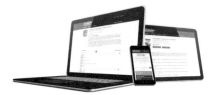

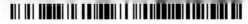

Printed in the United States
by Baker & Taylor Publisher Services